Current Concept in Cartilage Treatment

Mehmet E. Erdil • Mehmet Emin Şimşek
Taha Kizilkurt • Musa Ugur Mermerkaya
Mustafa Akkaya
Editors

Current Concept in Cartilage Treatment

Springer

Editors
Mehmet E. Erdil
Private Orthopaedic Practice
Istanbul, Türkiye

Taha Kizilkurt
Orthopaedics and Traumatology
Istanbul University
Istanbul, Türkiye

Mustafa Akkaya
Department of Orthopaedics
and Traumatology
Faculty of Medicine
Yuksek Ihtisas University
Ankara, Türkiye

Mehmet Emin Şimşek
Orthopaedics and Traumatology
Lokman Hekim University
Ankara, Türkiye

Musa Ugur Mermerkaya
Orthopaedics and Traumatolgy
Memorial Hospital
Ankara, Türkiye

ISBN 978-3-032-27098-6 ISBN 978-3-032-27099-3 (eBook)
https://doi.org/10.1007/978-3-032-27099-3

This Springer imprint is published by the registered company Springer Nature Switzerland AG
The registered company address is: Gewerbestrasse 11, 6330 Cham, Switzerland

Foreword

The treatment of cartilage lesions still represents one of the most challenging issues for the orthopedic surgeon. Articular cartilage is a highly specialized tissue whose unique structure provides the biomechanical properties necessary for smooth joint function and load distribution. However, these same biological characteristics are associated with a very limited intrinsic capacity for healing and regeneration. As a result, cartilage injuries often tend to persist or progress over time, potentially leading to degenerative joint changes and significantly affecting patients' quality of life. For this reason, the diagnosis and management of cartilage lesions require an increasingly careful, informed, and patient-specific approach.

Over the past decades, significant advances in scientific research and technological development have led to the introduction of a wide range of therapeutic strategies for the treatment of cartilage defects. From bone marrow stimulation techniques to osteochondral transplantation procedures, and more recently to solutions based on tissue engineering and regenerative medicine, the spectrum of available treatment options has expanded considerably. Nevertheless, the growing number of techniques and indications can make the selection of the most appropriate treatment strategy for each individual patient particularly complex.

In this context, the present volume, *Current Concept in Cartilage Treatment,* aims to provide a comprehensive and up-to-date overview of cartilage lesions and the currently available treatment strategies. Through the contributions of experts in the field, this book systematically reviews the different surgical and biological approaches, describing their underlying principles, indications, advantages, and limitations. The goal is to offer readers a clear and structured understanding of the current state of the art in cartilage treatment.

The reading and study of this book will help orthopedic surgeons and all professionals involved in joint preservation to gain greater awareness of the therapeutic possibilities available today. Ultimately, the purpose of this volume is to help guide the reader through this complex and rapidly evolving field, providing practical and scientifically grounded knowledge to support informed decision-making in the management of cartilage lesions.

Clinica Ortopedica e Traumatologica 2, IRCCS Istituto Ortopedico Rizzoli
Bologna, Italy

Stefano Zaffagnini

Preface

Articular cartilage pathology remains one of the most challenging areas in contemporary orthopaedics and regenerative medicine. The intrinsic avascular structure of cartilage and its limited capacity for self-repair continue to hinder the achievement of consistent and durable clinical outcomes. Despite these biological constraints, recent decades have witnessed substantial progress driven by advances in molecular biology, biomaterials, tissue engineering, and surgical techniques. These developments have contributed to a gradual shift from purely mechanical approaches toward biologically oriented and patient-specific treatment strategies.

In this rapidly evolving field, there is a clear need for comprehensive resources that not only summarize current knowledge but also critically evaluate emerging evidence and ongoing controversies. This book has been developed with the aim of providing such a resource. Rather than functioning as a traditional textbook, it offers an integrated and up-to-date perspective on cartilage biology, pathology, and treatment, with particular emphasis on bridging fundamental science and clinical application.

A distinctive feature of this volume is its international and multidisciplinary authorship. Contributions from experienced orthopaedic surgeons and scientists from Türkiye are combined with those of internationally recognized experts actively involved in cartilage research and clinical practice. This collaborative structure allows the presentation of diverse perspectives, reflecting variations in clinical practice, research methodologies, and healthcare systems, thereby enhancing both the scientific depth and global relevance of the content.

This work has been developed under the auspices of the **Turkish Society of Sports Injuries, Arthroscopy and Knee Surgery (TUSYAD) Cartilage Committee** and represents the first internationally published book arising from this initiative. As such, it marks an important step in the development of coordinated academic efforts within this field and highlights the value of structured collaboration in advancing orthopaedic science.

The scope of the book is deliberately comprehensive. It includes chapters addressing the fundamental aspects of cartilage biology, biomechanics, and pathophysiology, as well as translational research linking experimental findings with clinical practice. In addition, current treatment strategies are discussed in detail, ranging from non-operative management to advanced surgical techniques and emerging regenerative therapies. While evidence-based principles form the foundation of the discussions, the limitations of the available evidence and the role of clinical experience are also acknowledged.

Beyond serving as a reference source, this book is intended to support critical thinking and encourage further research. By bringing together contributions from different academic traditions and healthcare environments, it aims to provide a broader understanding of cartilage treatment and to facilitate international scientific dialogue.

We would like to express our sincere appreciation to all contributing authors for their valuable contributions and commitment to this project. We also thank the Turkish Society of Sports Injuries, Arthroscopy and Knee Surgery (TUSYAD) Cartilage Committee for its support and leadership, and Springer for providing the platform to disseminate this work to the international community.

It is our expectation that this book will serve as a useful reference for orthopaedic surgeons, researchers, and healthcare professionals involved in cartilage repair and regeneration, and that it will contribute to the ongoing development of this field.

Istanbul, Türkiye — Mehmet E. Erdil
Ankara, Türkiye — Mehmet Emin Şimşek
Istanbul, Türkiye — Taha Kızılkurt
Ankara, Türkiye — Musa Ugur Mermerkaya
Ankara, Türkiye — Mustafa Akkaya
2026

Contents

1 **Anatomy, Histology, and Osteochondral Unit of Healthy Cartilage and the Effect of Synovial Membrane** 1
Muge Kirac, Yigit Umur Cirdi, Alp Er Tunga Bolukbasi, and Safa Gursoy

2 **Subchondral Treatment Options in Cartilage Lesions** 9
Reha N. Tandogan and Tahir Ozturk

3 **Radiological Imaging of Chondral and Osteochondral Lesions** 25
Ufuk Arzu, İsmail Tarık Atasoy, and Gökhan Polat

4 **Classification of Cartilage Lesions** 31
Ali Said Nazligül and Mustafa Akkaya

5 **Treatment Algorithm for Cartilage Lesions and Current Directives in Clinical Practices** 37
Özer Öztürk and Tekin Kerem Ülkü

6 **Scaffold Applications in the Treatment of Cartilage Lesions** 45
Lorenzo Zanasi, Alberto Grassi, Luca Andriolo, Stefano Zaffagnini, and Giuseppe Filardo

7 **Microfracture in Cartilage Treatment and Its Effect on Healing** 65
Taha Kızılkurt, İsmail Tarık Atasoy, and Mehmet Aşık

8 **Osteochondral Autograft Transfer (OATS and Mosaicplasty) in Cartilage Treatment**. 73
Mehmet Emin Şimşek and Rıfat Şahin

9 **Autologous Chondrocyte Implantation and Matrix-Induced Autologous Chondrocyte Implantation**. 85
Erkan Alkan and M. Ugur Mermerkaya

10 **Third-Generation GACI (Gel-Based Autologous Chondrocyte Implantation)** 95
Niyazi Ercan, Sancar Alp Ovalı, and Ramazan Akmeşe

11 **Particulated Cartilage Applications in Cartilage Treatment** . . . 105
Andriolo Luca, Grassi Alberto, Zanasi Lorenzo, Filardo Giuseppe, and Zaffagnini Stefano

12 **Bone Marrow Aspirate Concentrate and Hyaluronic Acid-Based Scaffold Applications and the Healing Cycle** 115
Zirvecan Güneş and Gazi Huri

13 **Cartilage Treatment with Adipose Mesenchymal Stem Cells** 133
Simone Orazi, Angelo Boffa, Luca Andriolo, Alessandro Di Martino, and Stefano Zaffagnini

14 **Articular Cartilage Preservation Surgeries** 143
Matteo Innocenti and Mattia Chirico

15 **Osteochondral Allograft Transplantation for Cartilage Repair and the Healing Cycle** 163
Gokhan Meric and Behic Celik

16 **Use of 3D Bioprinters in Cartilage Repair and Engineering** 169
Feza Korkusuz and Batuhan Erhan Aktaş

17 **Differences in the Treatment of Cartilage Lesions According to Anatomic Localizations** 195
Fatih Karaaslan, Turan Cihan Dülgeroğlu, and Yavuz Kocabey

18 **Cell and Gene Therapy for Cartilage Regeneration** 217
Sevil Köse, Çağla Zübeyde Köprü, and Petek Korkusuz

19 **Inflammatory and Metabolic Cartilage Diseases** 235
Bilgehan Çatal

20 **Physical Therapy, Rehabilitation, and Return to Sports After Cartilage Surgery** 253
Defne Kaya Utlu

21 **Atlas of Cartilage** 261
Mehmet E. Erdil and Bahattin Kemah

About the Editors

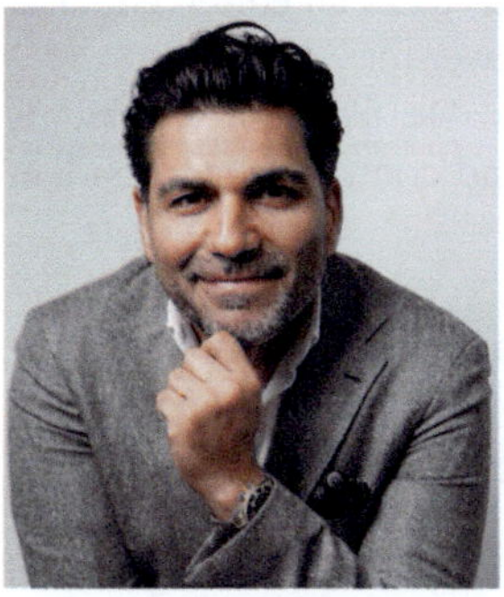

Mehmet E. Erdil is a Professor of Orthopaedics and Traumatology based in Istanbul and the founder of Orthomax Clinic. He previously held faculty positions at Acıbadem University, Istanbul Medipol University, and Bezmialem Vakıf University. He earned his MD and completed residency at Istanbul University, followed by a research fellowship at the University of Pittsburgh in Sports Medicine. His clinical focus includes knee surgery, cartilage repair, meniscus pathology, sports injuries, and arthroplasty. He has authored numerous scientific publications, contributed to orthopaedic textbooks, and serves on editorial boards and scientific committees.

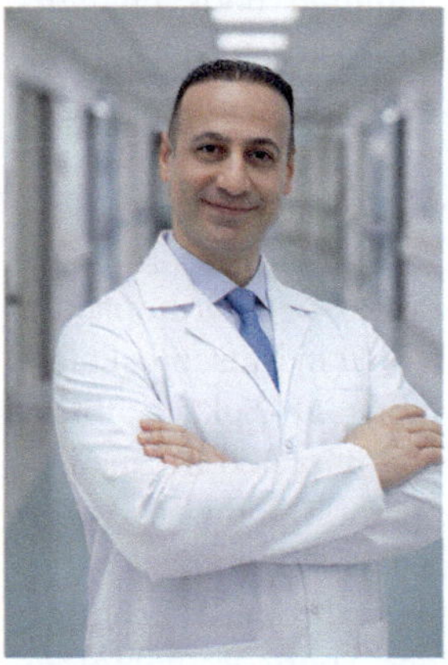

Mehmet Emin Şimşek is a Professor of Orthopaedics and Traumatology at Lokman Hekim University in Ankara. He completed medical school at Erciyes University and residency at Ankara Yıldırım Beyazıt University. His main fields include knee surgery, cartilage restoration, meniscal pathology, sports injuries, and arthroplasty. He has published widely in international journals, contributed book chapters, and participates in the editorial process of an international textbook. Dr. Şimşek serves on scientific committees of national orthopaedic societies, lectures at national and international meetings, and is active in cadaveric surgical training.

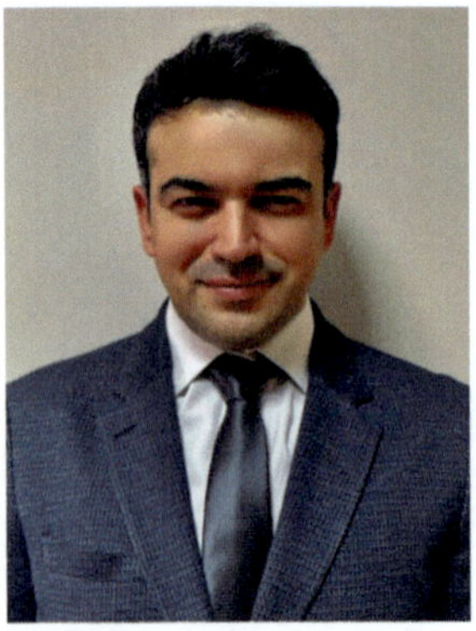

Taha Kızılkurt is an Associate Professor of Orthopaedics and Traumatology at Istanbul University, Istanbul Faculty of Medicine. He obtained his medical degree from Marmara University and completed residency at Istanbul University, later earning national board certification from TOTEK. His clinical and academic interests include sports traumatology; knee, shoulder, and hip surgery; arthroscopy; hip preservation; fracture management; and joint reconstruction. He has authored numerous international publications and textbook chapters and serves as an editor, editorial board member, and reviewer for

orthopaedic journals. He frequently presents at scientific meetings and contributes to resident training.

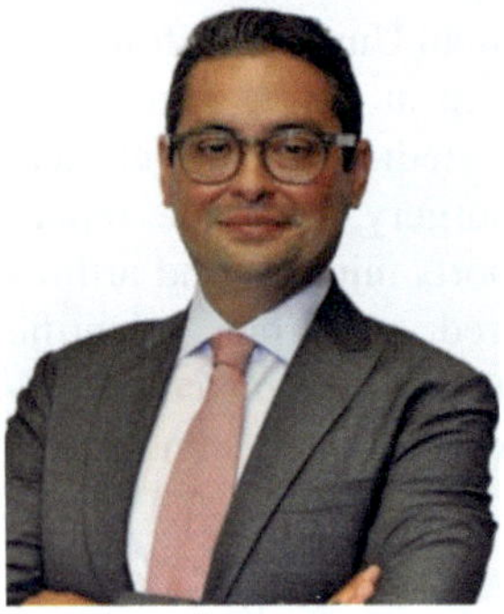

M. Uğur Mermerkaya is a Professor of Orthopaedics and Traumatology at Memorial Ankara Hospital. He graduated from Hacettepe University Faculty of Medicine and completed residency at the same institution. He pursued advanced training in sports traumatology and arthroscopic surgery in Munich and Zurich. His clinical focus includes trauma surgery, sports injuries, arthroscopic procedures, and primary and revision arthroplasty. Prof. Mermerkaya has published extensively, authored book chapters, and served as speaker and instructor at national and international courses. He previously served on the board of TUSYAD and is a member of multiple orthopaedic societies.

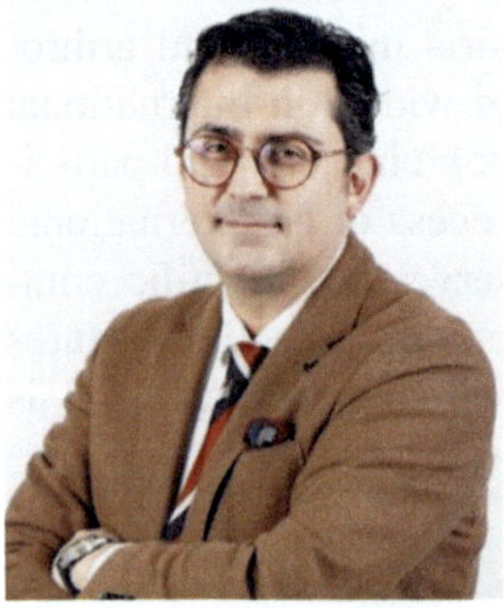

Mustafa Akkaya is a Professor of Orthopaedics and Traumatology with a PhD in Musculoskeletal and Regenerative Medicine at Yuksek Ihtisas University in Ankara. He completed his medical training, residency, and doctoral studies at Ankara Yıldırım Beyazıt University. His clinical expertise includes knee and hip arthroplasty, complex revision surgery, infections, sports traumatology, and regenerative orthopaedics. He has published extensively in high-impact journals and contributed chapters to leading textbooks. Prof. Akkaya has participated in EU-funded projects, holds a patented surgical instrument, and completed fellowships at renowned centers including Helios ENDO Klinik, ATOS Clinic, and Rizzoli Institute. He serves on editorial boards and contributes to academic and professional societies.

Anatomy, Histology, and Osteochondral Unit of Healthy Cartilage and the Effect of Synovial Membrane

1

Muge Kirac, Yigit Umur Cirdi,
Alp Er Tunga Bolukbasi, and Safa Gursoy

1.1 Introduction

Cartilage is a specialized type of connective tissue that is found in many parts of the body, including the joints. It is composed of a matrix of collagen fibers and proteoglycans. The collagen fibers provide strength and support, while the proteoglycans provide cushioning and shock absorption. The proteoglycans are negatively charged, and they attract water molecules. This attraction of water molecules helps maintain cartilage hydration and supports its cushioning function.

Chondrocytes and their precursor cells, chondroblasts, are the only cells found in cartilage. Chondrocytes organize themselves into clusters of cells called cell nests located within lacunae. Developing from the embryonic mesenchyme, chondroblasts first appear as clusters of vacuolated cells with a rounded morphology. Cartilage growth occurs in two ways. Interstitial growth occurs by the proliferation of chondroblasts within the existing matrix, whereas appositional growth occurs through the development of new chondroblasts from the perichondrium. Cartilage tissue maintains a production and degradation cycle throughout life, and composition changes over time. Surrounding factors and pressure vectors shape the surface geometry and topological features at the morphogenesis phase [1]. Destruction of the cartilage tissue generally results in loss of function and diseases eventually.

There are three types of cartilage: hyaline cartilage, fibrocartilage, and elastic cartilage. Hyaline cartilage is the most common cartilage. Articular cartilage is the connective tissue that covers the bone surface in diarthrodial joints and is composed of hyaline cartilage. Together with synovial fluid, it facilitates low-friction joint motion. As articular cartilage is avascular, alym-

Our article is original and is not under consideration by other journals. Also, the material in the article has not been published previously, and all our authors agree as to the content. All authors in this study were fully involved in the study and preparation of the manuscript and that the material within has not been and will not be submitted for publication elsewhere. All authors in this study, their immediate family, and any research foundation with which they are affiliated have not received any financial payments or other benefits from any commercial entity related to the subject of this article. Ethical Committee approval was also obtained.

M. Kirac
Faculty of Medicine, Department of Orthopaedics and Traumatology, Acibadem Mehmet Ali Aydınlar University, Istanbul, Turkey

Y. U. Cirdi (✉) · S. Gursoy
Faculty of Medicine, Department of Orthopaedics and Traumatology, Acibadem Mehmet Ali Aydınlar University, Istanbul, Turkey

Department of Orthopaedics and Traumatology, Acibadem Atasehir Hospital, Istanbul, Turkey

A. E. T. Bolukbasi
Department of Orthopaedics and Traumatology, Acibadem Atasehir Hospital, Istanbul, Turkey

M. E. Erdil et al. (eds.), *Current Concept in Cartilage Treatment*,
https://doi.org/10.1007/978-3-032-27099-3_1

phatic, and aneural tissue, oxygen and nutrients are supplied to the chondrocytes by diffusion predominantly from the synovial fluid [2].

The osteochondral unit is the basic functional unit of a joint. It is composed of the articular cartilage, the subchondral bone, and the synovial fluid. While articular cartilage provides a smooth, gliding surface for the bones to articulate against, the subchondral bone provides support for the articular cartilage and helps distribute loads across the joint. The synovial membrane covers the inner part of the joint capsule, and it produces synovial fluid, which nourishes the articular cartilage and helps to remove waste products. The synovial membrane also contains macrophages and lymphocytes, which help to defend the joint against infection.

A comprehensive understanding of healthy cartilage anatomy, histology, and the osteochondral unit may guide the development of innovative procedures for cartilage-related disorders and improve the quality of life of affected individuals.

1.2 Anatomy and Histology of Healthy Cartilage

Cartilage is a hard, semi-transparent, elastic, and flexible specialized connective tissue. There are three types of cartilage: hyaline cartilage, fibrocartilage, and elastic cartilage. Cartilage does not contain blood vessels, nerves, or lymph vessels. Cells acquire their nourishment from the adjacent connective tissues via diffusion across the matrix.

Hyaline cartilage is the most common cartilage and is found in the articular surfaces, the nose, larynx, trachea, bronchi, ribs, and the developing skeleton. Hyaline cartilage is a highly specialized tissue uniquely designed for load distribution with a smooth, low-friction articulating surface. It also serves as a temporary template for skeletal development. The hyaline cartilage consists of chondrocytes, type 2 collagen, and extracellular matrix, including water, proteoglycans, glycoproteins, and lipids. Aggrecan is the main proteoglycan of the cartilage tissue, mostly found in articular cartilage to withstand compression forces. Continuous synthesis of the aggrecan in healthy cartilage is mainly induced by insulin-like growth factor (IGF) [3].

Articular cartilage is the tissue covering the bone surface covered with hyaline cartilage at the ends of the diarthrodial joints. The free surface of the structure is oriented towards the joint cavity, while the opposite surface is connected to the subchondral bone. Together with synovial fluid, articular cartilage facilitates low-friction motion between joint surfaces. The thickness and cell density of the tissue vary between different joints, and in humans it is thickest over the ends of the femur and tibia, measuring from 2 to 4 mm.

The hyaline cartilage surface is surrounded by the perichondrium, a zone of transition between the surrounding connective tissue and the cartilage. The perichondrium consists of two layers: the outer fibrous layer and the inner chondrogenic cell layer. However, there is no perichondrium in articular cartilage. As articular cartilage is avascular, alymphatic, and aneural tissue, oxygen and nutrients are supplied to the chondrocytes by diffusion predominantly from the synovial fluid. Since articular cartilage is avascular and cannot form a fibrin clot, its healing and repair capacity is limited. Therefore, injuries to articular cartilage are challenging to treat and restore because of its complex structure and limited intrinsic healing capacity (Chap. 21, Fig. 21.1).

The matrix of hyaline cartilage is arranged in a three-dimensional network. There is a strong connection of the mechanical characteristics of the cartilage tissue and composition of the extracellular matrix (ECM) and biomechanical function. The composition of the ECM varies widely with the localization in the body. Articular cartilage ECM consists of 65–80% water, 10–20% collagens, 12% proteoglycans, and 2% glycoproteins [4]. There are more than 15 collagen subtypes present, but type II collagen plays a major role in articular cartilage; the other minor collagen subtypes constitute the fibril meshwork. There is also type VI collagen found in the ECM with subtle amounts of type IX and XI collagen. Type IX collagen interacts with type II collagen to improve biomechanical resilience and type XI collagen to adjust thickness [5]. The collagen fibers are arranged in bundles that run in different directions. This arrangement of collagen fibers gives hyaline cartilage its strength and flexibility [6].

Articular cartilage is composed of four horizontal layers: superficial, transitional, deep, and calcified cartilage zones (Fig. 1.1) [7, 8]. The zonal arrangement holds functional significance, with variations in zone sizes observed across different joints and species. Cells in different layers exhibit variations in their dimensions, morphology, and metabolic functioning. Cell density in adult humans is greatest near the articular surface and diminishes as distance from the surface increases. Additionally, cell density declines in every zone of the tissue as age progresses. The collagen content is most abundant in the surface zone but decreases by 20% in the middle and deep zones. The content of proteoglycan is at its minimum in the superficial zone and increases by up to 50% in the middle and deep zones.

Superficial (Tangential) Layer: The superficial layer is accountable for facilitating smooth motion and providing lubrication, constituting around 10–20% of the articular cartilage. The articular cartilage is at its thinnest in this zone. Consisting of flattened chondrocytes, it possesses a high water concentration, a low proteoglycan content, and tightly packed layers of collagen fibers that are uniformly thin. The zone consists of two collagen layers: a thin fibrillary lamina splendens layer devoid of cells and a cellular layer containing flattened chondrocytes [9, 10]. The outermost layer (lamina splendens) is composed of a thin layer of small fibrils devoid of chondrocytes, and these fine fibrils are aligned in parallel to the articular surface. The cellular layer is composed of compacted chondrocytes and collagen fibers that are aligned parallel to the articular surface. The precise arrangement of the outermost layer dictates the mechanical characteristics of the tissue and can also serve as an obstacle for the movement of large molecules, such as antibodies, from the synovial fluid to the cartilage. The outermost layer usually exhibits fast green staining exclusively, while safranin-O staining is absent [11].

Transitional (Intermediate or Middle) Layer: The cartilage is important for facilitating the transition between the shearing forces acting on the superficial layer and the compression forces acting on the deeper layers. It constitutes approximately 40–60% of the cartilage. The structure consists of spherical chondrocytes enclosed by extracellular matrix. The collagen fibers exhibit a disorganized pattern, while the concentration of proteoglycan is elevated. In the transitional zone, when the safranin-O staining initially becomes visible,

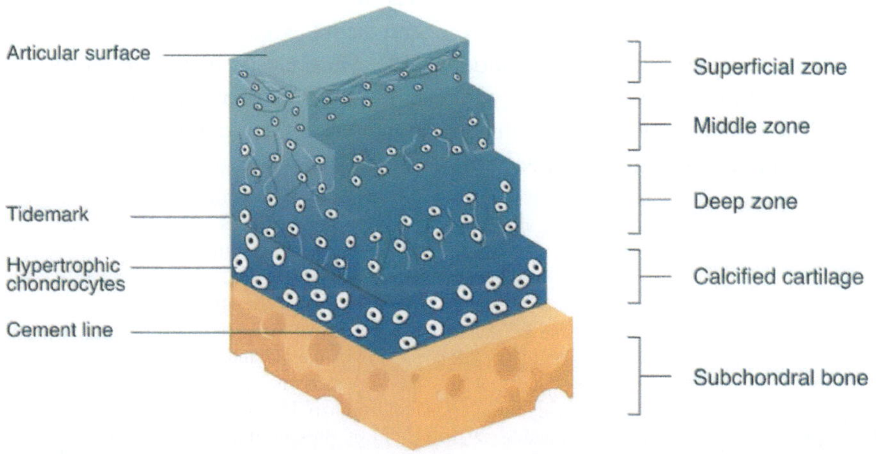

Fig. 1.1 The histologic structure of an osteochondral unit

the cells exhibit a rounded or oval shape and appear to be randomly distributed [11]. Conversely, in the deeper region, the cells are organized in short columns.

Deep (Radial or Radiate) Layer: The deep layer constitutes around 30% of the articular cartilage and is responsible for distributing stresses and resisting compression. Typically, large chondrocytes are clustered together in radial columns and positioned at a right angle to the surface. The cell density is the lowest out of the four layers. The collagen fibrils are oriented perpendicular to the surface of the joint. This area has the greatest concentration of proteoglycan and the lowest concentration of water.

The tidemark is a narrow, basophilic line that is typically visible in a slide stained with hematoxylin and eosin. It serves as the demarcation between the mineralized and unmineralized areas and acts as a boundary between the deep zone and the calcified zone.

Calcified Zone: The calcified zone is distinguished by the presence of rounded chondrocytes situated in uncalcified lacunae and the lack of proteoglycans. The collagen fibers are oriented perpendicular to the articular surface and firmly attached to a calcified matrix. The function of this structure is to provide support for bones, and it is made up of circular chondrocytes that are found in non-calcified lacunae. The collagen fibrils are oriented orthogonally to the articular surface.

The interterritorial matrix constitutes about 90% of the composition and is not fused with chondrocytes. The chondrocytes located in the transitional and deep layers of the articular cartilage are closely connected to their territorial matrices. The collagen fibrils in the interterritorial matrix have a larger diameter compared to those in the territorial matrix. The collagen fibrils in the superficial zone are aligned parallel to the articular surface, whereas in the transitional zone, they are arranged randomly, and in the deep zone they are directed perpendicular to the surface.

Articular cartilage is primarily composed of water, making up approximately 65–80% of its total composition. The proteoglycan aggregates undergo swelling because of water absorption, which allows cartilage to resist compressive forces. The wet weight of cartilage primarily consists of water (60–80%) and macromolecules (20–40%), such as collagens, proteoglycans, and noncollagenous proteins. Collagens account for 50–60% of the weight of cartilage when it is dry, while proteoglycans account for 30% of the weight.

Fibrocartilage is located in the intervertebral discs, temporomandibular joint disc, knee meniscus, sternoclavicular joint disc, pubic symphysis, and attachment points of the tendon and ligament to the bone. It has great tensile strength. It lacks perichondrium.

Elastic cartilage is covered with perichondrium and is found in the outer ear, auditory tube, and epiglottis. Due to its special matrix, it has flexibility and the ability to maintain its original shape after applied force. The elastin molecule has the ability to elongate when force is applied and recoil when the force vector is withdrawn [12]. Thus, elastic fibers can return to their original shape after being stretched. Chondrocytes are relatively bigger compared to hyaline cartilage (Fig. 1.2).

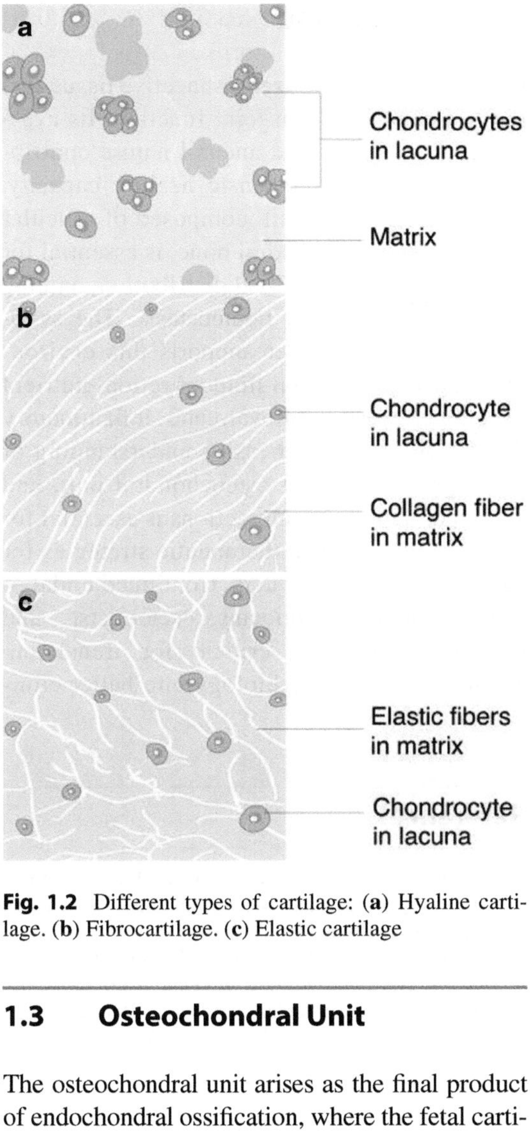

Fig. 1.2 Different types of cartilage: (**a**) Hyaline cartilage. (**b**) Fibrocartilage. (**c**) Elastic cartilage

1.3 Osteochondral Unit

The osteochondral unit arises as the final product of endochondral ossification, where the fetal cartilage "anlagen" is diminished by endochondral ossification after birth, leaving permanent articular cartilage at the ends of fully developed long bones. The osteochondral unit is the basic unit of a joint. It is composed of the articular cartilage, the subchondral bone, and the synovial fluid. Articular cartilage provides a smooth, low-friction surface that enables movement between opposing joint surfaces. The collagen fibers provide strength and support, while the proteoglycans provide cushioning and shock absorption. The subchondral bone provides support for the articular cartilage and helps to distribute loads across the joint [13].

The subchondral bone is the layer of bone that lies beneath the articular cartilage. It is composed of a dense network of trabeculae, type I collagen, and hydroxyapatite [14]. The osteochondral unit is a complex structure that is essential for the proper function of a joint. Understanding the anatomy and physiology of the osteochondral unit provides insight into the mechanisms underlying joint injury and degenerative joint disorders.

The main functions of the osteochondral unit include the following:

- Provides a smooth, low-friction surface that enables movement between opposing joint surfaces
- Provides support for the articular cartilage
- Helps to distribute loads across the joint
- Provides nutrients and oxygen to the articular cartilage
- Helps to remove waste products from the articular cartilage

The osteochondral unit is a vital component of the musculoskeletal system. However, it is also susceptible to injury and degeneration. This can lead to pain, stiffness, and decreased range of motion.

There are a number of treatment options available for osteochondral injuries. These include non-surgical treatments, such as physical therapy and medication, and surgical treatments, such as cartilage repair and replacement. The choice of treatment should be guided by the severity of the injury, patient-specific factors, and functional demands.

1.4 Effect of Synovial Membrane

The synovial membrane is a thin, vascular membrane that lines the joint capsule. It produces synovial fluid, which nourishes the articular cartilage and helps to remove waste products. The synovial membrane also contains macrophages and lymphocytes, which help to defend the joint against infection. The synovial membrane is a dynamic tissue that is constantly changing. It responds to changes in the environment, such as inflammation, infection, and injury.

The synovial membrane consists of two layers: (1) a superficial layer that lines the entire joint capsule, tendon sheath, and bursa, which consists of macrophages and fibroblasts and (2) a deep layer that communicates with blood and lymphatic vessels. Synovial membrane cells secrete an ultrafiltrate that contains lubricant molecules, mainly proteoglycan-4 and hyaluronan [15], called synovial fluid, allowing for frictionless movement, especially in diarthrodial joints. Additionally, cellular communication is achieved via cytokines secreted from the synovial membrane of the joint [16].

The superficial layer of the synovial membrane is rich in macrophages. In inflammatory arthritis such as rheumatoid arthritis (RA), the superficial layer is prominently thickened, and CD68+ macrophages migrate superficially [17]. By understanding the function of the synovial membrane, we can better understand the causes of joint pain and inflammation. For instance, joint effusion in osteoarthritis is caused by the overproduction of the synovial fluid secondary to damaged cartilage wear and mechanical stimulation. It is actually a reaction to compensate for disturbed osteochondral and synovial interaction.

The synovial membrane influences cartilage through several mechanisms:

The synovial membrane produces synovial fluid, which provides nutrients and oxygen to the articular cartilage.

The synovial membrane helps to remove waste products from the articular cartilage.

The synovial membrane secretes hyaluronan-rich fluid to facilitate ambulation.

The synovial membrane can become infected, which can also damage the articular cartilage.

Maintenance of the intact non-adherent surface [17].

1.5 Conclusion

Cartilage is a specialized connective tissue that plays a central role in joint function. Its avascular, alymphatic, and aneural nature contributes to its limited intrinsic healing capacity. The osteochondral unit, composed of articular cartilage and subchondral bone, is essential for smooth joint motion, load distribution, and the maintenance of joint homeostasis. The synovial membrane further supports this environment through synovial fluid secretion, nutrient exchange, waste removal, and inflammatory regulation. A comprehensive understanding of cartilage biology, the osteochondral unit, and synovial membrane interactions is essential for developing improved therapeutic strategies for cartilage-related disorders. Continued collaboration among clinicians, scientists, and researchers will be critical for translating advances in cartilage biology into better clinical outcomes.

References

1. Wong M, Carter DR. Articular cartilage functional histomorphology and mechanobiology: a research perspective. Bone. 2003;33(1):1–13.
2. Zhou S, Cui Z, Urban JPG. Factors influencing the oxygen concentration gradient from the synovial surface of articular cartilage to the cartilage-bone interface: a modeling study. Arthritis Rheum. 2004;50(12):3915–24.
3. van der Kraan PM, van Caam APM, Blaney Davidson EN, van den Bosch MHJ, van de Loo FAJ. Growth factors that drive aggrecan synthesis in healthy articular cartilage. Role for transforming growth factor-β? Osteoarthr Cartil Open. 2024;6(2):100459.
4. Chen S, Fu P, Wu H, Pei M. Meniscus, articular cartilage, and nucleus pulposus: a comparative review of cartilage-like tissues in anatomy, development, and function. Cell Tissue Res. 2017;370(1):53–70.
5. Armiento AR, Alini M, Stoddart MJ. Articular fibrocartilage—why does hyaline cartilage fail to repair? Adv Drug Deliv Rev. 2019;146:289–305.
6. Loy BN, Zimel M, Gowda AL, Tooley TR, Maerz T, Bicos J, et al. A biomechanical and structural comparison of articular cartilage and subchondral bone of the glenoid and humeral head. Orthop J Sports Med. 2018;6(7):2325967118785854.

7. Huber M, Trattnig S, Lintner F. Anatomy, biochemistry, and physiology of articular cartilage. Investig Radiol. 2000;35(10):573.
8. Sophia Fox AJ, Bedi A, Rodeo SA. The basic science of articular cartilage: structure, composition, and function. Sports Health. 2009;1(6):461–8.
9. Minns RJ, Steven FS. The collagen fibril organization in human articular cartilage. J Anat. 1977;123(Pt 2):437–57.
10. Lane JM, Weiss C. Review of articular cartilage collagen research. Arthritis Rheum. 1975;18(6):553–62.
11. Nakagawa Y, Muneta T, Otabe K, Ozeki N, Mizuno M, Udo M, et al. Cartilage derived from bone marrow mesenchymal stem cells expresses lubricin in vitro and in vivo. PLoS One. 2016;11(2):e0148777.
12. Scott JE. Elasticity in extracellular matrix 'shape modules' of tendon, cartilage, etc. A sliding proteoglycan-filament model. J Physiol. 2003;553(Pt 2):335–43.
13. Lepage SIM, Robson N, Gilmore H, Davis O, Hooper A, St. John S, et al. Beyond cartilage repair: the role of the osteochondral unit in joint health and disease. Tissue Eng Part B Rev. 2019;25(2):114–25.
14. Arvidson K, Abdallah BM, Applegate LA, Baldini N, Cenni E, Gomez-Barrena E, et al. Bone regeneration and stem cells. J Cell Mol Med. 2011;15(4):718–46.
15. Hui AY, McCarty WJ, Masuda K, Firestein GS, Sah RL. A systems biology approach to synovial joint lubrication in health, injury, and disease. Wiley Interdiscip Rev Syst Biol Med. 2012;4(1):15–37.
16. Hyc A, Osiecka-Iwan A, Niderla-Bielinska J, Jankowska-Steifer E, Moskalewski S. Pro- and anti-inflammatory cytokines increase hyaluronan production by rat synovial membrane in vitro. Int J Mol Med. 2009;24(4):579–85.
17. Smith MD. The normal synovium. Open Rheumatol J. 2011;5:100–6.

Subchondral Treatment Options in Cartilage Lesions

2

Reha N. Tandogan and Tahir Ozturk

2.1 Introduction

Osteoarthritis (OA) affects millions worldwide and is an important healthcare problem. Previously thought to be a disease involving only articular cartilage, recent studies have shown that subchondral bone plays an important role in the pathogenesis and progression of the disease [1]. There is a complex interaction between cartilage and subchondral bone during the disease process, which has led researchers to consider subchondral bone as a new target in the treatment of OA [2]. This chapter will focus on the structure and interaction of articular cartilage and subchondral bone and will review the current status of subchondral interventions in treating early OA.

2.2 Structure of Articular Cartilage Subchondral Bone

2.2.1 Articular Cartilage

Articular cartilage is a complex tissue devoid of blood vessels, lymphatics, and nerve endings and has a limited potential for regeneration. Chondrocytes make up less than 10% of the cartilage volume and are responsible for the synthesis and homeostasis of the extracellular matrix (ECM). Chondrocytes respond to mechanical, electrical, and chemical stimuli by changing their metabolism and synthesis of ECM. ECM is composed of water (65–80% of wet weight), collagen (10–20% of wet weight), proteoglycans (10–15% of wet weight), and other minor non-collagenous proteins and glycoproteins [3]. Type II collagen is predominant, making up 90–95% of all collagenous material. Type I, IV, V, VI, IX, & XI collagen are present in lesser amounts and contribute to the structure and elasticity of cartilage [4, 5].

Proteoglycans are glycosylated protein monomers of glycosaminoglycan (GAG) chains attached to a protein core. GAGs interact with hyaluronic acid (HA) chains through link proteins to form large proteoglycan clusters. The primary proteoglycan in articular cartilage is aggrecan. Other significant GAGs are HA, chondroitin sulfate, keratan sulfate, and dermatan sulfate. The high-density sulfate anions in aggrecan attract cations in the water, contributing to the osmotic properties of the cartilage. Proteoglycans are elastic macromolecules. Collagen fibers and proteoglycan aggregates collectively provide compression resistance to cartilage [6].

The articular cartilage is organized into several zones with regional differences and thicknesses [7]. These are the superficial (tangential), middle (intermediate, transitional), and deep (radial

R. N. Tandogan (✉)
Cankaya Orthopedics & Cankaya Hospital Ankara, Ankara, Turkey
e-mail: rtandogan@ortoklinik.com

T. Ozturk
Memorial Bahcelievler Hospital, Istanbul, Turkey

M. E. Erdil et al. (eds.), *Current Concept in Cartilage Treatment*,
https://doi.org/10.1007/978-3-032-27099-3_2

zones) [8]. Chondrocytes in various layers differ in density, shape, size, and metabolic activity. Cell density is higher in the superficial zone and decreases with age and distance from the joint. The superficial zone is a thin layer of densely organized collagen fibrils parallel to the articular surface. Chondrocytes in the superficial zone are flattened, with lower proteoglycan content. Since this zone is in contact with the synovial fluid, it plays an essential role in maintaining the lubrication and elastic properties of the tissue. The middle zone is the widest, with thicker and randomly arranged collagen fibrils and rounder chondrocytes. The middle zone has the highest proteoglycan content and is an anatomical and functional transition between the other two zones. It is the first line of defense against compressive forces. The deep zone is composed of collagen fibers perpendicular to the subchondral bone, with chondrocytes arranged along the axis of these fibers. The proteoglycan content is high, and water content and cell density are low. This zone significantly contributes to the compressive resistance of the cartilage during body movement [4, 8]. The tidemark separates the deep zone from the calcified zone. This wavy, irregular band of fibrils connects the non-calcified layers to the calcified layer and resists shear forces. Small gaps in the tidemark provide channels for nutrients. The deepest layer is the calcified cartilage; this is partly mineralized and acts as a transition zone between the subchondral bone and cartilage. The calcified zone is composed of rounded chondrocytes in uncalcified lacunae. Proteoglycans are absent; collagen fibers are thick and perpendicular to the articular surface, anchoring the cartilage to the subchondral bone [9].

2.2.2 Normal Subchondral Bone

Subchondral bone consists of two anatomical structures: the bone plate and the subchondral trabeculae. The subchondral bone plate is a finely porous and resilient cortical structure adjacent to calcified cartilage. Nerves and vessels pass through its pores, branching into the calcified cartilage. Subchondral trabeculae, located under the subchondral bone plate, play an essential role in load absorption, structural support, and nutrient supply to the cartilage [10].

The subchondral bone dynamically adapts to the mechanical forces applied to the joint through remodeling. However, subchondral bone and cartilage show different capacities for mechanical adaptation. While cartilage tries to maintain functional status in response to mechanical damage, the surrounding ECM's repair capacity is less than that of subchondral bone. Subchondral bone responds to mechanical loading by remodeling and can re-establish normal physiological conditions [11].

2.3 Changes in Subchondral Bone in OA

Distinct microstructural changes occur in the subchondral bone at different OA stages. Increased subchondral bone turnover and resorption are observed in early OA, while subchondral bone sclerosis is seen in the later stages. During initial cartilage degeneration in early OA, the subchondral bone plate becomes thinner and more porous. Separation increases and trabecular thickness decreases in the subchondral trabeculae [12].

In contrast, late-stage OA is characterized by thickening of the subchondral bone plate and trabeculae, along with decreased bone marrow diameter due to sclerosis. Additionally, non-calcified cartilage thickens after degeneration [13]. Despite the increased bone volume, high bone turnover and decreased calcium-to-collagen ratio result in insufficient bone mineralization and a decreased elastic modulus of bone. As a result, the bone becomes more susceptible to deformation under mechanical loads [14].

2.4 Interaction of Subchondral Bone and Cartilage

Abnormal cellular interactions contribute to disease progression in OA, affecting the subchondral bone. These interactions involve osteoclasts, osteoblasts, osteocytes, and endothelial cells, leading to disordered remodeling and angiogenesis [12, 13]. Articular cartilage repair in early-stage OA reduces excessive mechanical loads on the subchondral bone, leading to insufficient loading and an increase in the expression rate of receptor activator of nuclear factor RANKL and osteoprotegerin (OPG) in osteocytes. A higher RANKL/OPG ratio promotes excessive osteoclastogenesis and enhanced bone resorption activity [15].

Areas of overactive remodeling and micro-damage are commonly observed in subchondral bone in OA patients and animal models [16]. Osteocytes at sites of micro-damage undergo apoptosis, while neighboring apoptotic cells increase the expression of pro-osteoclastic molecules in the early stages of OA, regulating the disease [17]. Osteocytes also regulate osteoblast mineralization through the activation of the Wnt signaling pathway. Progressive cartilage destruction in OA leads to increased mechanical loading, resulting in a rise in the production of Wnt proteins and reduced secretion of sclerostin (SOST) by osteocytes. These factors contribute to osteoblast activation and bone formation in OA's progressive and late stages [18].

Transforming growth factor-β1 (TGF-β1) released by osteocytes increases osteoblast-mediated bone anabolic metabolism in progressive OA. TGF-β1 supports osteoblast activity and remineralization by activating the Smad2/3 pathway in the subchondral bone. Simultaneously, osteoclastic bone resorption provides increased levels of active TGF-β1 in the subchondral bone, attracting osteoprogenitors to remodeling areas via Smad2/3, forming osteoid islets [19].

Abnormal mechanical stress in osteoblasts triggers a metabolism characterized by the rise expression of interleukin (IL) 6, prostaglandin E2 (PGE2), matrix metalloproteinases (MMPs) 3, 9, 13, and RANKL, and reduced production of OPG (Ni G-X et al.). IL-6 and PGE2 stimulate osteoclast formation by inhibiting OPG secretion and increasing RANKL production. PGE2 increases IL-6 secretion through a positive feedback cycle, ensuring osteoclast differentiation within the OPG/RANKL/RANK system [20].

The interaction between osteoblasts, osteoclasts, and type H endothelial cells (ECs) contributes to angiogenesis and remodeling of the subchondral bone [21]. Type H ECs, surrounded by osterix-expressing osteoprogenitors, stimulate the proliferation and differentiation of osteoprogenitor cells by producing endocrine factors such as platelet-derived growth factor (PDGF)-A, TGF-β1, and fibroblast growth factor (FGF)-1, thus facilitating local bone formation [22]. Intercellular communication between type H ECs via the Notch/delta-like protein 4 (DLL4) signaling pathway induces Noggin production, further stimulating osteoprogenitor differentiation [23]. Type H ECs also regulate bone remodeling by stimulating osteoclast migration and differentiation through the production of RANKL and MMP-9 [24]. Osteoblast-derived SLIT3 and TGF-β1 raise the number of type H ECs by acting as pro-angiogenic factors [25]. TGF-β1 produced from osteoclastic resorption primarily drives subchondral angiogenesis in early-stage OA, while PDGF-BB produced from preosteoclasts plays a relatively dominant role in angiogenic and osteogenic differentiation in late-stage OA (Fig. 2.1) [26].

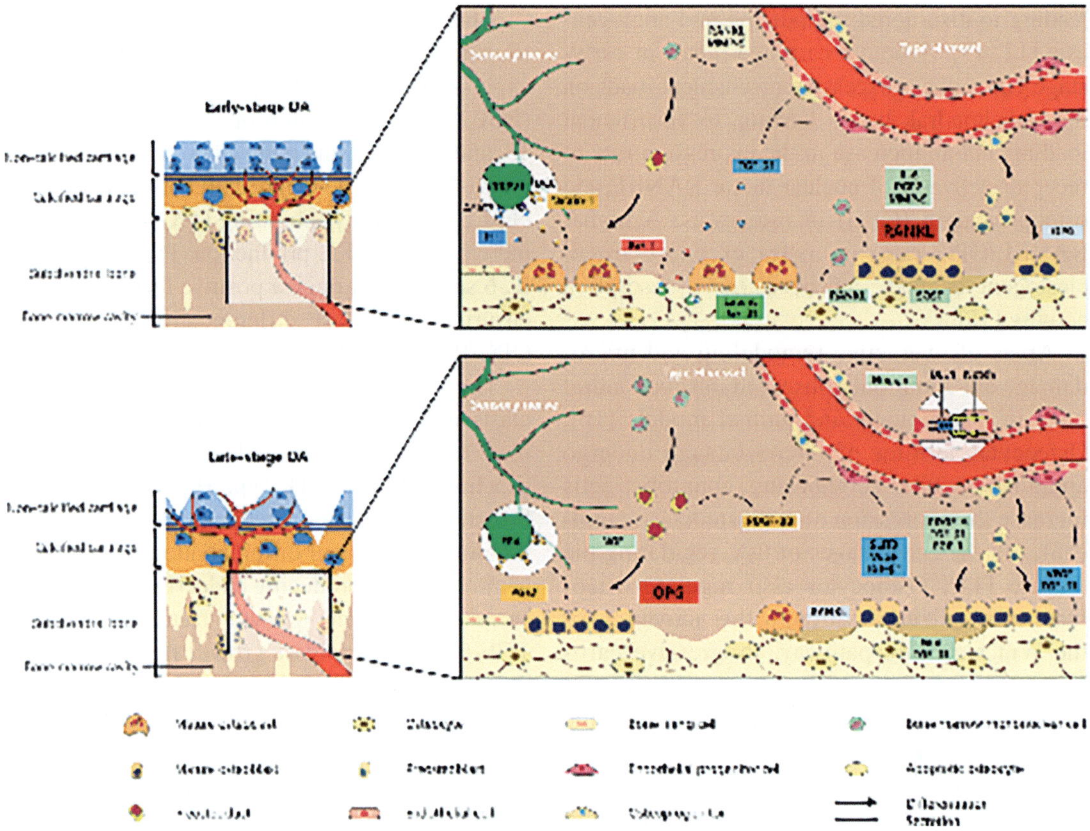

Fig. 2.1 Interaction of subchondral bone and cartilage [20] (https://creativecommons.org/licenses/by/4.0/. This material is available under Public License. This figure is cited from an open-access article distributed under the Creative Commons Attribution 4.0 Unported (CC BY 4.0) license, which allows others to copy, redistribute, rearrange, transform, and build upon this work for any purpose, provided they cite the original work. This figure has not changed; access to article with this link/URI is https://ard.bmj.com/content/80/4/413.long, https://doi.org/10.1136/annrheumdis-2020-218089)

2.5 Bone Marrow Lesions in OA

Subchondral bone marrow lesions (BML's) are found in up to 66% of symptomatic OA knees. The dimensions of BMLs are variable; more than one-third may still be present within 2 years. Structural changes in OA affect the entire joint, including the subchondral bone, and BML's are associated with pain, directly influencing OA's prognosis and treatment outcomes [27].

BMLs are diagnosed using magnetic resonance imaging (MRI) and appear hypo-intense on T1-weighted images. They exhibit a hyper-intense appearance on fluid-sensitive images, such as T2-weighted, proton density, moderately fat-suppressed, and short tau inversion recovery (STIR) images (Fig. 2.2) [28]. The pathogenesis of BMLs in OA is thought to be micro-fractures at the osteochondral junction, allowing extrusion of synovial fluid or diffusion of soluble factors into the subchondral bone, resulting in the appearance of BML. BMLs are not exclusive to OA and can be observed in other traumatic, vascular, and inflammatory processes; therefore, other potential causes should be excluded [27]. BML's associated with OA, without visible fracture lines in the subchondral area, are linked to structural changes such as loss of osteochondral integrity, fibrosis, cysts, and depletion of de novo cartilage [29].

The exact cause of BMLs is unclear, but several risk factors have been identified for their

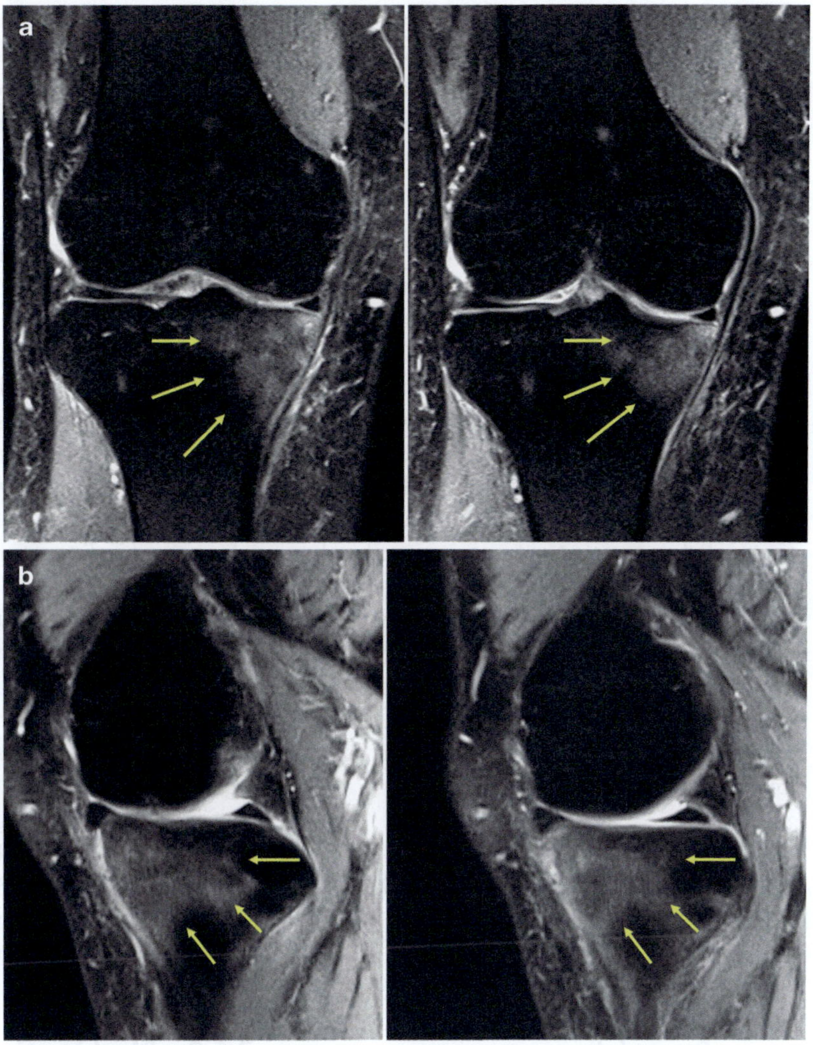

Fig. 2.2 T-2 fat-suppressed MRI sequences depicting BML in the medial tibial condyle in a 72-year-old male patient after a prolonged hike. (**a**) Coronal images; (**b**) Sagittal images, arrows outlining the extent of BML. No avascular necrosis or collapse is seen

presence and progression. Biomechanical factors, such as lower extremity malalignment, is a significant contributing factor. Varus tibiofemoral alignment, which leads to increased stress in the medial compartment, forms BML's with the adduction moment [30]. Treatments that redistribute load, such as orthoses or high tibial osteotomy, can reduce the size of BML's [31]. Obesity, dietary lipid intake, and high physical activity are other risk factors contributing to the formation of BMLs [32].

Patients with BMLs are two to five times more likely to experience knee pain than those without. The presence and size of BML's are associated with pain, especially during weight-bearing activities. Reduction in BML size may lead to regression in pain [33]. BMLs can predict OA progression, particularly cartilage loss, both structurally and radiographically. The presence and size of BML's in the medial compartment of the knee and varus tibiofemoral alignment are strongly associated with progressive loss in adjacent cartilage and are considered strong predictors of total knee replacement [34].

The association of BML's with the progression of OA has been well documented. In a study of 256 knees, Felson et al. have shown that patients with medial BML's were 6.5 times more likely to progress compared to patients without BML's [35]. This risk was 6.1 times higher for lateral lesions. The location of BMLs was correlated with the alignment of the limb, where varus knees had BMLs in the medial and valgus knees in the lateral compartment. A longitudinal MRI study of 217 knees showed that increased BML size was associated with increased loss of cartilage over time [34]. Furthermore, a BML predicted the progression of cartilage damage in asymptomatic subjects, indicating that BMLs may be a precursor to OA [36]. Compared to patients without BMLs, patients with BML and OA were 8.95 times more likely to need a joint replacement, and this risk was increased in patients with larger lesions [37].

Targeting BMLs is a new treatment approach, aiming to rapidly improve symptoms, delay structural degenerative progression, and reduce the need for joint replacement surgery [27]. Previous attempts to reduce BML's focused on reducing subchondral bone turnover (using bisphosphonates or strontium ranelate) or addressing biomechanical stresses that contribute to pain (such as patellofemoral support or high tibial osteotomy) [38, 39].

2.6 Targeting the Subchondral Bone in the Treatment of OA

2.6.1 Regulation of Abnormal Subchondral Bone Remodeling

The current treatment for OA remains relatively conservative and primarily focuses on pain management. However, effective treatment methods that can alter the spontaneous progression of OA and address inflammation by supporting the recovery of damaged chondrocyte function are still lacking. Targeting the abnormal subchondral bone in OA shows promise as a potential therapeutic approach, and various treatment strategies have been evaluated, primarily aimed at correcting abnormal subchondral bone remodeling.

Classical anti-resorptive agents such as bisphosphonates have been evaluated for their efficacy in treating OA. Different doses of risedronate did not significantly improve symptoms or delay radiological progression in patients with OA [40]. Alendronate treatment has improved pain scores and specific biochemical markers in patients with OA [41]. Intravenous zoledronic acid did not significantly improve OA patients' cartilage volume loss or pain scores [42]. Other antiresorptive agents, such as OPG, cathepsin K (CTSK) inhibitors, and strontium ranelate, have demonstrated potential protective effects on cartilage in animal studies [38, 43, 44].

Bioactive oral calcitonin has positively affected joint pain and biochemical markers of bone and cartilage destruction in OA patients. Calcitonin, which targets subchondral bone remodeling, has shown beneficial effects in phase III trials by supporting chondrocyte anabolism by binding to receptors on human OA chondrocytes [45].

Enhanced osteoclast activity in subchondral bone leads to overactivation of the TGF-β1 signaling pathway. Targeting subchondral TGF-β1 has been identified as a potential pharmacological approach for OA. In a mice anterior cruciate ligament transection (ACLT) model, it was found that implantation of alginic acid with a TGF-β1 antibody or deletion of Tgfbr2 prevented phosphorylation of Smad2/3 in osteoblastic precursor cells, resulting in improvements in bone parameters and cartilage structure [46].

2.6.2 Blocking the Connection with Subchondral H-Type Vessels

The formation of subchondral H-type vessels contributes to the progression of OA by creating a connection between the subchondral bone and articular cartilage. Animal studies have demonstrated that blocking the formation of H-type vessels can reduce cartilage destruction and subchondral bone loss in OA models [47]. Bevacizumab, an antibody that inhibits vascular endothelial growth factor (VEGF), attenuates the formation of subchondral type H vessels, thereby inhibiting chondrocyte hypertrophy and OA progression [48].

In addition to VEGF, other secretory factors produced by osteoclasts or osteoblasts in the subchondral bone microenvironment, such as TGF-β1, platelet-derived growth factor-BB (PDGF-BB), and SLIT3, promote subchondral angiogenesis. Antagonists targeting these molecules show potential as therapeutic interventions for OA. Halofuginone, a small molecule compound, inhibits Smad2/3-dependent TGF-β1 signaling. By targeting this pathway, halofuginone can reduce the formation of H-type vessels and prevent cartilage degradation by restoring the coupling of subchondral bone remodeling [47].

2.6.3 Improvement of Pain Associated with OA by Subchondral Bone Regulation

Osteoclasts, responsible for bone resorption, cause an acidic microenvironment by secreting H+ ions, which can induce bone pain in animal models. Acidosis triggers the expression and activation of the acid-sensing receptor known as transient receptor potential vanilloid 1 (TRPV1) in the dorsal root ganglion (DRGs). Activation of TRPV1 leads to the influx of extracellular calcium, followed by the activation of calmodulin-dependent protein kinase II (CaMKII) and the transcription factor cAMP-responsive element-binding protein (CREB), resulting in the activation of calcitonin gene-related peptide (CGRP), a molecule associated with pain [49, 50].

Acid-sensing ion channel 3 (ASIC3) is also implicated in hyperalgesia through increased calcium influx in OA models [51]. Furthermore, in animal model studies of OA, PGE2 synthesized by osteoblasts in response to low bone density upregulates the voltage-gated sodium channel Nav1.8, leading to increased sodium influx in subchondral nociceptive neurons and contributing to skeletal allodynia [52].

Current guidelines for managing OA pain recommend using non-steroidal anti-inflammatory drugs (NSAIDs), paracetamol, opioids, and corticosteroids. Additionally, inhibitors and antagonists targeting pain-related molecules show promise. Inhibition of cyclooxygenase 2 (COX-2), Nav1.8, EP4 receptors, TRPV1, and ASIC3 has effectively reduced nociceptive signals and calcium influx, thus reducing OA-related pain in animal models. Tanezumab, a specific inhibitor, is a promising treatment option [51–53].

2.7 Subchondral Interventions in OA

Primary treatment of painful BMLs in patients with early OA is conservative with a period of rest, partial weight-bearing, and anti-inflammatory drugs. Cryotherapy and isometric exercises are also helpful. Most patients respond to conservative measures by 3 weeks. However, the BMLs take much longer to subside in MRI scans. The authors advocate a follow-up visit at 3 weeks to monitor the effect of conservative treatment, followed by a visit at 6 weeks and an MRI scan at 4–6 months. Patients with significant pain despite adequate conservative management for 6–8 weeks may be candidates for subchondral interventions.

2.7.1 Subchondral Cement Injection for OA

Subchondral injection of bioactive bone cement, also known as "Subchondroplasty," has been used to treat painful BML in patients with knee OA. This procedure provides mechanical support to the subchondral bone and overlying cartilage.

The site of the injection in the tibia or femur is determined preoperatively using MRI scans, and the procedure is usually performed using fluoroscopic guidance, aiming for an injection 10–15 mm below the joint surface. Multi-fenestrated cannulae that allow for 360-degree cement extrusion are used for injection (Fig. 2.3). Commercially available guides have also been described to target the area of BML. Concurrent arthroscopic debridement and treatment of meniscal tears is usually performed. Arthroscopy is also useful to check for intra-articular leakage of the cement and removal of this material from the joint to prevent synovitis and loose body for-

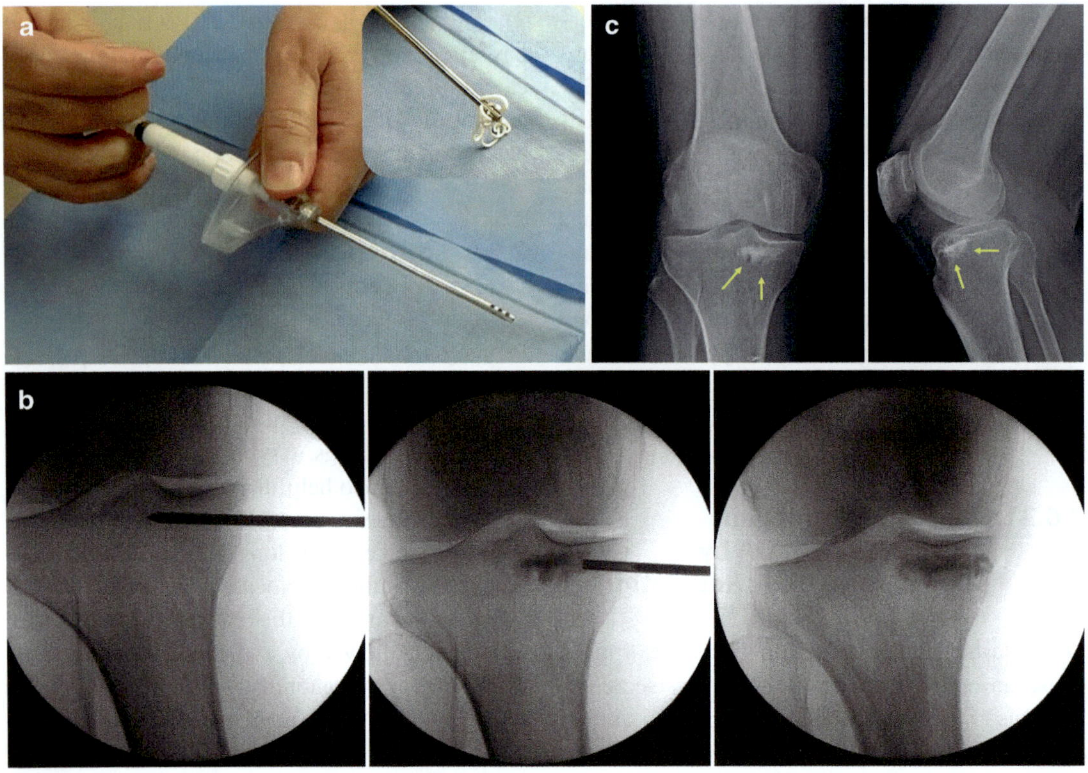

Fig. 2.3 Subchondral cement injection for painful BML unresponsive to conservative treatment for the patient depicted in Fig. 2.2; (**a**) Proprietary multi-fenestrated cannula developed for circumferential injection of cement; (**b**) Injection of bioactive cement into the medial tibial plateau under fluoroscopic guidance; (**c**) One-year X-ray showing no progression of disease and partial resorption of cement

mation. Intra-articular leakage is more common in the distal femur since most injection sites require a trans-articular trajectory (Fig. 2.4). Most studies on subchondral cement injection have reported on femoral and tibial BMLs; however, favorable outcomes with reduction of pain and improvement in functional scores have also been reported in patellar lesions [54]. Commercially available calcium phosphate bone cements have varying mechanical properties, working and setting times, and penetration properties; the surgeon should be aware of these to avoid technical problems [55]. Although the cement used in subchondral injections is thought to be biodegradable, injected cement material may persist in the bone for several years [56]. The resorption seen after 2 years in canine studies may not be applicable to humans [57]. However, no technical issues or adverse outcomes have been reported in patients undergoing total knee arthroplasty following subchondral cement injection [58].

Immediate weight-bearing as tolerated is allowed in the postoperative period, although a single crutch may be needed for balance and pain control. Pain may worsen in the early postoperative period but usually subsides in a few days. Early range of motion and quadriceps strengthening exercises are accompanied by cryotherapy. Unrestricted activity may be allowed after 6 weeks.

Most studies on the clinical outcomes of subchondral cement injection are Level 4 studies, and high-quality RCTs are missing [59]. Up to 90% of patient satisfaction rates have been shown in a systematic review of 765 patients in 17 studies [59]. Another systematic review of 10 studies involving 540 patients followed up for 6 months

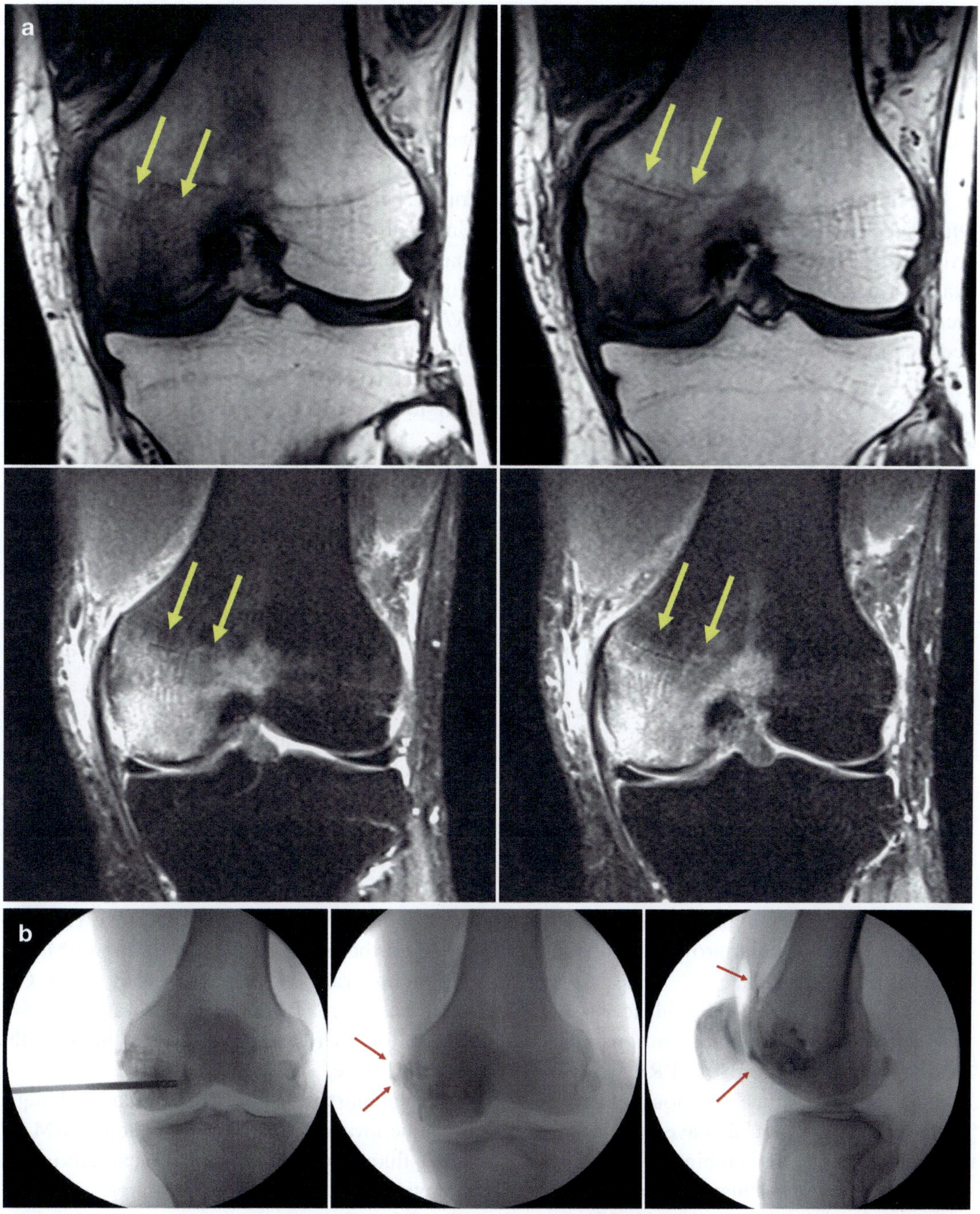

Fig. 2.4 Intra-articular cement leakage during femoral subchondral cement injection; (**a**) Preoperative T-1 and T-2 fat-suppressed MRI images showing a large BML in the medial femoral condyle; (**b**) Fluoroscopic images during subchondral cement injection showing intra-articular leakage, which was removed during arthroscopy

to 7 years has shown significant improvements in quality of life and pain relief. Conversion to total knee arthroplasty was reported in 14–30% of the patients at 2 years [60]. Risk factors for conversion to knee arthroplasty are age >50 and grade 4 cartilage lesions [61]. Poor outcomes have been reported in patients with advanced OA [62]. The effect of subchondral cement injection on the natural history of OA is unclear, but a disease-modifying effect is not expected. The arrest of radiographic progression of OA has not been reported.

The most frequent complication associated with subchondral cement injection is intra-articular leakage; serious complications such as avascular necrosis and osteomyelitis are rare. An increase in bone marrow edema and pain has been reported in case reports [59].

2.7.2 Subchondral Platelet-Rich Plasma Injections

Intra-articular platelet-rich plasma (PRP) is widely used in the symptomatic treatment of knee OA [63]. In a randomized controlled trial of 45 knees, in addition to providing symptomatic relief, intra-articular PRP injections also decreased the severity of subchondral BML's [64]. Subchondral/intraosseous PRP injection is a novel concept and is usually combined with an intra-articular injection (PRP or hyaluronic acid). The mechanism of action of PRP in subchondral bone is thought to be its anti-inflammatory effect and reduction of oxidative stress, thereby creating a favorable biological environment that positively impacts bone remodeling and fibro-neuro-vascular growth of subchondral bone [65].

There is limited clinical evidence to suggest the superiority of combined intra-osseous and intra-articular injection of PRP over intra-articular injection alone. Previous studies by Su et al. and Sanchez et al. have shown superior clinical outcomes of combined PRP injections compared to intra-articular PRP/HA, which was sustained for up to 18 months [66, 67]. In contrast, a randomized controlled trial of 50 patients found no significant benefit of additional intra-osseous PRP to intra-articular injections in terms of pain relief and functional outcomes at six months follow-up [68]. Another study by the same group found a significant reduction in erythrocyte sedimentation rate (ESR), C-reactive protein (CRP), and bone/cartilage turnover biomarkers in both isolated and combined PRP groups compared to saline [69].

A recent systematic review of 5 studies, including 112 patients, analyzed the outcomes of combined intra-osseous injections of PRP and found better Western Ontario and McMaster Universities Arthritis Index (WOMAC) scores than isolated intra-articular PRP injections. However, benefits in the visual analog scale (VAS) and Knee Injury and Osteoarthritis Outcome Scores (KOOS) were equivocal [70].

In conclusion, the addition of subchondral PRP to intra-articular injections can provide benefits in the symptomatic treatment of OA. However, robust clinical evidence on this matter is lacking, and further randomized controlled trials are needed to confirm efficacy.

2.7.3 Subchondral Injection of Bone Marrow Aspirate Concentrate

Bone Marrow Aspirate Concentrate (BMAC) has been utilized as a source of mesenchymal stem cells for the surgical treatment of cartilage defects or intra-articular injections in OA. It has the advantage of being a minimally manipulated procedure that can easily be performed as a single step at the point of care without regulatory constraints or the need for expensive cell cultures. Furthermore, the concentration of MSC's in subchondral bone decreases with age & OA [71]. Therefore, BMAC could be an attractive option for its regenerative effects in the subchondral bone.

The authors utilize a two-cannulae technique of saline lavage followed by injection of BMAC under fluoroscopic guidance to clear debris and necrotic adipocytes from the area of BML (Fig. 2.5).

A systematic review of 14 clinical studies involving intra-articular injection of BMAC for OA found symptomatic improvement. However, this was not sustained at long-term follow-up [72]. Hernigou et al. have followed 200 knees with subchondral BMAC injections for an average of 13 years. They were able to show an

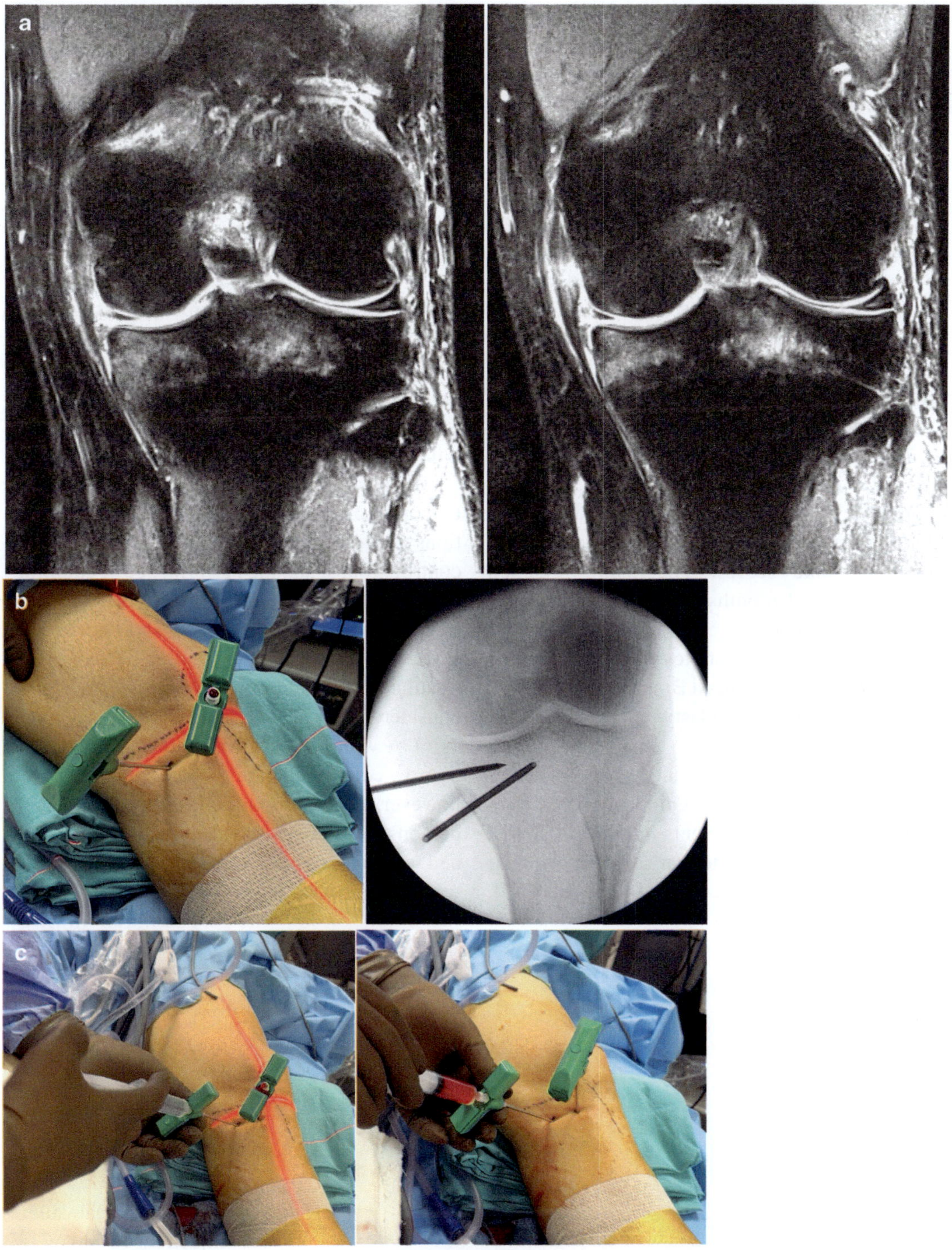

Fig. 2.5 Lavage followed by subchondral BMAC injection in a 67-year-old patient; (**a**) Coronal T-2 fat-suppressed MRI images depicting medial tibial BML and degenerative medial meniscus tear; (**b**) Placement of cannulae under fluoroscopic control; (**c**) Lavage followed by BMAC injection; the second cannula is blocked to avoid leakage of BMAC during injection

increase in cartilage thickness and a reduction in the size of BML's on MRI scans in the involved compartment following subchondral treatment. Conversion to knee arthroplasty was needed in 20% of the patients [71]. The same group analyzed 140 patients with bilateral end-stage knee OA, with one knee undergoing TKA while the other received a subchondral BMAC injection during surgery [73]. At the 10-year follow-up, 18% of the injected knees had required conversion to arthroplasty. BML's larger than 3 cm^2, younger age, and severe malalignment were independent risk factors for conversion to knee replacement [73].

In a more recent study, Kon et al. prospectively followed 30 patients for 24 months after a combined intra-articular-subchondral injection of BMAC. They found a significant reduction of BML and improvement in all pain and functional outcome scores. The pain worsened slightly after 12 months, and a failure rate of 13% was reported [74].

Another treatment strategy is to combine BMAC with Demineralized Bone Matrix (DBM), the so-called "Osteobioplasty" procedure. This treatment has been used to treat pre-collapse avascular necrosis of the hip and has been adapted to the BML's of the knee. Significant decreases in pain scores and improvements in IKDC & SF-12 scores have been reported in 20 patients with painful BML's at one-year follow-up [75]. Resolution of BML's was seen in 75% of the cases, with survivorship of 93% at 1 year [75]. Long-term outcomes of this intervention have not been reported.

Several technical points should be considered to increase the number of MSCs in BMAC [76]. The iliac crest has a higher number of MSCs compared to the tibia and femur and should be the donor site of choice. Multiple small-volume syringes, aspirating bone marrow from different locations in the crest, have a higher yield of nucleated cells compared to a single aspiration site. It is important to report the number of nucleated cells in the concentrate since higher cell counts have been associated with better outcomes.

The small number of studies reporting on the outcomes of subchondral BMAC have the limitations of short follow-up in most cases, absence of control groups, and the performance of additional procedures such as arthroscopy or DBM and lumping together of traumatic and degenerative BMLs confounding the results. However, the treatment is safe, minimally invasive, and can be considered in younger patients with K-L grade 1–3 OA with painful BMLs. Resolution of bone marrow edema and pain is consistently observed; however, disease-modifying effects need to be demonstrated (Fig. 2.6). Bone-on-bone arthritis and extremes of leg alignment are associated with inferior outcomes.

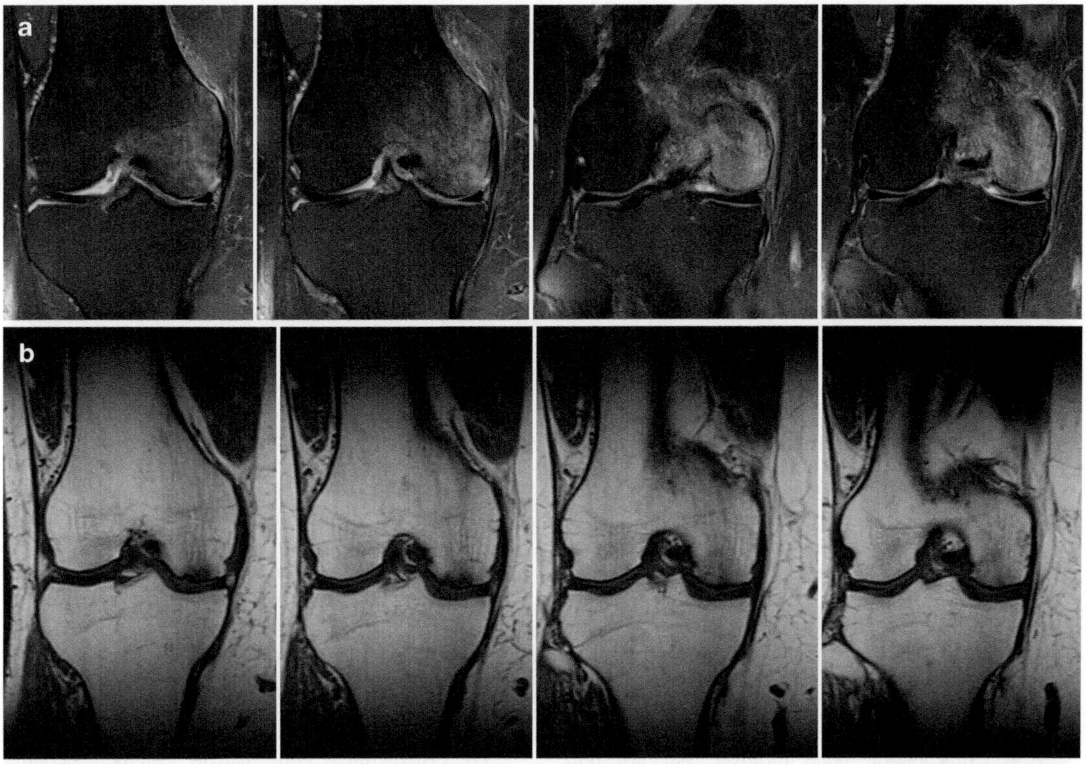

Fig. 2.6 One-year follow-up of a patient with BML of the medial femoral condyle treated with subchondral lavage and BMAC injection; (**a**) Preoperative T-2 MRI sequences demonstrating extensive BML; (**b**) One-year follow-up T-1 MRI sequences show dramatic resolution of BML. A small area of subchondral avascular necrosis without collapse can be observed; the patient is asymptomatic

2.8 Conclusions

Subchondral bone has emerged as the new frontier in cartilage damage. Treatment methods targeting the area either alone or in combination with intra-articular injections have the possibility to provide symptomatic relief. However, disease-modifying effects have yet to be demonstrated.

Acknowledgements None.

Funding Statement This work did not receive any specific grant from any funding agency in the public, commercial or not-for-profit sector.

References

1. Sharma AR, Jagga S, Lee S-S, Nam J-S. Interplay between cartilage and subchondral bone contributing to pathogenesis of osteoarthritis. Int J Mol Sci. 2013;14:19805–30.
2. Kwan Tat S, Lajeunesse D, Pelletier J-P, Martel-Pelletier J. Targeting subchondral bone for treating osteoarthritis: what is the evidence? Best Pract Res Clin Rheumatol. 2010;24:51–70.
3. Chen FH, Rousche KT, Tuan RS. Technology insight: adult stem cells in cartilage regeneration and tissue engineering. Nat Clin Pract Rheumatol. 2006;2:373–82.
4. Sophia Fox AJ, Bedi A, Rodeo SA. The basic science of articular cartilage: structure, composition, and function. Sports Health. 2009;1:461–8.

5. Shoulders MD, Raines RT. Collagen structure and stability. Annu Rev Biochem. 2009;78:929–58.
6. Mescher A. Junqueira's Basic Histology Text & Atlas, 14th ed. 2016
7. Chen S, Fu P, Wu H, Pei M. Meniscus, articular cartilage and nucleus pulposus: a comparative review of cartilage-like tissues in anatomy, development and function. Cell Tissue Res. 2017;370:53–70.
8. Buckwalter JA, Mow VC, Ratcliffe A. Restoration of injured or degenerated articular cartilage. J Am Acad Orthop Surg. 1994;2:192–201.
9. Huber M, Trattnig S, Lintner F. Anatomy, biochemistry, and physiology of articular cartilage. Investig Radiol. 2000;35:573–80.
10. Goldring SR, Goldring MB. Changes in the osteochondral unit during osteoarthritis: structure, function and cartilage-bone crosstalk. Nat Rev Rheumatol. 2016;12:632–44.
11. Day JS, Van Der Linden JC, Bank RA, Ding M, Hvid I, Sumner DR, Weinans H. Adaptation of subchondral bone in osteoarthritis. Biorheology. 2004;41:359–68.
12. Bettica P, Cline G, Hart DJ, Meyer J, Spector TD. Evidence for increased bone resorption in patients with progressive knee osteoarthritis: longitudinal results from the Chingford study. Arthritis Rheum. 2002;46:3178–84.
13. Klose-Jensen R, Hartlev LB, Boel LWT, Laursen MB, Stengaard-Pedersen K, Keller KK, Hauge E-M. Subchondral bone turnover, but not bone volume, is increased in early stage osteoarthritic lesions in the human hip joint. Osteoarthr Cartil. 2015;23:2167–73.
14. Hügle T, Geurts J. What drives osteoarthritis?-synovial versus subchondral bone pathology. Rheumatology (Oxford). 2017;56:1461–71.
15. Cabahug-Zuckerman P, Frikha-Benayed D, Majeska RJ, Tuthill A, Yakar S, Judex S, Schaffler MB. Osteocyte apoptosis caused by Hindlimb unloading is required to trigger osteocyte RANKL production and subsequent resorption of cortical and trabecular bone in mice femurs. J Bone Miner Res. 2016;31:1356–65.
16. Lacourt M, Gao C, Li A, Girard C, Beauchamp G, Henderson JE, Laverty S. Relationship between cartilage and subchondral bone lesions in repetitive impact trauma-induced equine osteoarthritis. Osteoarthr Cartil. 2012;20:572–83.
17. Kennedy OD, Laudier DM, Majeska RJ, Sun HB, Schaffler MB. Osteocyte apoptosis is required for production of osteoclastogenic signals following bone fatigue in vivo. Bone. 2014;64:132–7.
18. Li J, Xue J, Jing Y, Wang M, Shu R, Xu H, Xue C, Feng J, Wang P, Bai D. SOST deficiency aggravates osteoarthritis in mice by promoting sclerosis of subchondral bone. Biomed Res Int. 2019;2019:7623562.
19. Dai G, Xiao H, Liao J, Zhou N, Zhao C, Xu W, Xu W, Liang X, Huang W. Osteocyte TGFβ1-Smad2/3 is positively associated with bone turnover parameters in subchondral bone of advanced osteoarthritis. Int J Mol Med. 2020;46:167–78.
20. Liu X-H, Kirschenbaum A, Yao S, Levine AC. Interactive effect of interleukin-6 and prostaglandin E2 on osteoclastogenesis via the OPG/RANKL/RANK system. Ann N Y Acad Sci. 2006;1068:225–33.
21. Zhu S, Bennett S, Kuek V, Xiang C, Xu H, Rosen V, Xu J. Endothelial cells produce angiocrine factors to regulate bone and cartilage via versatile mechanisms. Theranostics. 2020;10:5957–65.
22. Hasegawa T, Tsuchiya E, Abe M, Amizuka N. Cellular interplay of bone cells and vascular endothelial cells in bone. Clin Calcium. 2016;26:677–82.
23. Ramasamy SK, Kusumbe AP, Wang L, Adams RH. Endothelial Notch activity promotes angiogenesis and osteogenesis in bone. Nature. 2014;507:376–80.
24. Romeo SG, Alawi KM, Rodrigues J, Singh A, Kusumbe AP, Ramasamy SK. Endothelial proteolytic activity and interaction with non-resorbing osteoclasts mediate bone elongation. Nat Cell Biol. 2019;21:430–41.
25. Sanchez C, Mazzucchelli G, Lambert C, Comblain F, DePauw E, Henrotin Y. Comparison of secretome from osteoblasts derived from sclerotic versus non-sclerotic subchondral bone in OA: a pilot study. PLoS One. 2018;13:e0194591.
26. Xie H, Cui Z, Wang L, et al. PDGF-BB secreted by preosteoclasts induces angiogenesis during coupling with osteogenesis. Nat Med. 2014;20:1270–8.
27. Walsh DA, Sofat N, Guermazi A, Hunter DJ. Osteoarthritis bone marrow lesions. Osteoarthr Cartil. 2023;31:11–7.
28. Roemer FW, Frobell R, Hunter DJ, Crema MD, Fischer W, Bohndorf K, Guermazi A. MRI-detected subchondral bone marrow signal alterations of the knee joint: terminology, imaging appearance, relevance and radiological differential diagnosis. Osteoarthr Cartil. 2009;17:1115–31.
29. Koushesh S, Shahtaheri SM, McWilliams DF, Walsh DA, Sheppard MN, Westaby J, Haybatollahi SM, Howe FA, Sofat N. The osteoarthritis bone score (OABS): a new histological scoring system for the characterisation of bone marrow lesions in osteoarthritis. Osteoarthr Cartil. 2022;30:746–55.
30. Beckwée D, Vaes P, Shahabpour M, Muyldermans R, Rommers N, Bautmans I. The influence of joint loading on bone marrow lesions in the knee: a systematic review with meta-analysis. Am J Sports Med. 2015;43:3093–107.
31. Choi HG, Kim JS, Yoo HJ, Jung YS, Lee YS. The fate of bone marrow lesions after open wedge high tibial osteotomy: a comparison between knees with primary osteoarthritis and subchondral insufficiency fractures. Am J Sports Med. 2021;49:1551–60.
32. Lim YZ, Wang Y, Wluka AE, Davies-Tuck ML, Hanna F, Urquhart DM, Cicuttini FM. Association of obesity and systemic factors with bone marrow lesions at the knee: a systematic review. Semin Arthritis Rheum. 2014;43:600–12.
33. Aso K, Shahtaheri SM, McWilliams DF, Walsh DA. Association of subchondral bone marrow lesion localization with weight-bearing pain in people with

knee osteoarthritis: data from the osteoarthritis initiative. Arthritis Res Ther. 2021;23:35.
34. Hunter DJ, Zhang Y, Niu J, Goggins J, Amin S, LaValley MP, Guermazi A, Genant H, Gale D, Felson DT. Increase in bone marrow lesions associated with cartilage loss: a longitudinal magnetic resonance imaging study of knee osteoarthritis. Arthritis Rheum. 2006;54:1529–35.
35. Felson DT, McLaughlin S, Goggins J, LaValley MP, Gale ME, Totterman S, Li W, Hill C, Gale D. Bone marrow edema and its relation to progression of knee osteoarthritis. Ann Intern Med. 2003;139:330–6.
36. Wluka AE, Wang Y, Davies-Tuck M, English DR, Giles GG, Cicuttini FM. Bone marrow lesions predict progression of cartilage defects and loss of cartilage volume in healthy middle-aged adults without knee pain over 2 yrs. Rheumatology (Oxford). 2008;47:1392–6.
37. Scher C, Craig J, Nelson F. Bone marrow edema in the knee in osteoarthrosis and association with total knee arthroplasty within a three-year follow-up. Skeletal Radiol. 2008;37:609–17.
38. Pelletier J-P, Roubille C, Raynauld J-P, Abram F, Dorais M, Delorme P, Martel-Pelletier J. Disease-modifying effect of strontium ranelate in a subset of patients from the phase III knee osteoarthritis study SEKOIA using quantitative MRI: reduction in bone marrow lesions protects against cartilage loss. Ann Rheum Dis. 2015;74:422–9.
39. Centeno C, Cartier C, Stemper I, Dodson E, Freeman M, Azuike U, Williams C, Hyzy M, Silva O, Steinmetz N. The treatment of bone marrow lesions associated with advanced knee osteoarthritis: comparing intraosseous and intraarticular injections with bone marrow concentrate and platelet products. Pain Physician. 2021;24:E279–88.
40. Bingham CO, Buckland-Wright JC, Garnero P, et al. Risedronate decreases biochemical markers of cartilage degradation but does not decrease symptoms or slow radiographic progression in patients with medial compartment osteoarthritis of the knee: results of the two-year multinational knee osteoarthritis structural arthritis study. Arthritis Rheum. 2006;54:3494–507.
41. Nishii T, Tamura S, Shiomi T, Yoshikawa H, Sugano N. Alendronate treatment for hip osteoarthritis: prospective randomized 2-year trial. Clin Rheumatol. 2013;32:1759–66.
42. Aitken D, Laslett LL, Cai G, Hill C, March L, Wluka AE, Wang Y, Blizzard L, Cicuttini F, Jones G. A protocol for a multicentre, randomised, double-blind, placebo-controlled trial to compare the effect of annual infusions of zoledronic acid to placebo on knee structural change and knee pain over 24 months in knee osteoarthritis patients—ZAP2. BMC Musculoskelet Disord. 2018;19:217.
43. Kadri A, Ea HK, Bazille C, Hannouche D, Lioté F, Cohen-Solal ME. Osteoprotegerin inhibits cartilage degradation through an effect on trabecular bone in murine experimental osteoarthritis. Arthritis Rheum. 2008;58:2379–86.
44. Connor JR, LePage C, Swift BA, Yamashita D, Bendele AM, Maul D, Kumar S. Protective effects of a cathepsin K inhibitor, SB-553484, in the canine partial medial meniscectomy model of osteoarthritis. Osteoarthr Cartil. 2009;17:1236–43.
45. Karsdal MA, Byrjalsen I, Alexandersen P, Bihlet A, Andersen JR, Riis BJ, Bay-Jensen AC, Christiansen C, CSMC021C2301/2 investigators. Treatment of symptomatic knee osteoarthritis with oral salmon calcitonin: results from two phase 3 trials. Osteoarthr Cartil. 2015;23:532–43.
46. Zhen G, Wen C, Jia X, et al. Inhibition of TGF-β signaling in mesenchymal stem cells of subchondral bone attenuates osteoarthritis. Nat Med. 2013;19:704–12.
47. Lu J, Zhang H, Cai D, et al. Positive-feedback regulation of subchondral H-type vessel formation by chondrocyte promotes osteoarthritis development in mice. J Bone Miner Res. 2018;33:909–20.
48. Nagai T, Sato M, Kutsuna T, Kokubo M, Ebihara G, Ohta N, Mochida J. Intravenous administration of anti-vascular endothelial growth factor humanized monoclonal antibody bevacizumab improves articular cartilage repair. Arthritis Res Ther. 2010;12:R178.
49. Nagae M, Hiraga T, Yoneda T. Acidic microenvironment created by osteoclasts causes bone pain associated with tumor colonization. J Bone Miner Metab. 2007;25:99–104.
50. Yoneda T, Hiasa M, Nagata Y, Okui T, White F. Contribution of acidic extracellular microenvironment of cancer-colonized bone to bone pain. Biochim Biophys Acta. 2015;1848:2677–84.
51. Izumi M, Ikeuchi M, Ji Q, Tani T. Local ASIC3 modulates pain and disease progression in a rat model of osteoarthritis. J Biomed Sci. 2012;19:77.
52. Zhu J, Zhen G, An S, et al. Aberrant subchondral osteoblastic metabolism modifies NaV1.8 for osteoarthritis. elife. 2020;9:e57656.
53. Chen J, Li J, Li R, Wang H, Yang J, Xu J, Zha Z. Efficacy and safety of Tanezumab on osteoarthritis knee and hip pains: a meta-analysis of randomized controlled trials. Pain Med. 2017;18:374–85.
54. Huddleston HP, Cregar WM, Alzein MM, Vadhera AS, Wong SE, Yanke AB. Outcomes of patellar subchondroplasty surgery: a case series. J Knee Surg. 2023;36:941–8.
55. Colon DA, Yoon BJV, Russell TA, Cammisa FP, Abjornson C. Assessment of the injection behavior of commercially available bone BSMs for Subchondroplasty® procedures. Knee. 2015;22:597–603.
56. Fokter SK, Kuhta M, Hojnik M, Ledinek Ž, Kostanjšek R. Tissue integration of calcium phosphate compound after subchondroplasty: 4-year follow-up in a 76-year-old female patient. Bioengineering (Basel). 2023;10:208.
57. Brimmo OA, Bozynski CC, Cook CR, Kuroki K, Sherman SL, Pfeiffer FM, Stoker AM, Cook JL. Subchondroplasty for the treatment of posttraumatic bone marrow lesions of the medial femoral

condyle in a pre-clinical canine model. J Orthop Res. 2018;36:2709–17.
58. Yoo JY, O'Malley MJ, Matsen Ko LJ, Cohen SB, Sharkey PF. Knee arthroplasty after subchondroplasty: early results, complications, and technical challenges. J Arthroplast. 2016;31:2188–92.
59. Nairn LN, Subramaniam M, Ekhtiari S, Axelrod DE, Grant JA, Khan M. Safety and early results of subchondroplasty® for the treatment of bone marrow lesions in osteoarthritis: a systematic review. Knee Surg Sports Traumatol Arthrosc. 2021;29:3599–607.
60. Tran Y, Pelletier-Roy R, Merle G, Aubin C-É, Nault M-L. Subchondroplasty in the treatment of bone marrow lesion in early knee osteoarthritis: a systematic review of clinical and radiological outcomes. Knee. 2022;39:279–90.
61. Wood DS, Paulson S, Nolan JR, Spanyer J, Harm RG, Heis FT. What factors are associated with conversion to knee arthroplasty after subchondroplasty? Clin Orthop Relat Res. 2023;481:1543–50.
62. Chatterjee D, McGee A, Strauss E, Youm T, Jazrawi L. Subchondral calcium phosphate is ineffective for bone marrow edema lesions in adults with advanced osteoarthritis. Clin Orthop Relat Res. 2015;473:2334–42.
63. ESSKA Consensus Project—Injectable Orthobiologics in Knee OA—Part 1, PRP. https://cdn.ymaws.com/www.esska.org/resource/resmgr/docs/consensus_projects/orbit_consensus_complete2022.pdf
64. Lin W, Xie L, Zhou L, Zheng J, Zhai W, Lin D. Effects of platelet-rich plasma on subchondral bone marrow edema and biomarkers in synovial fluid of knee osteoarthritis. Knee. 2023;42:161–9.
65. Delgado D, Garate A, Vincent H, Bilbao AM, Patel R, Fiz N, Sampson S, Sánchez M. Current concepts in intraosseous platelet-rich plasma injections for knee osteoarthritis. J Clin Orthop Trauma. 2019;10:36–41.
66. Su K, Bai Y, Wang J, Zhang H, Liu H, Ma S. Comparison of hyaluronic acid and PRP intra-articular injection with combined intra-articular and intraosseous PRP injections to treat patients with knee osteoarthritis. Clin Rheumatol. 2018;37:1341–50.
67. Sánchez M, Delgado D, Pompei O, Pérez JC, Sánchez P, Garate A, Bilbao AM, Fiz N, Padilla S. Treating severe knee osteoarthritis with combination of intra-osseous and intra-articular infiltrations of platelet-rich plasma: an observational study. Cartilage. 2019;10:245–53.
68. Barman A, Prakash S, Sahoo J, Mukherjee S, Maiti R, Roy SS. Single intra-articular injection with or without intra-osseous injections of platelet-rich plasma in the treatment of osteoarthritis knee: a single-blind, randomized clinical trial. Injury. 2022;53:1247–53.
69. Barman A, Bandyopadhyay D, Mohakud S, Sahoo J, Maiti R, Mukherjee S, Prakash S, Roy SS, Viswanath A. Comparison of clinical outcome, cartilage turnover, and inflammatory activity following either intra-articular or a combination of intra-articular with intra-osseous platelet-rich plasma injections in osteoarthritis knee: a randomized, clinical trial. Injury. 2023;54:728–37.
70. Patel S, Rajnish RK, Baburaj V, Kumar P, Sharma S, Kumar V. Intraosseous infiltration of platelet-rich plasma for knee osteoarthritis: a systematic review of literature and limited meta-analysis. Indian J Orthop. 2022;56:1847–57.
71. Hernigou P, Delambre J, Quiennec S, Poignard A. Human bone marrow mesenchymal stem cell injection in subchondral lesions of knee osteoarthritis: a prospective randomized study versus contralateral arthroplasty at a mean fifteen year follow-up. Int Orthop. 2021;45:365–73.
72. Cavallo C, Boffa A, Andriolo L, Silva S, Grigolo B, Zaffagnini S, Filardo G. Bone marrow concentrate injections for the treatment of osteoarthritis: evidence from preclinical findings to the clinical application. Int Orthop. 2021;45:525–38.
73. Hernigou J, Vertongen P, Rasschaert J, Hernigou P. Role of scaffolds, subchondral, intra-articular injections of fresh autologous bone marrow concentrate regenerative cells in treating human knee cartilage lesions: different approaches and different results. Int J Mol Sci. 2021;22:3844.
74. Kon E, Boffa A, Andriolo L, Di Martino A, Di Matteo B, Magarelli N, Trenti N, Zaffagnini S, Filardo G. Combined subchondral and intra-articular injections of bone marrow aspirate concentrate provide stable results up to 24 months. Knee Surg Sports Traumatol Arthrosc. 2023;31:2511–7.
75. Kasik CS, Martinkovich S, Mosier B, Akhavan S. Short-term outcomes for the biologic treatment of bone marrow edema of the knee using bone marrow aspirate concentrate and injectable demineralized bone matrix. Arthrosc Sports Med Rehabil. 2019;1:e7–e14.
76. Pasculli RM, Kenyon CD, Berrigan WA, Mautner K, Hammond K, Jayaram P. Mesenchymal stem cells for subchondral bone marrow lesions: from bench to bedside. Bone Rep. 2022;17:101630.

3 Radiological Imaging of Chondral and Osteochondral Lesions

Ufuk Arzu, İsmail Tarık Atasoy, and Gökhan Polat

Although plain radiography, computerized tomography (CT), and bone scan may be helpful in the detection of chondral and osteochondral lesions, MRI is the only imaging modality that will provide a comprehensive assessment of all these issues [1].

3.1 Plain Radiography

Direct radiography is diagnostic only in the presence of large and extensive loss of articular cartilage or narrowing of the joint space. It has limited sensitivity in the demonstration of chondral and osteochondral pathologies [2]. Plain radiographs may demonstrate acute osteochondral fractures due to acute trauma. In the chronic setting, central osteophyte formation may occur at the site of an overlying chondral defect. Also, radiographs demonstrate the development of subchondral cystic changes, displaced loose bodies, and unstable fragments [1].

Radiographs should be performed weight-bearing to give a more relevant assessment of alignment. Also, loss of joint space may also be more pronounced or only present during weight-bearing.

In 1959, Berndt and Harty classified talar dome osteochondral lesions due to plain radiography [3]. In the 1980s, computerized tomography and magnetic resonance imaging began to be applied for the chondral and osteochondral lesions (Fig. 3.1).

U. Arzu
Department of Orthopedics and Traumatology, Faculty of Medicine, Marmara University Pendik Training and Research Hospital, Istanbul, Turkey

İ. T. Atasoy · G. Polat (✉)
Department of Orthopedics and Traumatology, Istanbul Faculty of Medicine, Istanbul University, Istanbul, Turkey

M. E. Erdil et al. (eds.), *Current Concept in Cartilage Treatment*,
https://doi.org/10.1007/978-3-032-27099-3_3

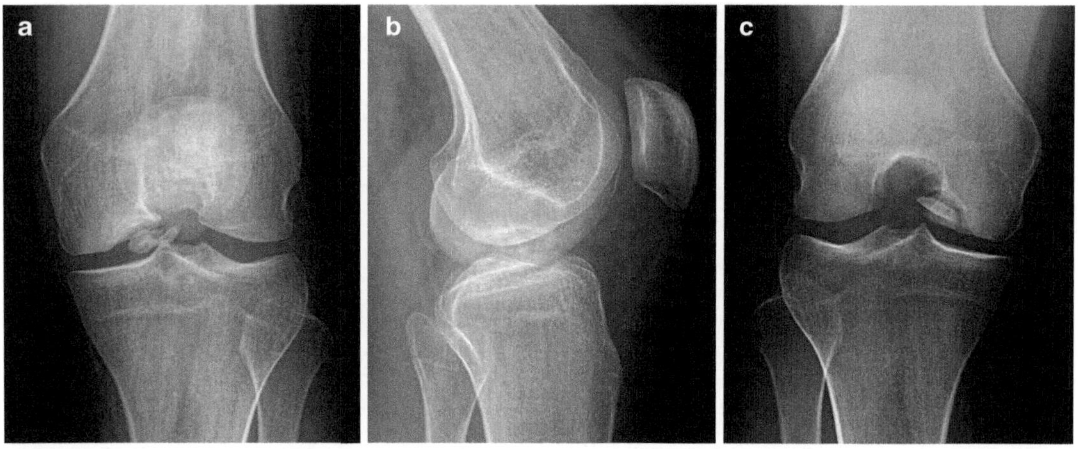

Fig. 3.1 Osteochondral lesion posterolateral to the medial condyle of the distal femur, plain radiography images. (**a**) AP View. (**b**) Lateral View. (**c**) Rosenberg View

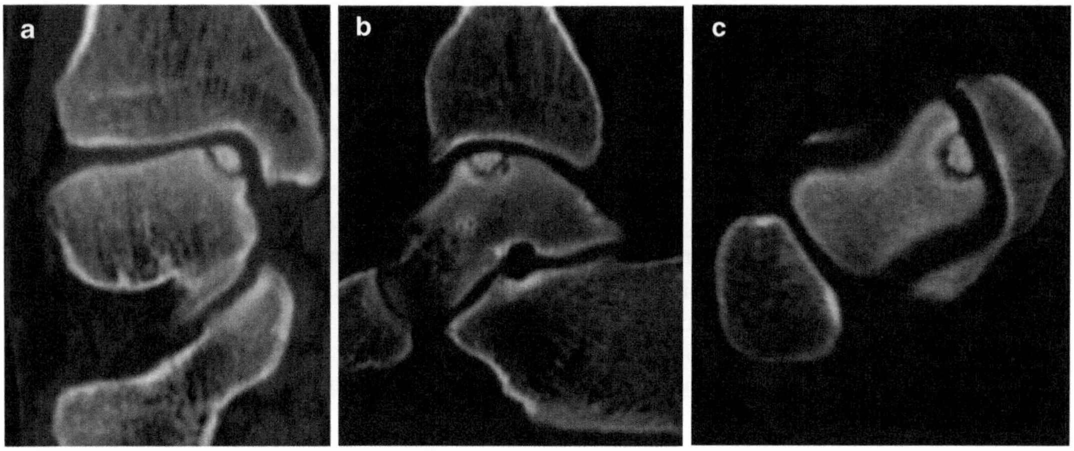

Fig. 3.2 Traumatic osteochondral lesion of the talus located laterally, computerized tomography images. (**a**) AP Plane. (**b**) Lateral Plane. (**c**) Axial Plane

3.2 Computerized Tomography (CT)

In the acute setting of the trauma, CT can demonstrate the osteochondral fractures. In the chronic setting, CT can show us the presence of subchondral sclerosis and cystic changes or central osteophytes and displaced ossified loose bodies (Fig. 3.2). CT is superior to MRI in demonstrating small cracks in the subchondral plate associated with cystic change, which may allow propulsion of synovial fluid into the cyst [1]. However, CT will not show us any bone marrow edema or the chondral surfaces.

Modern multislice CT can be reconstructed in any plane and also into 3-D images. CT arthrography will provide a detailed assessment of the chondral surfaces and may be used as an alternative when MRI is contraindicated [4]. However, using ionized radiation and its invasive nature are disadvantages of CT arthrography. CT arthrography is also used for cartilage imaging [5], and the introduction of spiral CT has enabled thin, overlapping sections with excellent secondary sagittal and coronal reformations to be obtained, resulting in a revival of CT arthrography for the assessment of intra-articular lesions, including articular cartilage [6, 7] (Fig. 3.2).

3.3 Magnetic Resonance Imaging (MRI)

Magnetic resonance imaging provides a noninvasive assessment of the chondral surfaces, subchondral bone, joint fluid, capsule, and ligaments. MRI is the best imaging method for assessment of chondral and osteochondral lesions at the present (Fig. 3.3).

3.3.1 Normal Articular Cartilage

Healthy hyaline cartilage has uniform thickness, a smooth surface, and a homogeneous signal in MR sections. When a chondral lesion is detected, its localization, severity, and size should be described in detail.

3.3.2 Chondral Contusion, Delamination, and Fracture

Traumatic lesions are often sharp-edged, single, solitary, focal defects. The traumatic lesion, which develops as a result of tensile and rotational forces, is usually a full-thickness or high-grade partial cartilage damage or an osteochondral lesion involving the underlying subchondral bone. It may be accompanied by edema or fracture of the subchondral bone. After these traumatic processes, chondral delamination, flap-type lesions, and chondral fissures may occur. Chondral delamination is a more rare lesion. In this injury, the calcified zone is separated from the noncalcified zone. If there is no displacement, it can be quite subtle. These lesions become more conspicuous if there is adjacent subchondral bone marrow edema. Sometimes bone marrow edema does not accompany the chondral lesion.

There are studies that show that blunt trauma to articular cartilage produces profound changes in histologic, biomechanical, and ultrastructural changes in the absence of surface disruption [8, 9]. Acute traumatic chondral fractures are relatively common [10]. They are typically seen as a linear focus of high signal on fat-supressed sequencing at the medial or lateral margin of the talar dome on coronal sequencing, sagittal in orientation, breaching the chondral surface [11] (Fig. 3.4).

3.3.3 Acute Osteochondral Injury

In 1959, Berndt and Harty described four stages in acute impactional injury of the talar dome [3].

- Stage 1: compression fracture of subchondral bone, with intact chondral surface and subchondral plate.
- Stage 2: partially detached osteochondral fragment, breaching the articular cartilage and subchondral plate.
- Stage 3: completely detached in situ osteochondral fragment, with breach of the chondral surface and subchondral plate.
- Stage 4: detached, migrated osteochondral fragment.

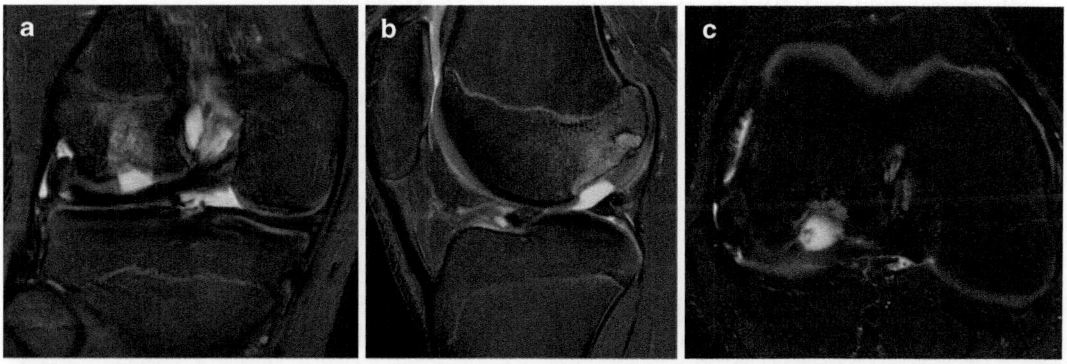

Fig. 3.3 Preoperative magnetic resonance imaging (MRI) slices of a right knee showing an osteochondral lesion and surrounding bone marrow edema in the lateral femoral condyle (**a**) AP Plane. (**b**) Lateral Plane. (**c**) Axial Plane

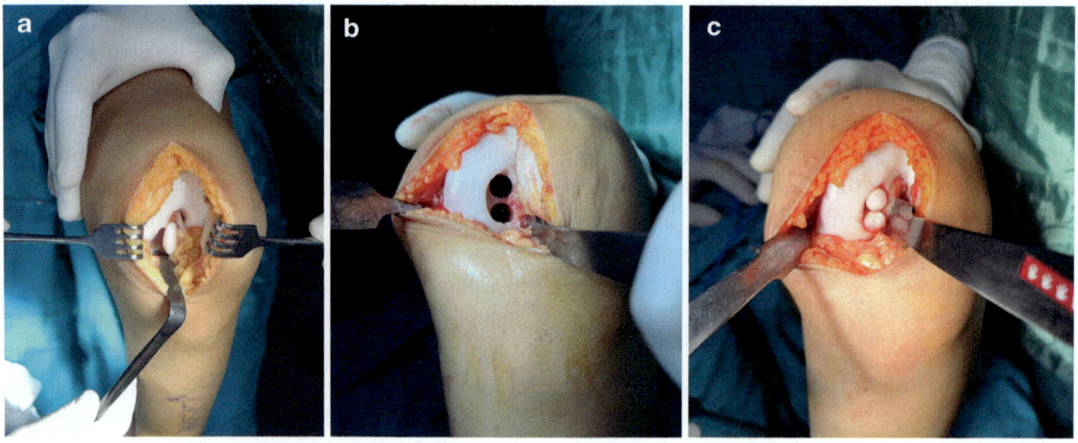

Fig. 3.4 Intraoperative images of a mosaicplasty surgical procedure: (**a**) Exposure of the lesion showing osteochondral fragment. (**b**) Preparation of the defect area for the implantation of cylindrical osteochondral plugs. (**c**) Final view showing implanted cylindrical osteochondral plugs

This staging system for the acute injury has been widely adopted as a radiographic and arthroscopic classification, but its clinical use is limited because it does not correlate with prognosis and does not guide management [1]. Also, this classification is not giving any ideas about the status of the articular surface, bone marrow, or any possible subchondral cystic changes. There are differences of bone marrow edema secondary to the trauma between osteoarthritis. The histologic findings in posttraumatic bone marrow edema correlate with microfracture and hemorrhage in animal studies [12]. However, in areas of bone marrow edema in osteoarthritis, trabecular remodeling, marrow necrosis, and fibrosis may be determined [13].

Transchondral, transosseous fractures are usually appreciable on MRI; however, the osseous component of the injury may be relatively inconspicuous on MRI when compared with a CT scan [1].

3.3.4 Subchondral Cysts

Post-traumatic bone marrow edema, due to poor blood supply to the talar dome and poor healing potential, predisposes to the development of focal areas of ischemic/devascularized subchondral bone where resorption of subchondral trabeculae, replacement with fibrotic tissue, and subsequent formation of cystic change may occur [14]. Due to the pressure of the joint, synovial fluid may be forced in to the subchondral bone through a crack in the presence of the chondral surface. These cystic changes may vary from predominately fibrotic to predominately fluid content [15]. Just like transchondral or transosseous fractures, MRI has limited use in small cracks in the subchondral plate associated with cystic changes. In the presence of such a situation, it can be evaluated with CT (Fig. 3.5).

3.3.5 Unstable Chronic Osteochondral Lesions: Chronic Osteochondral Defects

The displacement of the osteochondral lesion may occur at the time of an acute trauma or may develop as a complication of an osteochondral lesion [1]. The criteria of stability for diagnosis of instability of an osteochondral lesion are the presence of a line of high signal on proton density (PD) or fat-suppressed PD sequencing breaching the chondral surface, subchondral plate, and extending along the interface between the osteochondral fragment and the base of the osteochondral fragment [11, 16, 17].

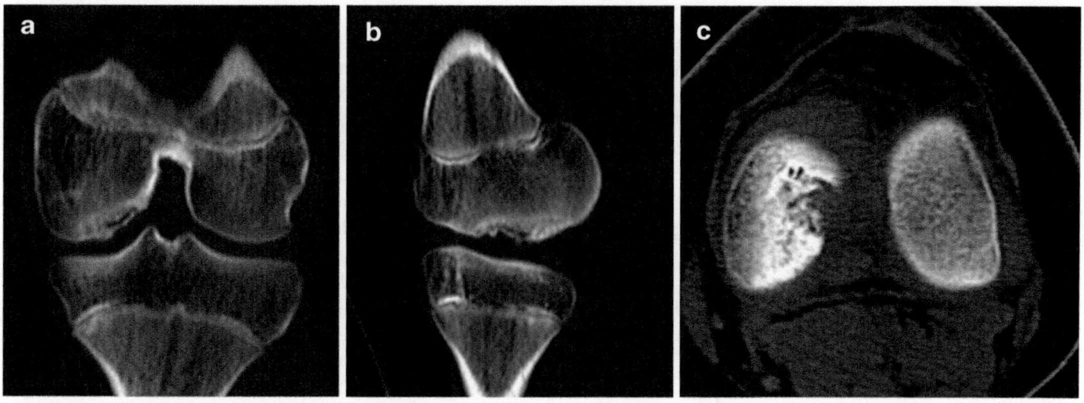

Fig. 3.5 Computerized tomography images showing an osteochondral lesion and underlying subchondral cystic changes. (**a**) AP Plane. (**b**) Lateral Plane. (**c**) Axial Plane

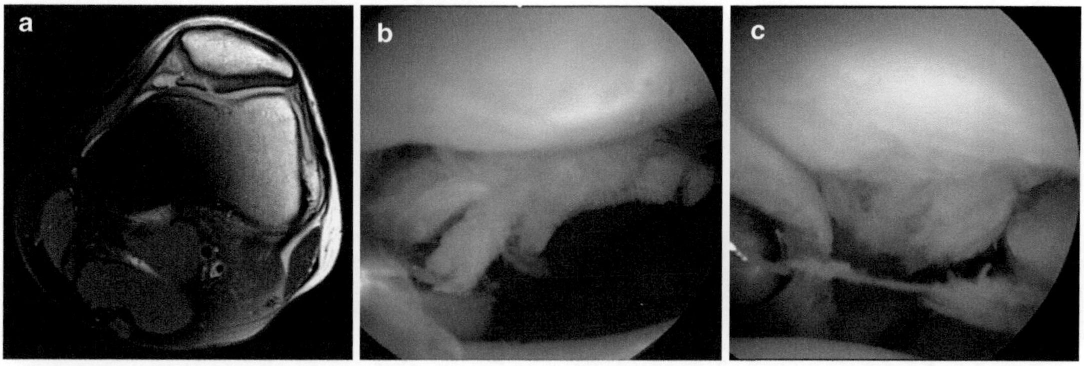

Fig. 3.6 Arthroscopic surgical treatment of an osteochondral lesion in the knee. (**a**) Preoperative magnetic resonance imaging (MRI) slices of the left knee medial patellar surface showing the chondral fragment. (**b**) Pure chondral nature of the fragment can be seen. (**c**) Image showing lesion area after the debridement

Displaced osteochondral fragments are usually readily identified on MRI. Fragments may be seen adjacent to the osteochondral defect, in the anterior or posterior recess, or within the syndesmotic recess [1] (Fig. 3.6).

References

1. Linklater JM. Imaging of talar dome chondral and osteochondral lesions. Top Magn Reson Imaging. 2010;21(1):3–13.
2. Loomer R, Fisher C, Lloyd-Smith R, Sisler J, Cooney T. Osteochondral lesions of the talus. Am J Sports Med. 1993;21(1):13–9.
3. Berndt AL, Harty M. Transchondral fractures (osteochondritis dissecans) of the talus. JBJS. 1959;41(6):988–1020.
4. Schmid MR, Pfirrmann CWA, Hodler J, Vienne P, Zanetti M. Cartilage lesions in the ankle joint: comparison of MR arthrography and CT arthrography. Skeletal Radiol. 2003;32:259–65.
5. Reiser M, Karpf PM, Bernett P. Diagnosis of chondromalacia patellae using CT arthrography. Eur J Radiol. 1982;2(3):181–6.
6. Vande Berg BC, Lecouvet FE, Poilvache P, Jamart J, Materne R, Lengele B, et al. Assessment of knee cartilage in cadavers with dual-detector spiral CT arthrography and MR imaging. Radiology. 2002;222(2):430–6.
7. Vande Berg BC, Lecouvet FE, Poilvache P, Maldague B, Malghem J. Spiral CT arthrography of the postoperative knee. In: Seminars in musculoskeletal radiology. New York: Thieme Medical Publishers; 2002. p. 47–56.
8. Thompson RC Jr, Oegema TR Jr, Lewis JL, Wallace L. Osteoarthrotic changes after acute transarticular load. An animal model. JBJS. 1991;73(7):990–1001.

9. Donohue JM, Buss D, Oegema TR Jr, Thompson RC Jr. The effects of indirect blunt trauma on adult canine articular cartilage. JBJS. 1983;65(7):948–57.
10. Loren GJ, Ferkel RD. Arthroscopic assessment of occult intra-articular injury in acute ankle fractures. Arthrosc J Arthrosc Relat Surg. 2002;18(4):412–21.
11. Mintz DN, Tashjian GS, Connell DA, Deland JT, O'Malley M, Potter HG. Osteochondral lesions of the talus: a new magnetic resonance grading system with arthroscopic correlation. Arthrosc J Arthrosc Relat Surg. 2003;19(4):353–9.
12. Ryu KN, Jin W, Ko YT, Yoon Y, Oh JH, Park YK, et al. Bone bruises: MR characteristics and histological correlation in the young pig. Clin Imaging. 2000;24(6):371–80.
13. Zanetti M, Bruder E, Romero J, Hodler J. Bone marrow edema pattern in osteoarthritic knees: correlation between MR imaging and histologic findings. Radiology. 2000;215(3):835–40.
14. Elias I, Jung JW, Raikin SM, Schweitzer MW, Carrino JA, Morrison WB. Osteochondral lesions of the talus: change in MRI findings over time in talar lesions without operative intervention and implications for staging systems. Foot Ankle Int. 2006;27(3):157–66.
15. Linklater J. Ligamentous, chondral, and osteochondral ankle injuries in athletes. In: Seminars in musculoskeletal radiology. New York: Thieme Medical Publishers; 2004. p. 81–98.
16. De Smet AA, Fisher DR, Burnstein MI, Graf BK, Lange RH. Value of MR imaging in staging osteochondral lesions of the talus (osteochondritis dissecans): results in 14 patients. AJR Am J Roentgenol. 1990;154(3):555–8.
17. O'Connor MA, Palaniappan M, Khan N, Bruce CE. Osteochondritis dissecans of the knee in children: a comparison of MRI and arthroscopic findings. J Bone Jt Surg Br. 2002;84(2):258–62.

Classification of Cartilage Lesions

4

Ali Said Nazligül and Mustafa Akkaya

Hyaline cartilage is found in all synovial joints of the body, and the articular cartilage integrity plays a critical role in maintaining normal joint function. Articular cartilage injuries are very common and affect a large proportion of the world population. Articular cartilage damage encompasses a spectrum of disease types ranging from focal defects to advanced degenerative diseases of the articular cartilage [1]. Diagnosis and classification of articular cartilage lesions is critical because of the ever-increasing number of cartilage lesions being identified and the complexity of their clinical presentation. Treatment of articular cartilage lesions is challenging because cartilage has a limited ability to heal spontaneously [2]. There are numerous techniques for treating cartilage lesions and varying prognoses for different treatment options. However, there is no consensus on which lesions to treat or which treatment method is appropriate for a particular lesion. Therefore, different classification systems for cartilage lesions have been developed to ensure an objective evaluation and to assess the results of the treatments performed.

The criteria used to classify cartilage lesions should properly define the lesion and provide guidance on treatment options and prognosis. The classification systems developed today rely on both magnetic resonance imaging (MRI) and arthroscopic images. Among these, classification systems based on arthroscopic images are considered the gold standard for classifying cartilage lesions. Although considered the gold standard, these classification systems can sometimes fall short because of the difficulty in identifying deep-seated lesions with arthroscopy.

Numerous methods have been developed to evaluate the characteristics of cartilage lesions using magnetic resonance imaging (MRI) (Boston Leeds Osteoarthritis Knee Score-BLOKS, Whole-organ Magnetic Resonance Imaging Score (WORMS), Area Measurement And Depth & Underlying Structures (AMADEUS) Score, and MRI Osteoarthritis Knee Score) or by arthroscopic assessment (Outerbridge, International Cartilage Regeneration and Joint Preservation Society, Bauer-Jackson) [1, 3–8] [Outerbridge, 1961 #3]. While each of these systems differs in the range of scores and delineation criteria between grades, the lesion characteristics assessed are relatively similar across grading systems. Articular cartilage lesion characteristics that are assessed include depth, size, location, and number.

A. S. Nazligül
Department of Orthopedics and Traumatology, Ankara Sincan Training and Research Hospital, Ankara, Turkey

M. Akkaya (✉)
Department of Orthopedics and Traumatology, Faculty of Medicine, Yuksek Ihtisas University, Ankara, Türkiye

M. E. Erdil et al. (eds.), *Current Concept in Cartilage Treatment*,
https://doi.org/10.1007/978-3-032-27099-3_4

Arthroscopic imaging and arthroscopic examination are the gold standard for the diagnosis of chondral lesions. However, arthroscopic evaluation remains subjective and superficial. Therefore, MRI is increasingly being used as a non-invasive diagnostic method for chondral lesions, providing information on tissue changes that occur prior to radiographic changes. MRI-based methods are continuously improving to accurately assess articular cartilage and subchondral bone. Several semiquantitative MR scoring systems have been developed to assess various joint structures, including articular cartilage, such as WORMS, BLOKS, and AMADEUS. MRI-based classification systems have also shown satisfactory results compared to ICRS classification [9, 10].

Among the various classification systems for cartilage lesions, the following are the most commonly used ones based on arthroscopic images.

1. Outerbridge Classification.
2. International Cartilage Regeneration and Joint Preservation Society (ICRS) Classification.

Among the various MRI-based scoring systems for cartilage lesions, the following is quick and easy-to-use [10].

3. Area Measurement and Depth & Underlying Structures (AMADEUS) Score

4.1 Outerbridge Classification

Outerbridge published a paper on the etiology of chondromalacia patella in 1961 and subsequently developed his own classification system for chondromalacia patella [3, 11, 12]. The Outerbridge classification system, initially developed for chondromalacia of the patella, has been eventually extended to provide a practical, reproducible classification system for all cartilage lesions [13].

The Outerbridge classification system, based on images obtained during arthroscopy or open surgery, assigns a grade between 0 and IV to the cartilage lesion. Grade 0 indicates normal cartilage. Grade I chondral lesions must be confirmed by examination with an instrument such as a probe, and evidence of softening and swelling with a probe indicates a grade I chondral lesion according to the Outerbridge classification system. Grade II chondral lesions are described as partial-thickness defects with surface fissures. Grade II chondral lesions are less than 1.5 cm in diameter and do not extend to the subchondral bone (Fig. 4.1). Grade III chondral lesions are larger than 1.5 cm in diameter and extend to the subchondral bone. The most severe chondral lesions are Grade IV lesions (Fig. 4.1). Grade IV lesions have chondral damage with completely exposed subchondral bone (Fig. 4.1) [3, 11, 12].

Outerbridge classification	
Grade 0	Normal cartilage tissue
Grade I	Cartilage softening and swelling (determined by examination with a probe)
Grade II	Partial-thickness defect and surface fissures (<1.5 cm and not reaching the subchondral bone)
Grade III	Deep fissures (>1.5 cm and reaching the subchondral bone)
Grade IV	Chondral damage with an exposed subchondral bone

Various studies have evaluated the reliability of the Outerbridge classification system. The study by Lasmar et al. compared the Outerbridge and FSA schemes and found no difference in interobserver or intraobserver reliability [14]. The Outerbridge classification was successfully used in a study by Bateman et al., who reported on the results of arthroscopic treatment of labral tears in older athletes [15]. In another study, the Outerbridge classification was again used with success to classify and evaluate cartilage lesions in the hip joint [16]. In another study by Curl WW et al., attempting to evaluate cartilage lesions of the knee also successfully used the Outerbridge classification system [17].

Although the Outerbridge classification is easily applicable and commonly used, it also has some limitations. The main limitation is the lack of consistency and reproducibility between clinicians. The general interobserver and intraobserver reliability of the Outerbridge classification system is fair to substantial [18, 19]. However, some studies have reported that there is a rela-

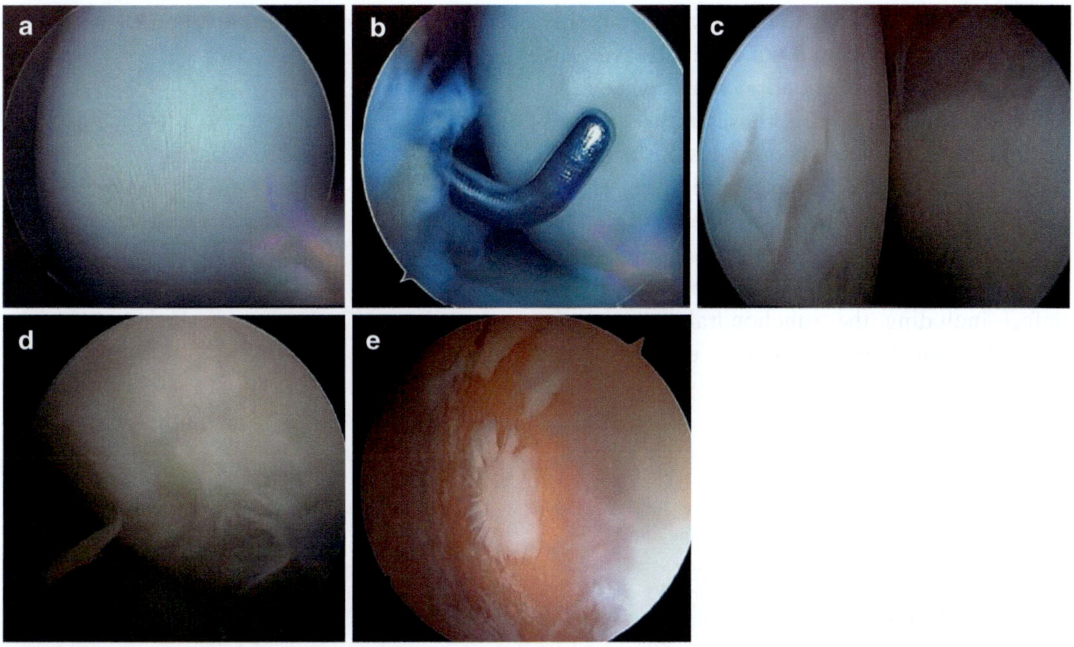

Fig. 4.1 Outerbridge classification arthroscopic image examples: (**a**) Normal; (**b**) Grade I; (**c**) Grade II; (**d**) Grade III; (**e**) Grade IV

tionship between a surgeon's experience and the Outerbridge classification, which affects the reliability of this classification system [19]. There is no clear relationship between the Outerbridge classification system and prognosis. Although the Outerbridge classification system is still the most commonly used classification system for grading cartilage lesions, it does not provide the surgeon with any guidance for treatment decisions and provides little prognostic information (Fig. 4.1).

4.2 ICRS Classification

In 2003, the International Cartilage Regeneration and Joint Preservation Society proposed an arthroscopy-based classification system [1]. This classification system was originally developed to address the need for standardized and universally accepted classification systems in cartilage pathology and to classify the severity of traumatic cartilage lesions but was later applied in a similar way to assess articular cartilage degeneration. This classification system, which can also be used for focal cartilage lesions, is based on depth. In this classification system, categorization is done after performing debridement around the chondral lesion.

The ICRS classification system considers several factors, including the size, depth, location, and surrounding cartilage condition of the lesion. The ICRS classification system uses a grading scale from 0 to IV, where each grade represents a different severity of cartilage injury and has subgroups under grades 1, 3, and 4. Grade 0 means normal, healthy cartilage without any signs of damage. Grade 1 includes near-normal cartilage and is divided into two subgroups, with grade 1A describing superficial lesions and softening of the cartilage tissue and grade 1B describing superficial tears and lacerations. Grade 2 chondral lesions include those that affect less than 50% of the cartilage thickness; there are no subgroups for grade 2 lesions. Grade 3 lesions in the ICRS classification system represent severe cartilage abnormalities that affect more than 50% of the cartilage thickness. Grade 3 lesions are divided into four subgroups. Grade 3A lesions are those that do not reach the calcified layer, while grade 3B lesions reach the calcified layer. Grade 3C chondral lesions are those that extend beyond the calcified layer but do not reach the subchondral bone, and grade 3D chondral lesions are those with cartilage delamination. Grade 4 chondral lesions describe injuries with full-thickness cartilage lesions, exposing the subchondral bone completely. Grade 4 chondral lesions are further subdivided into 4A and 4B. Grade 4A describes a cartilage defect including the subchondral bone plate, and 4B a cartilage defect with exposed deep subchondral bone [1] (Fig. 4.2).

ICRS classification [1]	
Grade 0	Normal cartilage
Grade 1	Nearly normal cartilage
Grade 1A	Superficial lesion (soft indentation)
Grade 1B	Superficial fissures and cracks
Grade 2	Lesions involving less than 50% of cartilage thickness
Grade 3	Lesions involving more than 50% of cartilage thickness
Grade 3A	Lesions that do not reach the calcified layer
Grade 3B	Lesions that reach the calcified layer
Grade 3C	Lesions that extend beyond the calcified layer but not the subchondral bone
Grade 3D	Cartilage delamination
Grade 4	Full-thickness cartilage lesion
Grade 4A	Lesion exposing the superficial subchondral bone
Grade 4B	Lesion exposing the deep subchondral bone

There are various studies that evaluate the reliability of the ICRS classification system. Dwyer et al. found high interobserver and intraobserver reliability and high correlation with histologic assessment of depth, demonstrating the validity of the ICRS classification system [20]. In another study, Niemeyer et al. compared arthroscopic ICRS grading of cartilage lesions with grading at arthrotomy and found 80.9% consensus between arthroscopic and open grading [21]. The fact that arthroscopic assessments are subjective is considered to be one of the limitations of these two classification systems. Another limitation of these classifications is that they cannot give a clear idea about the deep subchondral layers since arthroscopic assessment is only superficial.

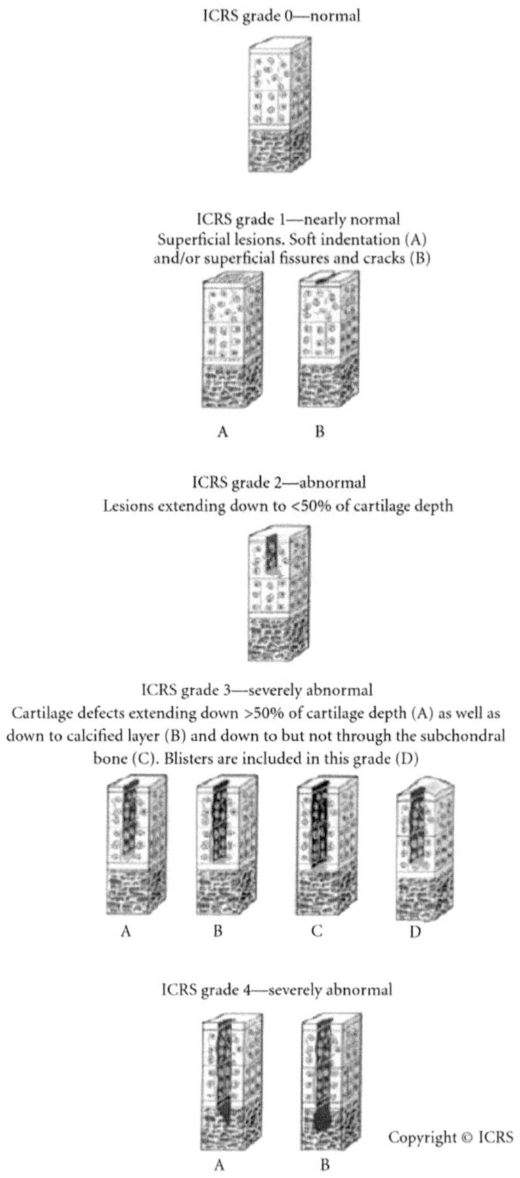

Fig. 4.2 ICRS classification. (Reprinted with permission from the ICRS Cartilage Injury Evaluation Package)

4.3 AMADEUS Score

There are several MRI-based classification systems for the evaluation and assessment of knee osteoarthritis, but there is a lack of robust classification systems for the untreated focal cartilage lesion of the knee [22, 23]. In 2017, Jungmann et al. developed a simple MRI-based scoring system to quantify the severity of osteochondral defects in the knee [8]. The AMADEUS score was developed to assess the severity of a cartilage defect to guide the treatment decision and prognosis of preoperatively detected focal chondral lesions during MRI of the knee joint.

The AMADEUS scoring system has three separate parameters for evaluating a focal chondral or osteochondral defect. These parameters are cartilage defect area, depth of the defect, and presence of subchondral bone defects/cysts and bone marrow edema–like lesions (BME).

The sum of all values gives the total AMADEUS score, which ranges from 0 to 100. A score of 100 means that the cartilage and bone are intact (no osteochondral defect). The worst score is 0, representing the most severe cartilage defect.

The AMADEUS code is 3- or 4-digit code that can be specified by adding all the characteristics. The first digit represents the cartilage defect area. Cartilage defect size is measured in 2 planes, and the defect area is calculated. Defects are divided into 5 groups: ≤1 cm^2 (35 points), >1 to ≤2 cm^2 (30 points), >2 to ≤4 cm^2 (20 points), >4 to ≤6 cm^2 (10 points), and >6 cm^2 (0 points). If there is no defect, the score is 40 points. The second digit of the AMADEUS code indicates the depth of the defect. The presence of a strong signal change in the cartilage is coded as "a" (15 points). Defects with partial thickness are coded as "b" (10 points), and cartilage defects with full thickness are coded as "c" (0 points). If there is no defect, this corresponds to 20 points. The third digit of the AMADEUS code provides information about the subchondral bone. If the subchondral bone has no defects, this is coded as "A" (30 points). The presence of a subchondral bone defect or pathology requiring treatment, such as subchondral cysts or necrosis, is coded as "B" (20 points). If the lesion depth is more than 5 mm, it is coded as "C" (0 points). In addition, the presence of bone marrow edema, defined as poorly demarcated T1-hypointense and IM-FS-hyperintense signal within the trabecular bone adjacent to the defect, is coded as "E" (0 points; 10 points if no BME is present). If BME is present, the digit "E" is added to the digit "A", "B", or "C" [8].

Area measurement and depth and underlying structures (AMADEUS) score [8]

AMADEUS feature	Points	AMADEUS feature	Points
Defect size		*Subchondral bone defect*	
No defect	40	A. No defect	30
≤1 cm^2	35	B. Bony defect/ cyst ≤5 mm depth	20
>1 to ≤2 cm^2	30	C. Nony defect/ cyst >5 mm depth	0
>2 to ≤4 cm^2	20		
>4 to ≤6 cm^2	10	D. No defect-associated BME	10
>6 cm^2	0	E. Defect-associated BME	0
Defect depth			
(n) No defect	20		
(a) Signal alteration	15		
(b) Partial-thickness defect	10		
(c) Full-thickness defect	0		
AMADEUS total score		100	
AMADEUS grade		(0 worst, 100 best)	
Grade I		>75	
Grade II		>50 and ≤75	
Grade III		>25 and ≤50	
Grade IV		≤25	

In young, active patients with cartilage lesions, the joint-sparing treatment of cartilage lesions represents a challenge for orthopedic surgeons. No consensus has yet been reached between the various classification systems that have been developed for cartilage lesions. Arthroscopic imaging and arthroscopic examination are the gold standard for the diagnosis of cartilage lesions [22]. However, since arthroscopic assessment remains subjective and superficial, MRI is increasingly being used as a non-invasive diagnostic method for chondral lesions, and new classification systems are continuously being developed as technology advances.

References

1. Brittberg M, Winalski CS. Evaluation of cartilage injuries and repair. J Bone Joint Surg Am. 2003;85-A Suppl 2:58–69.
2. Jackson DW, Lalor PA, Aberman HM, Simon TM. Spontaneous repair of full-thickness defects of articular cartilage in a goat model. A preliminary study. J Bone Joint Surg Am. 2001;83(1):53–64.
3. Outerbridge RE. The etiology of chondromalacia patellae. J Bone Joint Surg Br. 1961;43-B:752–7.
4. Hunter DJ, Lo GH, Gale D, Grainger AJ, Guermazi A, Conaghan PG. The reliability of a new scoring system for knee osteoarthritis MRI and the validity of bone marrow lesion assessment: BLOKS (Boston Leeds osteoarthritis knee score). Ann Rheum Dis. 2008;67(2):206–11.
5. Hunter DJ, Guermazi A, Lo GH, Grainger AJ, Conaghan PG, Boudreau RM, et al. Evolution of semi-quantitative whole joint assessment of knee OA: MOAKS (MRI osteoarthritis knee score). Osteoarthr Cartil. 2011;19(8):990–1002.
6. Peterfy CG, Guermazi A, Zaim S, Tirman PF, Miaux Y, White D, et al. Whole-organ magnetic resonance imaging score (WORMS) of the knee in osteoarthritis. Osteoarthr Cartil. 2004;12(3):177–90.
7. Kornaat PR, Ceulemans RY, Kroon HM, Riyazi N, Kloppenburg M, Carter WO, et al. MRI assessment of knee osteoarthritis: Knee Osteoarthritis Scoring System (KOSS)--inter-observer and intra-observer reproducibility of a compartment-based scoring system. Skeletal Radiol. 2005;34(2):95–102.
8. Jungmann PM, Welsch GH, Brittberg M, Trattnig S, Braun S, Imhoff AB, et al. Magnetic resonance imaging score and classification system (AMADEUS) for assessment of preoperative cartilage defect severity. Cartilage. 2017;8(3):272–82.
9. Ellermann JM, Donald B, Rohr S, Takahashi T, Tompkins M, Nelson B, et al. Magnetic resonance imaging of osteochondritis dissecans: validation study for the ICRS classification system. Acad Radiol. 2016;23(6):724–9.
10. Heinz T, Meller F, Luetkens KS, Horas K, Schafer T, Rudert M, et al. Can the MRI based AMADEUS score accurately assess pre-surgery chondral defect severity according to the ICRS arthroscopic classification system? J Exp Orthop. 2022;9(1):83.
11. Outerbridge RE. Further studies on the etiology of chondromalacia patellae. J Bone Joint Surg Br. 1964;46:179–90.
12. Outerbridge RE, Dunlop JA. The problem of chondromalacia patellae. Clin Orthop Relat Res. 1975;110:177–96.
13. Noyes FR, Stabler CL. A system for grading articular cartilage lesions at arthroscopy. Am J Sports Med. 1989;17(4):505–13.
14. Lasmar NP, Lasmar RC, Vieira RB, de Oliveira JR, Scarpa AC. Assessment of the reproducibility of the OUTERBRIDGE and FSA classifications for chondral lesions of the knee. Rev Bras Ortop. 2011;46(3):266–9.
15. Bateman DK, Black EM, Lazarus MD, Abboud JA. Outcomes following arthroscopic repair of posterior labral tears in patients older than 35 years. Orthopedics. 2017;40(2):e305–e11.
16. Kemp JL, Makdissi M, Schache AG, Pritchard MG, Pollard TC, Crossley KM. Hip chondropathy at arthroscopy: prevalence and relationship to labral pathology, femoroacetabular impingement and patient-reported outcomes. Br J Sports Med. 2014;48(14):1102–7.
17. Curl WW, Krome J, Gordon ES, Rushing J, Smith BP, Poehling GG. Cartilage injuries: a review of 31,516 knee arthroscopies. Arthroscopy. 1997;13(4):456–60.
18. Amenabar T, Piriz J, Mella C, Hetaimish BM, O'Donnell J. Reliability of 3 different arthroscopic classifications for chondral damage of the acetabulum. Arthroscopy. 2015;31(8):1492–6.
19. Cameron ML, Briggs KK, Steadman JR. Reproducibility and reliability of the outerbridge classification for grading chondral lesions of the knee arthroscopically. Am J Sports Med. 2003;31(1):83–6.
20. Dwyer T, Martin CR, Kendra R, Sermer C, Chahal J, Ogilvie-Harris D, et al. Reliability and validity of the arthroscopic international cartilage repair society classification system: correlation with histological assessment of depth. Arthroscopy. 2017;33(6):1219–24.
21. Niemeyer P, Pestka JM, Erggelet C, Steinwachs M, Salzmann GM, Südkamp NP. Comparison of arthroscopic and open assessment of size and grade of cartilage defects of the knee. Arthroscopy. 2011;27(1):46–51.
22. Figueroa D, Calvo R, Vaisman A, Carrasco MA, Moraga C, Delgado I. Knee chondral lesions: incidence and correlation between arthroscopic and magnetic resonance findings. Arthroscopy. 2007;23(3):312–5.
23. Munk B, Madsen F, Lundorf E, Staunstrup H, Schmidt SA, Bolvig L, et al. Clinical magnetic resonance imaging and arthroscopic findings in knees: a comparative prospective study of meniscus anterior cruciate ligament and cartilage lesions. Arthroscopy. 1998;14(2):171–5.

5 Treatment Algorithm for Cartilage Lesions and Current Directives in Clinical Practices

Özer Öztürk and Tekin Kerem Ülkü

5.1 Introduction

Injuries of the cartilage may stem from excessive use, direct impact, misalignment, or rotational issues. Damage to the articular cartilage is frequent, as chondral injuries are found in 60% of knee arthroscopic surgeries. Although focal cartilage defects are prevalent and could exist in up to 63% of the general populace and 36% of athletes, most of them do not exhibit symptoms. Dealing with articular cartilage lesions poses a distinctive challenge, given their limited ability to heal, partly due to low chondrocyte turnover rates and avascularity. The widespread occurrence and substantial expense associated with chondral disease, spanning from minor focal defects to advanced osteoarthritis, carry significant financial implications for the healthcare system.

Orthopedic practitioners may encounter knee cartilage symptoms in diverse manifestations within their practice. Patients may present with complaints such as joint pain, swelling, and inability to bear weight. Cartilage deformation can lead to osteoarthritis and chondral defects in weight-bearing regions, putting them at risk of developing osteoarthritis.

Ö. Öztürk · T. K. Ülkü (✉)
Department of Orthopedic Surgery, Faculty of Medicine, Acibadem University, Istanbul, Turkey

5.2 Treatment

The treatment of cartilage repair is transitioning from being primarily within the domain of subspecialists to becoming more prevalent across the orthopedic community. Treatment options encompass arthroscopic debridement, abrasion arthroplasty, marrow-stimulation techniques like microfracture and subchondral drilling, osteochondral autograft transfer (OAT), osteochondral allograft transplantation (OCA), and autologous chondrocyte implantation (ACI) [1].

Reparative techniques are designed to encourage the generation of new fibrocartilage tissue by improving access to the vascular system and introducing new progenitor cells capable of chondrogenesis. This is achieved through procedures such as microfracture and drilling. Reconstructive techniques are geared toward filling the defect with either autologous, homologous, or other types of tissue, as exemplified by procedures such as autologous chondrocyte implantation (ACI) and osteochondral autologous transplantation (OAT).

5.2.1 Joint Debridement

The objective of this technique is to remove loose chondral tissues. Eliminating loose intra-articular tissue debris and inflammatory mediators produced by the synovial lining yields satisfactory

M. E. Erdil et al. (eds.), *Current Concept in Cartilage Treatment*,
https://doi.org/10.1007/978-3-032-27099-3_5

short-term outcomes for both acute and degenerative chondral lesions. Lavage typically offers short-term symptomatic relief. While suitable for older sedentary patients, the results are often inadequate for active populations.

5.2.2 Marrow-Stimulation Techniques: Microfracture and Drilling

The notion of marrow stimulation was initially proposed by Pridie in the 1950s. The fundamental theory behind its mechanism suggests that a clot develops within the defect due to blood and bone marrow released from small perforations made in the subchondral plate of the lesion bed [2]. Subchondral drilling and microfracture, both described techniques, are utilized for penetrating the subchondral bone. Their purpose is to stimulate the growth of fibrocartilage into the chondral defect.

5.2.2.1 Microfracture

At present, the microfracture technique stands as the favored approach for marrow stimulation. This process involves arthroscopic debridement of the cartilage defect down to the subchondral bone [3, 4]. A knife may be utilized to establish vertical walls in the adjacent healthy cartilage, while curettes are employed to remove the remaining tissue within the defect's margin. After preparing the defect, small curved awls or thin wire drills are employed to make perforations in the subchondral bone. These perforations leave a bone bridge of 3–4 mm between holes and reach a depth of 4 mm across the exposed surface of the lesion [5]. When conducted arthroscopically, it's necessary to reduce the fluid pressure in the knee to observe fat droplets emerging from the newly created holes. This observation indicates that the desired depth of penetration has been attained. The technique's popularity surged due to its perceived minimal morbidity, affordability, and promising initial outcomes as a primary cartilage procedure, particularly in young and active patients.

5.2.2.2 Subchondral Drilling

In this procedure, multiple drill holes are created in the subchondral bone, penetrating into the bone marrow to trigger a vascular response. Despite the perceived efficacy of this procedure, questions persist due to challenges such as limited access, risk of thermal necrosis, and uncertainties regarding long-term outcomes. Recent studies have suggested that drilling does not induce thermal injury. Hence, despite being less frequently utilized compared to microfracture, drilling represents another alternative technique within the realm of marrow-stimulating approaches.

5.2.3 Osteochondral Autograft Transfer (OAT)

Osteochondral autograft transfer (OAT) is a cartilage restoration procedure known for producing genuine hyaline articular cartilage. OAT involves using a patient's own bone and mature hyaline cartilage, transferring this tissue from a less weight-bearing region to repair a defect in a more weight-bearing area, typically as either a single large bone plug or multiple small plugs [6] (Fig. 5.1).

Achieving perpendicularity is crucial for the successful execution of OAT, whether performed via a mini-open incision or arthroscopically. Therefore, it is often more effectively achieved through an open approach. Even though some studies have demonstrated lower contact pressures medially, the lateral trochlea is most commonly used for OAT. However, the medial trochlea, being smaller, provides less tissue for harvest.

5.2.4 Osteochondral Allograft Transplantation (OCA)

Osteochondral allograft transplantation (OCA) involves using bone and hyaline cartilage harvested from a recently deceased donor within 28 days. Osteochondral allograft transplants are applied to address medium articular lesions (up

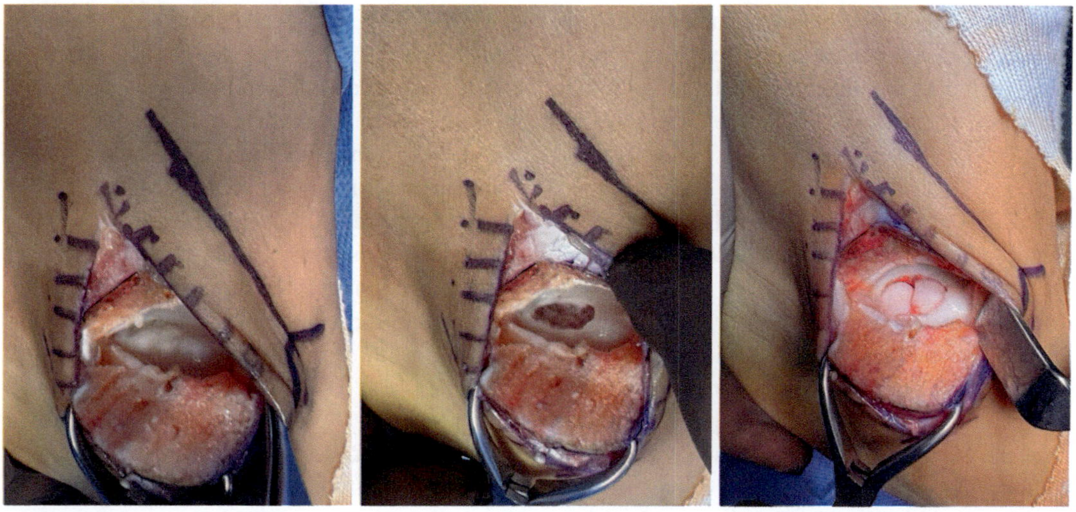

Fig. 5.1 Osteochondral lesion of the talus was treated with osteochondral autograft transfer via medial malleolus osteotomy

to 4 cm^2) in patients with relatively high activity levels [7].

In the initial stage, arthroscopy can be employed for diagnostic purposes and to accurately measure the size of the defect. Pre-cut OCA plugs are then implanted according to the OAT technique [8]. In cases requiring larger plugs, an arthrotomy is conducted to expose the defect, which is then sized using sizing tamps. It is crucial to ensure perpendicularity during this process.

5.2.5 Autologous Chondrocyte Implantation (ACI) and Matrix Autologous Chondrocyte Implantation (MACI)

Brittberg et al. reported autologous chondrocyte implantation (ACI) as an alternative treatment for articular cartilage injuries, resulting in a repair resembling hyaline cartilage. ACI is a two-stage procedure used to treat large full-thickness cartilage defects [9]. The first stage involves arthroscopic assessment of the chondral lesion and biopsy, with chondrocytes harvested from lesser weight-bearing articular surfaces of the knee, such as the lateral edge of the intercondylar notch or the superomedial trochlea [10]. The harvested cartilage specimens are sent to the laboratory for the isolation of chondrocytes from them.

The original ACI techniques entailed injecting the cultured cells beneath a collagen membrane or a periosteal patch. However, issues such as periosteal patch hypertrophy, high reoperation rates for debridement, and cell leakage had adverse effects on the overall outcomes of the ACI procedure. These issues led to the development of a third-generation MACI technique. Unlike its predecessors, the MACI technique involves culturing harvested chondrocytes for 3–4 weeks and then directly seeding the cells into a type-I/III collagen scaffold matrix [11]. This matrix is then fixed into the chondral defect using fibrin glue.

5.2.6 Bone Marrow Aspirate Concentrate Implantation (BMAC)

The BMAC method involves harvesting and concentrating mesenchymal progenitor cells, growth factors, and cytokines from autologous bone marrow obtained from the patient [12, 13]. This concentrated mixture is then injected into a focal chondral defect, forming a bioactive clot. Clot stabilization can be enhanced by combining it with fibrin glue or by placing a membrane. Bone marrow aspirate can be harvested from various sites, including the iliac crest, distal femur, proximal tibia, or calcaneus.

5.2.7 Autologous Matrix-Induced Chondrogenesis (AMIC)

Autologous matrix-induced chondrogenesis (AMIC) combines marrow stimulation techniques (MST) with a type I/III porcine collagen- or hyaluronan-based membrane [14]. Positioned over the MST defect, the patch serves as a scaffold, retaining bone marrow elements and enabling their maturation. This process facilitates the differentiation of these elements into chondrogenic cells (Fig. 5.2).

The procedure is usually conducted through arthrotomy, with marrow stimulation techniques performed in the standard manner. To mitigate the risk of dislodging the patch during knee range of motion, it should be slightly undersized so that its edges are not raised or proud.

5.2.8 Micronized Cartilage Extracellular Matrix (Biocartilage)

Micronized cartilage extracellular matrix is a desiccated acellular particulated cartilage allograft employed as a bioactive scaffold for addressing focal cartilage defects. It contains type II collagen, proteoglycans, and chondral growth factors. The procedure can be carried out either through an open approach or arthroscopically. It's essential to ensure thorough drying of the defect. Subsequently, the implant is mixed with an autologous blood solution in a 1:0.8 ratio, and the resulting mixture is introduced into the defect. This can be done manually for open procedures or using an arthroscopic device available with the device kit for arthroscopic procedures.

5.2.9 Particulated Juvenile Allograft Cartilage (PJAC)

Advancements in cartilage restoration techniques have led to the adoption of fresh particulated juvenile allograft chondrocytes for transplantation at the lesion site, aiming to replicate the native cartilaginous articular surface [15]. The primary graft material currently available for this procedure is the DeNovo NT Natural Tissue Graft (Zimmer, Warsaw, IN, USA), which comprises immature live chondrocyte cells within their native extracellular matrix, sourced from donors typically younger than 13 years old.

Fibrin adhesive serves to secure these cartilaginous pieces within the lesion. Its efficacy has been demonstrated in knee pathologies, such as high-grade cartilage lesions of the patella, femoral condyles, or trochlear groove, leading to swift and safe pain relief and improved outcomes in short-term follow-up. Nevertheless, the available

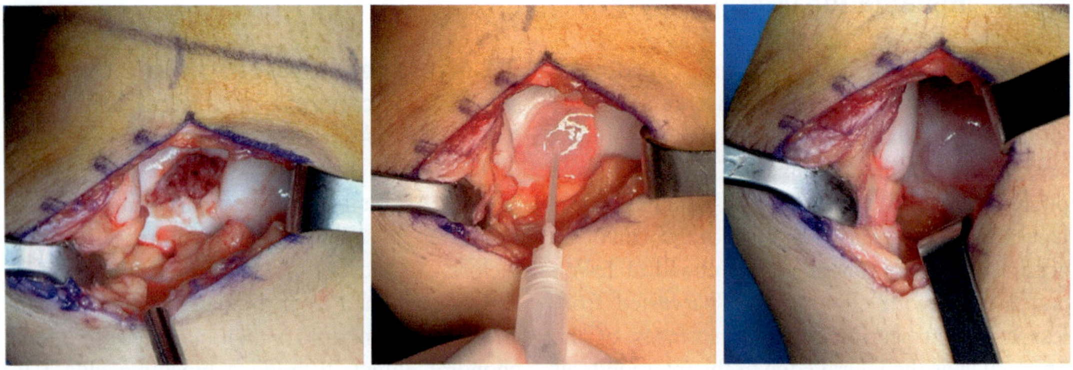

Fig. 5.2 An osteochondral lesion of the femoral condyle was treated with the AMIC procedure

data are limited to level IV evidence, with only small cohorts included.

5.2.10 Particulated Autologous Cartilage Implantation (PACI)

While PJAC utilizes particulated cartilage obtained from juvenile allografts, the use of particulated autologous cartilage implantation (PACI) involves utilizing particulated cartilage obtained from the patient's own tissue during the same surgical procedure.

Approximately 300 mg of cartilage without bone is harvested from the surgeon's chosen location, typically from the intercondylar notch, medial femoral trochlear ridge, or lateral femoral trochlear ridge.

After achieving hemostasis, a thin layer of fibrin glue is applied to the defect, followed by the even application of the cartilage paste across the defect. A second layer of fibrin glue is then applied to firmly secure the cartilage in place. Subsequently, the construct is secured to the top of the defect using small absorbable sutures and fibrin glue around the periphery.

5.2.11 Human Umbilical Cord Blood–Derived Mesenchymal Stem Cells (CARTISTEM)

CARTISTEM is a human allogeneic umbilical cord blood–derived mesenchymal stem cell (hUCB-MSC) utilized for treating degenerative or traumatic grade IV cartilage lesions of the knee.

The hUCB-MSCs are combined with a 1.5-mL sodium hyaluronate (HA) suspension. Next, multiple 5-mm drill holes, spaced 2 to 3 mm apart and 5 mm in depth, are created in the area of the cartilage defect. The hUCB-MSC-HA solution is then transplanted into each of these newly created drill holes.

5.3 Treatment Algorithm

Articular cartilage defects of the knee are prevalent. Treatment options vary from palliative approaches like debridement to reparative techniques such as marrow stimulation and restorative methods like osteochondral grafting and autologous chondrocyte implantation. All of these techniques lead to an improvement in clinical status compared to the preoperative state. Before undergoing any cartilage restoration procedure, it is advisable to consider non-operative treatment options.

Non-operative care options include weight loss, ice therapy, anti-inflammatory medications, bracing, physical therapy, and intra-articular injections (such as corticosteroids, hyaluronic acid, and biologics) [16]. Surgery is typically considered for patients who continue to experience pain, swelling, or functional limitations despite conservative measures, particularly in the presence of a focal chondral or osteochondral lesion [17]. Before the cartilage treatment, possible malalignment, ligament insufficiency, and concomitant meniscal deficiency are evaluated and, if necessary, addressed as part of the treatment plan [18]. When deciding on the appropriate cartilage restoration technique, the primary considerations are the patient's level of activity and the condition of the underlying subchondral bone.

Primary repair is performed for any chondral injury that is suitable for fixation. This includes addressing acute osteochondral fragments or unstable osteochondritis dissecans lesions either in situ or with repair. Patients with lesions that cannot be repaired primarily may benefit from alternative treatments. Marrow stimulation techniques are often considered a first-line treatment in such cases. These techniques are commonly employed for smaller lesions (<2.5 cm^2) or in patients with medium lesions (2.5–4 cm^2) and low physical or physiological demand levels. For small lesions in high-demand patients or cases where marrow stimulation has proven ineffective, treatment may involve the use of one or two 10-mm osteochondral autografts. For larger lesions (>4 cm^2), osteochondral allografting or autologous chondrocyte implantation is typically preferred. Autologous chondrocyte implantation is particularly advisable for younger patients with superficial lesions, as it avoids subchondral bone violation and minimizes the impact on future treatments such as osteochondral allograft transplantation. The treatment algorithm is summarized in Fig. 5.3 and detailed below.

5.3.1 Small Lesions (<2.5 cm^2)

Classical marrow stimulation techniques (MST) are considered the most cost-effective treatment for lesions smaller than <2.5 cm^2 [19]. Comparisons between osteochondral autograft transplantation (OAT) and MST have shown that OAT results in better long-term outcomes and increased patient activity levels [20]. In their study, Gudas et al. enrolled 60 competitive or highly trained athletes with symptomatic osteochondritis dissecans or full-thickness articular cartilage lesions. These patients were randomly assigned to receive either microfracture or osteochondral autograft transplantation (OAT). Patients treated with OAT exhibited a statistically significant better clinical outcome compared to those in the microfracture group, and also, both treatment techniques demonstrated a significant improvement from baseline scores [21]. However, evidence from randomized controlled trials (RCTs) comparing autologous chondrocyte implantation (ACI)/matrix-induced autologous chondrocyte implantation (MACI) and MST is inconsistent [22]. Typically, no significant differences are observed in short-term follow-up (<2 years) [23, 24]. In cases involving bone involvement, OAT and osteochondral allograft transplantation

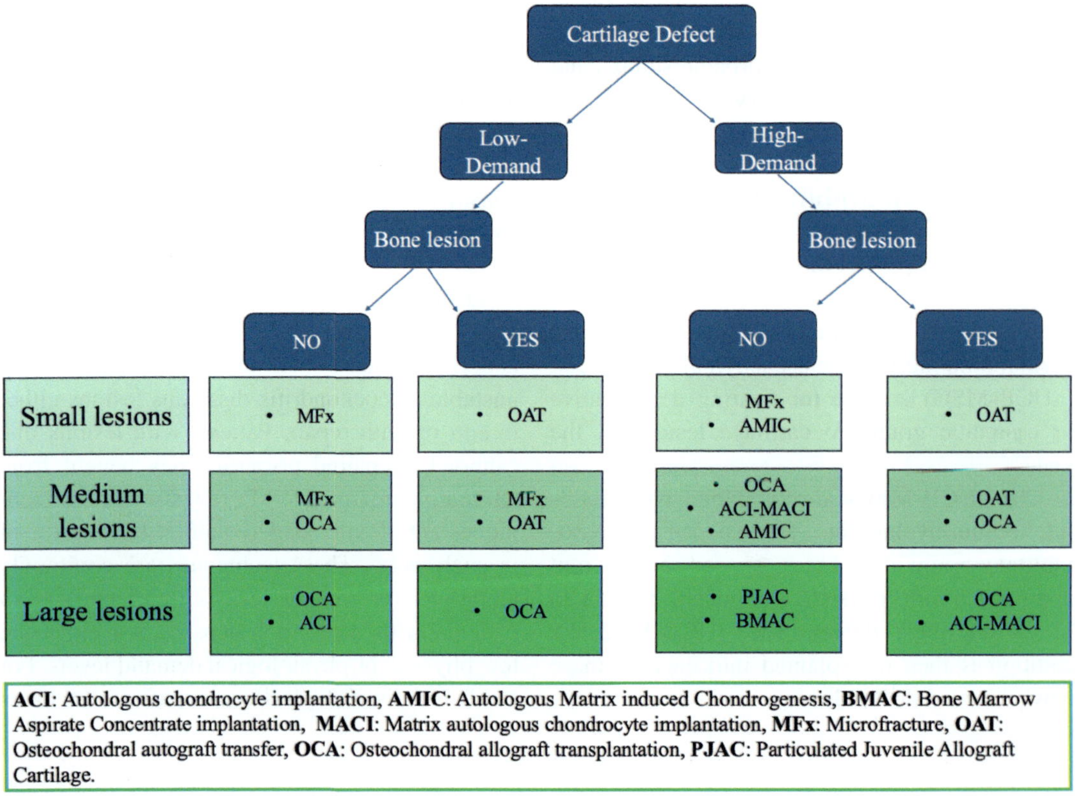

Fig. 5.3 Treatment algorithm for cartilage defect

(OCA) are the osteochondral procedures with the most evidence supporting their efficacy in treating small-sized cartilage defects [25].

5.3.2 Medium Lesions (2.5–4 cm^2)

For medium-sized lesions (2.5–4 cm^2) of the trochlea and femoral condyles, osteochondral allograft transplantation (OCA), osteochondral autograft transplantation (OAT), and autologous chondrocyte implantation (ACI)/matrix-induced autologous chondrocyte implantation (MACI) are the preferred first-choice procedures, supported by significant evidence in the literature [26, 27]. OAT offers advantages over ACI/MACI, such as lower cost, earlier weight-bearing/mobilization, and quicker return to sports. Conversely, ACI/MACI offers advantages over OAT, including the absence of donor site morbidity and preservation of underlying subchondral bone.

5.3.3 Large Lesions (>4 cm^2)

Surgical options for treating large cartilage defects (>4 cm^2) without bone involvement include autologous chondrocyte implantation (ACI)/matrix-induced autologous chondrocyte implantation (MACI), osteochondral allograft transplantation (OCA), particulated juvenile allograft chondrocyte implantation (PJAC), and bone marrow aspirate concentrate (BMAC) implantation [26, 28]. Focal cartilage defects, particularly in the femoral condyles, have shown successful long-term outcomes with both OCA and ACI/MACI. OCA is the preferred cartilage procedure for large defects (>4 cm^2) with underlying bone involvement, demonstrating durability and good to excellent functional outcomes in high-demand patients over long-term follow-up [29, 30]. If OCA is unavailable, ACI/MACI with bone grafting of the bone defect serves as an alternative solution. In their study, Bentley et al. compared mosaicplasty and autologous chondrocyte implantation (ACI) for the repair of symptomatic cartilage defects in 100 consecutive patients, with an average defect size of 4.66 cm^2. One year post-surgery, 88% of the lesions on the medial femoral condyle treated with ACI achieved excellent to good clinical results, compared to 74% treated with mosaicplasty ($P = 0.032$) [31].

References

1. Riboh JC, Cvetanovich GL, Cole BJ, Yanke AB. Comparative efficacy of cartilage repair procedures in the knee: a network meta-analysis. Knee Surg Sports Traumatol Arthrosc. 2017;25(12):3786–99.
2. Orth P, Gao L, Madry H. Microfracture for cartilage repair in the knee: a systematic review of the contemporary literature. Knee Surg Sports Traumatol Arthrosc. 2020;28(3):670–706.
3. Steadman JR, Briggs KK, Rodrigo JJ, Kocher MS, Gill TJ, Rodkey WG. Outcomes of microfracture for traumatic chondral defects of the knee: average 11-year follow-up. Arthroscopy. 2003;19(5):477–84.
4. Mithoefer K, Williams RJ 3rd, Warren RF, Potter HG, Spock CR, Jones EC, et al. The microfracture technique for the treatment of articular cartilage lesions in the knee. A prospective cohort study. J Bone Joint Surg Am. 2005;87(9):1911–20.
5. Mithoefer K, McAdams T, Williams RJ, Kreuz PC, Mandelbaum BR. Clinical efficacy of the microfracture technique for articular cartilage repair in the knee: an evidence-based systematic analysis. Am J Sports Med. 2009;37(10):2053–63.
6. Santos AL, Demange MK, Prado MP, Fernandes TD, Giglio PN, Hintermann B. Cartilage lesions and ankle osteoarthrosis: review of the literature and treatment algorithm. Rev Bras Ortop. 2014;49(6):565–72.
7. Cotter EJ, Hannon CP, Christian DR, Wang KC, Lansdown DA, Waterman BR, et al. Clinical outcomes of multifocal osteochondral allograft transplantation of the knee: an analysis of overlapping grafts and multifocal lesions. Am J Sports Med. 2018;46(12):2884–93.
8. Gross AE, Kim W, Las Heras F, Backstein D, Safir O, Pritzker KP. Fresh osteochondral allografts for posttraumatic knee defects: long-term followup. Clin Orthop Relat Res. 2008;466(8):1863–70.
9. Pestka JM, Bode G, Salzmann G, Südkamp NP, Niemeyer P. Clinical outcome of autologous chondrocyte implantation for failed microfracture treatment of full-thickness cartilage defects of the knee joint. Am J Sports Med. 2012;40(2):325–31.
10. Kreuz PC, Müller S, von Keudell A, Tischer T, Kaps C, Niemeyer P, et al. Influence of sex on the outcome of autologous chondrocyte implantation in chondral defects of the knee. Am J Sports Med. 2013;41(7):1541–8.
11. Filardo G, Vannini F, Marcacci M, Andriolo L, Ferruzzi A, Giannini S, et al. Matrix-assisted autologous chon-

drocyte transplantation for cartilage regeneration in osteoarthritic knees: results and failures at midterm follow-up. Am J Sports Med. 2013;41(1):95–100.
12. de Girolamo L, Schönhuber H, Viganò M, Bait C, Quaglia A, Thiebat G, et al. Autologous matrix-induced chondrogenesis (AMIC) and AMIC enhanced by autologous concentrated bone marrow aspirate (BMAC) allow for stable clinical and functional improvements at up to 9 years follow-up: results from a randomized controlled study. J Clin Med. 2019;8(3).
13. Fortier LA, Potter HG, Rickey EJ, Schnabel LV, Foo LF, Chong LR, et al. Concentrated bone marrow aspirate improves full-thickness cartilage repair compared with microfracture in the equine model. J Bone Joint Surg Am. 2010;92(10):1927–37.
14. Benthien JP, Behrens P. Autologous matrix-induced Chondrogenesis (AMIC): combining microfracturing and a collagen I/III matrix for articular cartilage resurfacing. Cartilage. 2010;1(1):65–8.
15. Wixted CM, Dekker TJ, Adams SB. Particulated juvenile articular cartilage allograft transplantation for osteochondral lesions of the knee and ankle. Expert Rev Med Devices. 2020;17(3):235–44.
16. Cvetanovich GL, Riboh JC, Tilton AK, Cole BJ. Autologous chondrocyte implantation improves knee-specific functional outcomes and health-related quality of life in adolescent patients. Am J Sports Med. 2017;45(1):70–6.
17. Meyer MA, McCarthy MA, Gitelis ME, Poland SG, Urita A, Chubinskaya S, et al. Effectiveness of lavage techniques in removing immunogenic elements from osteochondral allografts. Cartilage. 2017;8(4):369–73.
18. Ambra LF, Hinckel BB, Arendt EA, Farr J, Gomoll AH. Anatomic risk factors for focal cartilage lesions in the patella and trochlea: a case-control study. Am J Sports Med. 2019;47(10):2444–53.
19. Solheim E, Hegna J, Inderhaug E, Øyen J, Harlem T, Strand T. Results at 10-14 years after microfracture treatment of articular cartilage defects in the knee. Knee Surg Sports Traumatol Arthrosc. 2016;24(5):1587–93.
20. Solheim E, Hegna J, Inderhaug E. Long-term survival after microfracture and mosaicplasty for knee articular cartilage repair: a comparative study between two treatments cohorts. Cartilage. 2020;11(1):71–6.
21. Gudas R, Kalesinskas RJ, Kimtys V, Stankevicius E, Toliusis V, Bernotavicius G, et al. A prospective randomized clinical study of mosaic osteochondral autologous transplantation versus microfracture for the treatment of osteochondral defects in the knee joint in young athletes. Arthroscopy. 2005;21(9):1066–75.
22. Brittberg M, Recker D, Ilgenfritz J, Saris DBF. Matrix-applied characterized autologous cultured chondrocytes versus microfracture: five-year follow-up of a prospective randomized trial. Am J Sports Med. 2018;46(6):1343–51.
23. Knutsen G, Engebretsen L, Ludvigsen TC, Drogset JO, Grøntvedt T, Solheim E, et al. Autologous chondrocyte implantation compared with microfracture in the knee. A randomized trial. J Bone Joint Surg Am. 2004;86(3):455–64.
24. Van Assche D, Staes F, Van Caspel D, Vanlauwe J, Bellemans J, Saris DB, et al. Autologous chondrocyte implantation versus microfracture for knee cartilage injury: a prospective randomized trial, with 2-year follow-up. Knee Surg Sports Traumatol Arthrosc. 2010;18(4):486–95.
25. Pareek A, Reardon PJ, Maak TG, Levy BA, Stuart MJ, Krych AJ. Long-term outcomes after osteochondral autograft transfer: a systematic review at mean follow-up of 10.2 years. Arthroscopy. 2016;32(6):1174–84.
26. Hinckel BB, Thomas D, Vellios EE, Hancock KJ, Calcei JG, Sherman SL, et al. Algorithm for treatment of focal cartilage defects of the knee: classic and new procedures. Cartilage. 2021;13(1_suppl):473s–95s.
27. Riff AJ, Huddleston HP, Cole BJ, Yanke AB. Autologous chondrocyte implantation and osteochondral allograft transplantation render comparable outcomes in the setting of failed marrow stimulation. Am J Sports Med. 2020;48(4):861–70.
28. Chahla J, Hinckel BB, Yanke AB, Farr J, Bugbee WD, Carey JL, et al. An expert consensus statement on the management of large chondral and osteochondral defects in the patellofemoral joint. Orthop J Sports Med. 2020;8(3):2325967120907343.
29. Thomas D, Shaw KA, Waterman BR. Outcomes after fresh osteochondral allograft transplantation for medium to large chondral defects of the knee. Orthop J Sports Med. 2019;7(3):2325967119832299.
30. De Caro F, Bisicchia S, Amendola A, Ding L. Large fresh osteochondral allografts of the knee: a systematic clinical and basic science review of the literature. Arthroscopy. 2015;31(4):757–65.
31. Bentley G, Biant LC, Carrington RW, Akmal M, Goldberg A, Williams AM, et al. A prospective, randomised comparison of autologous chondrocyte implantation versus mosaicplasty for osteochondral defects in the knee. J Bone Joint Surg Br. 2003;85(2):223–30.

Scaffold Applications in the Treatment of Cartilage Lesions

6

Lorenzo Zanasi, Alberto Grassi, Luca Andriolo, Stefano Zaffagnini, and Giuseppe Filardo

6.1 Introduction

Knee chondral and osteochondral defects represent a major issue in orthopaedics due to the limited regenerative potential of the osteochondral (OC) unit. Articular cartilage is a tissue made of a single cell line (chondrocytes) embedded in an extracellular matrix (ECM). Despite these simple constituents, its structure is far from simple. Conventionally, it can be divided into three layers: a superficial zone, a middle zone, and a deep zone, each with specific architecture, cellular density, and ECM elements [1]. The transition from articular cartilage to bone, also known as the bone-cartilage interface, is not abrupt: underneath the deep cartilage zone lies a layer of calcified cartilage with a cement line [2]. Subchondral bone is the layer beneath the cement line, and it can be divided into subchondral bone plate and trabecular bone. Its microenvironment has been demonstrated to actively affect viscoelasticity [3, 4] and nutritional metabolism of articular cartilage [5], and is populated by several cells, such as osteoblasts, osteoclasts, osteocytes, chondrocytes, endothelial cells, and mesenchymal stem cells (MSCs) [6]. This OC interface is therefore a complex functional unit, with distinct gradients, properties, cells, and components that act cohesively with sophisticated crosstalk [7]. This organized structure may be disrupted by several conditions, including osteochondritis dissecans (OCD), trauma, and degenerative diseases, possibly leading to chondral or osteochondral lesions with consequent pain and function impairment [8]. These lesions, if left treated or inadequately managed, may enlarge and, ultimately, contribute to the development of osteoarthritis (OA) [9]. Due to low cellularity, lack of blood vessels, minimal chondrocytes' proliferative capacity, and low cell migration to damaged areas, articular cartilage is intrinsically unable to repair itself [1, 10, 11].

Several approaches have been developed to relieve pain, restore function, and possibly avoid or delay OA [12]. These strategies have rapidly evolved from surgical approaches aimed at inducing endogenous repair mechanisms (e.g., microfracture [13]) to regenerative techniques (e.g., autologous chondrocyte implantation [ACI] [14]) either with a cell-based or a cell-free approach (Chap. 21, Fig. 20.8). Both microfracture and ACI present limitations in terms of repair tissue

L. Zanasi · A. Grassi (✉) · L. Andriolo · S. Zaffagnini
Clinica Ortopedica e Traumatologica 2, IRCCS Istituto Ortopedico Rizzoli, Bologna, Italy
e-mail: lorenzo.zanasi@ior.it; alberto.grassi@ior.it; luca.andriolo@ior.it; stefano.zaffagnini@unibo.it

G. Filardo
Service of Orthopaedics and Traumatology, Department of Surgery, EOC, Lugano, Switzerland

Faculty of Biomedical Sciences, Università della Svizzera Italiana, Lugano, Switzerland
e-mail: giuseppe.filardo@usi.ch

M. E. Erdil et al. (eds.), *Current Concept in Cartilage Treatment*,
https://doi.org/10.1007/978-3-032-27099-3_6

quality [15, 16] and technical procedure, which fostered the development and introduction of scaffolds [17]. A scaffold is a three-dimensional structure made of biodegradable polymers that simulate the architectural characteristics of chondral and osteochondral tissues and thus facilitate tissue growth, cell proliferation, and differentiation. Different types of scaffolds have been described and applied in the clinical setting [18]. They can be used to cover the defect in order to stimulate new cartilage growth alone, or they can be combined with microfracture as a one-step procedure to entrap cells released from the subchondral bone and stimulate matrix formation. Scaffolds have also been used as augmentation to ACI, in a procedure known as matrix-assisted autologous chondrocyte transplantation (MACT), based on the seeding of expanded chondrocytes into a matrix scaffold, creating a bioengineered tissue that is later placed onto the chondral defect (Chap. 21, Fig. 20.10). This approach allows one to overcome the previous issues of patch hypertrophy, cell leakage, and extensive suturing and even allowed the development of an arthroscopic approach [19, 20]. Whether they are used alone, in combination with microfracture, or in cell--based procedures, scaffolds have become a widespread solution, and, in their various spectrum of forms, they represent a reference among treatments aiming to achieve cartilage regeneration.

The following chapter will offer a review of the basic science and clinical application of scaffolds for the treatment of chondral and osteochondral lesions, providing an overview of the current literature on the main clinically available products and procedures.

6.2 Rationale

Scaffolds provide a platform for cell survival, proliferation, and differentiation, thereby creating a favorable environment for tissue regeneration. In this light, scaffolds have become of paramount importance in regenerative medicine, with promising clinical results in the field of cartilage treatments [21]. They present several characteristics that must be taken into account, such as biocompatibility, biodegradability pattern, porosity, and durability. Each scaffold has a specific mechanism of action, architecture, thickness, and composition, often allowing for patient-tailored solutions [22]. Scaffolds for the articular surface can be classified into two major categories: chondral scaffolds and osteochondral scaffolds, depending on the anatomical structure they are mimicking. The first ones are monophasic scaffolds, i.e., a single material or composites with no internal structural variation, and have indications for pure cartilage lesions, with preserved subchondral bone. These primarily consist of natural polymers but can also be made of synthetic polymers or a combination of both (i.e., hybrid scaffolds). Natural polymers such as hyaluronic acid, collagen, chitosan, and alginate [23, 24] have poor biomechanical properties but are often used due to their high bioactivity, biocompatibility, and biodegradability to non-toxic components. Their composition with natural materials makes them similar to cartilage ECM, which mimics an ideal environment for cells, regulating chondrocytes' adhesion and differentiation [25, 26]. On the other hand, osteochondral scaffolds have been developed to target osteochondral lesions and were originally designed as monophasic scaffolds. However, since the OC interface is characterized by distinct layers, each with different biomechanical, biochemical, and morphological properties, monophasic scaffolds are unable to mimic the complexity of the native OC unit. This can lead to poor integration of the regenerated cartilage with the underlying subchondral bone and to inadequate defect repair [27]. To address this issue, biphasic and multiphasic scaffolds have been developed, where two or more different materials, composites, bioactive molecules, or architectures are implemented to create a depth-dependent variation in the scaffold properties and functionality. This better replicates the osteochondral interface environment and offers biochemical stimuli to the cells of each layer of the OC unit. The stimuli may either come from the scaffold material itself mimicking the native tissue, or be integrated into the scaffold as bioactive molecules (e.g., bone morphogenetic protein-2 or transforming growth factor-β) [22, 28–30]. Osteochondral scaffolds can be made of a combination of natural polymers, synthetic polymers (such as polycaprolactone, polylactic acid, and poly(lactic-co-glycolic) acid), or ceramics (such as hydroxyapatite or tricalcium phosphate), which are usually incorporated as composites for the bone layer regeneration given their chemical and structural similarity to the mineral phase of native bone [23, 31–35]. A growing body of literature supports the potential and the use of new osteochondral scaffolds in clinical practice, along with the most traditional cartilage scaffolds used for the treatment of articular surface lesions.

6.3 Indications

There is no official consensus on the use of scaffolds in chondral and osteochondral defects. However, overall in the literature the most accepted indications are the following:

- Symptomatic ICRS grade III–IV chondral or osteochondral defects
- Etiology: traumatic injuries, degenerative diseases, OCD
- Defect size: depending on the scaffold applied
- Age: younger than 60 years of age is recommended
- Body mass index (BMI): up to 30 kg/m^2

On the other hand, commonly accepted contraindications valid for all the available scaffolds are the following:

- Moderate or advanced osteoarthritis (OA)
- Uncorrected mechanical malalignment
- Joint instability
- Patients suffering from rheumatic diseases (e.g., Reiter syndrome, psoriatic arthritis, gout, ankylosing spondylitis) or arthritis secondary to other inflammatory diseases; active joint infection
- Patients with malignant neoplasms or uncontrolled systemic diseases (e.g., diabetes, thyroid disorders)

6.3.1 Consensus-Based Indications in Different Scenarios

The International Cartilage Regenerative & Joint Preservation Society (ICRS) set up a consensus process in 2020 to establish the appropriateness of scaffolds in different clinical scenarios (Fig. 6.1). The main finding shows that the use of scaffold-based procedures is considered appropriate by the experts in all cases of chondral or osteochondral lesions in knees without instability, malalignment, or meniscal deficiency and not affected by OA [36]. On the other hand, more controversial applications and contraindications were identified as well. In more detail, this expert consensus analyzed the following parameters:

- *Chondral vs. osteochondral scaffolds:* Among the different etiologies, OCD has often shown in the literature to be the most favorable condition to benefit from scaffold-based procedures, but not for all scaffolds. Although chondral scaffolds may be sufficient in shallow OCDs [37], this may not be true for deeper lesions, while osteochondral scaffolds were

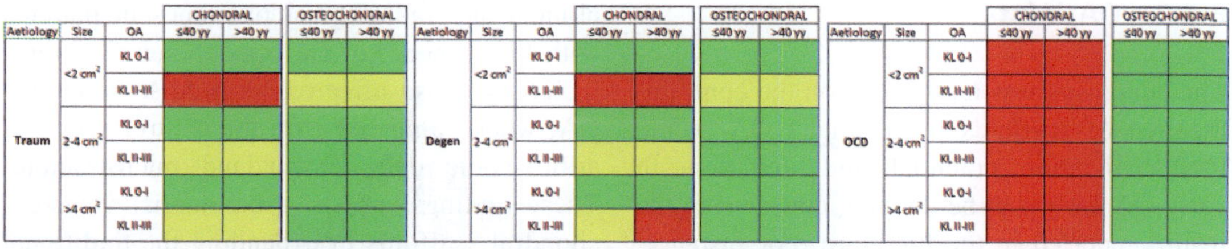

Fig. 6.1 Summary of appropriateness of indications for using chondral and osteochondral scaffolds in different scenarios (adapted from the ICRS RAND/UCLA Consensus [36])

always considered appropriate, except for OCD lesions in OA knees, where other options may be needed. The choice between chondral and osteochondral scaffolds in other aetiologies is mainly depth-dependent.

- *Sport activity level:* The importance of treating chondral or osteochondral defects was deemed appropriate regardless of the sport activity level, with both sports-active patients (who have higher functional requests) and sedentary patients benefitting from the procedure. On the other hand, the use of scaffolds in professional athletes, where many other factors have to be taken into consideration (e.g., return to sport, career duration, etc.) requires further investigation through specific high-level studies.
- *Defect size and OA joints:* Defect size was not a critical factor for treatment indication in non-OA knees; scaffold-based procedures were considered a suitable option even for small lesions, where other effective techniques are available (e.g., OAT, microfracture). However, in OA knees:
  - Chondral scaffolds were never considered appropriate
  - The use of osteochondral scaffolds was deemed uncertain in the case of small lesions (where the conservative treatment may be the more appropriate option)

    In bigger lesions, where little improvement can be expected from the conservative approach, osteochondral scaffolds were considered appropriate, with better results expected for younger patients (more controversial results emerged discussing OA joints in elderly patients)

6.3.2 OA Joints

The consensus was unanimous on the contraindication of scaffolds in advanced OA, while their application, potential, and limitations in early OA are yet to be defined, considering the results reported in the literature. For instance, the use of MACT as a salvage procedure in 41 patients with OA (Kellgren-Lawrence grade 2 or 3) showed poor results in a study by Andriolo et al. [38], with more than half of the patients experiencing failure at long-term follow-up. The total surgical and clinical failure rate was 59% at 15 years. According to the authors, the use of MACT in OA remains questionable. On the other hand, more promising results were shown when a multiphasic osteochondral scaffold (MaioRegen, Fin-ceramica Faenza SpA, Faenza, Italy) was implanted in 23 patients affected by early OA. The results of a study by Di Martino et al. [39] showed improvements in clinical scores at 12-month and 24-month follow-ups, with better results in patients younger than 40 years of age. The authors suggest such a solution may be a valid alternative after failure of conservative management for early OA patients with better results in younger patients (Chap. 21, Fig. 20.9). Later on, in 2019, the same group investigated this multilayer scaffold in 22 patients affected by early OA in terms of clinical outcomes at 5-year follow-up. Clinical results demonstrated significant improvement in the International Knee Documentation Committee (IKDC) subjective and objective scores and in Tegner scores, although the activity level never reached the pre-injury level. There was a 16.6% failure rate at the mid-term follow-up. The authors concluded that cell-free osteochondral scaffolds may offer a safe and valid solution in focal articular cartilage defects in early OA, offering stable clinical improvements with limited complication and failure rates [40]. Finally, in a recent multicenter randomized controlled trial (RCT) by Altschuler et al. [41], the use of an aragonite-based osteochondral scaffold (CARTIHEAL AGILI-C™, Smith+Nephew, Watford, UK; formerly CartiHeal Ltd, Israel) demonstrated superior clinical and radiological outcomes in patients with knee chondral and osteochondral lesions, including those affected by mild to moderate OA, when compared with the control group of arthroscopic debridement and microfracture. These findings support the potential of osteochondral scaffolds in expanding the traditional treatment indications to selected patients with early degenerative joint changes.

6.3.3 Complex or Borderline Cases

Among the complex cases not included in the consensus, several borderline situations have been studied and reported in the literature. For instance, the use of a biomimetic osteochondral scaffold (MaioRegen, Fin-ceramica Faenza SpA, Faenza, Italy) was evaluated in the treatment of late-stage knee osteonecrosis in 11 patients aged under 65 years. The results of a study by Berruto et al. [42] showed significant improvements in subjective IKDC and Lysholm knee scores at 2 years, while Visual Analogue Scale (VAS) values decreased. The Tegner activity scale showed no significant differences between pre-injury and 2-year follow-up. The study recorded two failures that required total knee arthroplasty. According to this study, given the satisfactory clinical results at medium-term follow-up, biomimetic osteochondral scaffolds could be an appropriate solution to treat late-stage osteonecrosis and postpone or even avoid the need for joint replacement procedures.

The same multilayer osteochondral scaffold was also evaluated by Filardo et al. [43] when applied in challenging knee lesions with concomitant treatment of comorbidities in 33 patients. These included history of intra-articular fracture, tibial plateau lesions, concurrent knee axial realignment procedures (Chap. 21, Fig. 20.9), meniscal scaffold or allograft implantation, and multiple articular surface lesions treated. The results were also compared with a group of 23 patients affected by such complex lesions and who were treated with a chondral scaffold. All clinical scores showed significant improvements, and the IKDC subjective score was higher with respect to the group treated with the chondral scaffold. The authors suggested osteochondral scaffolds may be used in combination with other procedures, providing encouraging results in complex cases that might otherwise require non-biological resurfacing.

6.4 Chondral Scaffolds

Scaffold-based regenerative procedures for the treatment of cartilage lesions can be broadly divided into two major categories: cell-free techniques, based on the use of biomaterials without cell seeding, and cell-based procedures, in which scaffolds are combined with cells [44]. In some cases, the same scaffold may be used for both approaches. The following paragraphs will describe how these scaffold-based procedures have been applied in the clinical practice.

6.4.1 Collagen-Based Scaffold Techniques

MACI® (autologous cultured chondrocytes on porcine collagen membrane, Vericel Corporation, Cambridge, MA, USA, formerly Matrix-induced Autologous Chondrocyte Implantation, Sanofi Biosurgery, Cambridge, MA, USA) was the first MACT procedure described. Cultured chondrocytes are seeded onto a type I/III collagen membrane cut to the desired shape and then fixed with fibrin glue. The procedure can also be performed arthroscopically: during a dry arthroscopy, a surgical sponge soaked in adrenaline is applied onto the subchondral bone to prevent bleeding of the prepared lesion bed. The membrane is then introduced into the knee through a large-bore arthroscopic cannula and placed onto the defect with the probe. Finally, fibrin glue is introduced into the defect and below the graft. Pressure on the membrane must be applied for at least 30 seconds for the fibrin glue to become active and thus to obtain further stability [45, 46].

The multicenter RCT SUMMIT (Superiority of MACI Implant Versus Microfracture Treatment) evaluated 144 patients at 5 years of follow-up for symptomatic cartilage defects of the knee. Five years after the treatment, the improvement in MACI over microfracture in Knee injury and Osteoarthritis Outcome Score (KOOS) pain and function was maintained and was statistically significant. Improvements in activities of daily living remained significantly better in MACI patients, with quality of life and other symptoms remaining higher in MACI patients but losing statistical significance relative to the results of the 2-year follow-up. MRI assessment showed improvement in defect filling for both treatments with no statistically significant differences between the two groups. The authors concluded that symptomatic cartilage knee defects 3 cm^2 or larger treated with MACI were clinically and statistically significantly improved at 5 years compared with microfracture [47]. These results confirmed previous studies, like the one of Basad et al. [48], who compared MACI with microfracture in an RCT in 60 patients with single, isolated chondral knee defects, reporting a statistically significant superiority of MACI at 2-year follow-up in all clinical scores. More recently, Bariè et al. [49] in an RCT evaluated the long-term outcomes of 21 patients who underwent MACI vs. ACI with a periosteum patch between 2006 and 2008, comparing patient satisfaction, clinical scores, and MRI evaluation. With the low number of participants available, no significant difference was noted between MACI and ACI at any time point. According to the authors, long-term results suggest that first- and third-generation ACI methods are equally effective treatments for isolated full-thickness cartilage defects of the knee.

AMIC® (Autologous Matrix-Induced Chondrogenesis, Geistlich Pharma AG, Switzerland) is a technique based on a cell-free bilayer collagen I/III membrane (ChondroGide®, Geistlich Biomaterials, Switzerland) as an augmentation for bone marrow stimulation procedures. The scaffold offers a deep layer allowing cell adhesion to the collagen fibers for proliferation and differentiation and a superficial cell-occlusive nonporous layer aiming at containing the clot in the defect, acting as a biological chamber that covers the defect. The surgical technique can be performed arthroscopically and begins with careful debridement of the defect. Subchondral bone is exposed through the use of a circular punch, making sure to create a smooth surface with perpendicular healthy cartilage borders. More punches can be used to shape larger defects. Several holes are performed through a 1.1 mm K-wire at 5 mm intervals into the subchondral bone. The membrane is then trimmed into the desired shape, and positioning is performed through dry arthroscopy, with the porous layer facing the subchondral bone. Alternatively, the scaffold can be implanted with an open approach, and the sizing can be obtained with a template-based approach through an aluminum foil. Fibrin glue is often used to fix the matrix, although sutures and other fixing devices can be used [50, 51].

Anders et al. [52] evaluated the efficacy and safety of AMIC® versus microfracture in a multicenter RCT that included 38 patients. The results showed improvements in clinical scores (modified Cincinnati and ICRS scores) at the 2-year follow-up, regardless of the treatment received. MRI evaluation of defect filling was satisfactory in most of the patients. Volz et al. [53], in a similar study, evaluated 47 patients treated with microfracture or AMIC® in a prospective multicenter clinical trial. Despite the comparable improvement after the first two years, the microfracture group showed a significant decline in clinical scores at 5-year follow-up while the AMIC® group maintained stable results, suggesting the superiority of AMIC® at long-term follow-up.

CaReS® (Cartilage Regeneration System, Arthro Kinetics, Krems, Austria) is a MACT procedure based on a three-dimensional hydrogel made of collagen type I. The cartilage defects are first trimmed using a metal punch, then the scaffolds, once loaded with cultured chondrocytes, are inserted through a punch 1 mm wider than the trimming one. Fibrin glue is applied onto the defect before inserting the scaffold. Since this scaffold is a hydrogel, it has the ability to release more than 50% of its water content, and the CaReS® implant is manufactured to be twice the height of the cartilage defect and has to be shaped accordingly [54]. Alternatively, this approach has been used as a cell-free procedure, as described by Roessler et al. [55], who evaluated 28 patients with large cartilage defects of the knee at 2-year follow-up. Results showed a significant improvement in IKDC and Tegner scores. At 24-month follow-up, the MRI assessment reported complete defect filling in 24 out of 28 patients. However, the results at 5-year follow-up showed an increased clinical failure rate, with 5 out of 28 patients (18%) requiring revision surgery and with a reduction in MOCART score between the 2-year and 5-year follow-up evaluations [56].

NovoCart® 3D (TETEC GmbH, Reutlingen, Germany) is a three-dimensional collagen–chondroitin sulfate scaffold embedded with autologous chondrocytes. The defect, once prepared and debrided, is filled with the soaked scaffold, which is then stabilized using intermittent sutures. Four to six darts can be used for additional fixing.

Müller et al. [57] evaluated 40 patients with knee cartilage defects treated with Novocart® 3D as first-line therapy and compared the results with 20 matched patients treated with ACI as second-line therapy after a previous treatment with bone marrow stimulation. According to the authors, both groups showed significant improvement at 36-month follow-up, although ACI after failed bone marrow stimulation led to worse clinical results. Niethammer et al. [58] evaluated the use of third-generation ACI with NovoCart® 3D in 84 patients with full cartilage knee defects at long-term follow-up: 41 athletic and 43 non-athletic patients were included with a mean follow-up of 8 years. All patients showed significant improvements postoperatively, and athletic patients demonstrated significantly better results in all clinical scores, with 96.4% being able to return to sport and over 50% returning to or surpassing their preinjury sports level. This procedure showed potential as a suitable treatment option for athletic patients with full-thickness cartilage knee defects. Still, while a return to sports activity is possible, it may sometimes require a shift from high-impact sports to less demanding activities.

Atelocollagen gel (ACC-01, Japan Tissue Engineering, Gamagori, Japan) is a scaffold applied within the ACI approach, used for traumatic knee cartilage defects and knee OCD with a defect area of over 4 cm^2. The cultured chondrocyte suspension is embedded in an atelocollagen gel solution and mixed thoroughly in order to obtain a jelly-like substance. The scaffold is then implanted into the defect through an arthrotomy after defect preparation. The surgical technique involves using a periosteal flap sutured over the defect.

Tohyama et al. [59], in a prospective multicenter study evaluated clinical and macroscopic outcomes in patients who underwent atelocollagen-associated ACI for the repair of full-thickness patellar or femoral condyle cartilage defects in 27 patients. At the 2-year follow-up, the Lysholm score significantly increased, while the ICRS grade for arthroscopic appearance was assessed as grade I (normal) in 24% of the patients and as grade II (nearly normal) in 68%. Two patients showed detachment of the graft. Later on, Takazawa et al. [60] evaluated clinical scores and MRI findings at 6-year follow-up in 14 patients: both results showed that the improvements at 1-year follow-up were stable 6 years after implantation. Finally, Kaibara et al. [61] evaluated 13 patients who underwent atelocollagen-based ACI from 2014 to 2018 with a mean final follow-up of 51 months, reporting significantly improved clinical scores and MRI findings.

6.4.2 Hyaluronic Acid-Based Scaffold Techniques

Hyalograft® C (Fidia Advanced Biopolymers Laboratories, Padua, Italy) is a scaffold used for MACT procedures. In this technique the cultured chondrocytes are seeded on Hyaff® 11 (a hyaluronic acid scaffold by Fidia Advanced Biopolymers Laboratories, Padua, Italy). This combination produces the bioengineered tissue Hyalograft® C, which can be implanted both arthroscopically or via an open procedure. In more detail, with a mini-arthrotomy approach, the defect is prepared and debrided, then the biomaterial is accurately shaped according to the lesion and simply placed onto it, with the use of fibrin glue or sutures mainly for large defects or patellofemoral joint lesions. When performed arthroscopically, a specific device is used to measure the lesion size, and a cannulated low-profile and low-speed drill is used to debride it through a K-wire with a safety stop at a 2 mm distance in order to avoid damage to the subchondral bone plate. The procedure can be repeated until the defect surface is fully prepared. At last, with a dedicated delivery system, the tissue-engineered patch shaped according to the stamp is transported through a cannula and positioned in the prepared area. The procedure is repeated until the defect is entirely filled. It is important to cover the prepared area as much as possible without covering the margin of the defect, but implanted stamps can be overlapped. This procedure has been withdrawn from the market for reasons unrelated to the clinical outcome, which showed good and long-lasting results [62–64].

Filardo et al. [65] evaluated the results of arthroscopic Hyalograft® C MACT at 7-year follow-up in 62 patients affected by chondral lesions of the femoral condyles. Results showed a statistically significant improvement in all clinical scores at 24-month follow-up that was stable at 84-month follow-up. An 11% failure was reported. Better results were reported in young active men, while degenerative lesions or patients who had previous surgery showed poorer results. Kon et al. [66] compared the use of Hyalograft® C with microfracture in 41 professional or competitive soccer players and evaluated them prospectively at 2 years and at a final 7.5-year follow-up. Microfracture allowed a faster recovery but presented a clinical deterioration over time, whereas arthroscopic MACT delayed the return of high-level male soccer players to competition but offered more durable clinical results. Similarly, Brix et al. [67] evaluated 53 patients treated with Hyalograft® C at a mean follow-up time of 9 years, including complex and salvage cases. Failure accounted for 22.6% of the patients, with the authors questioning its use for salvage cases. A meta-analysis by Everhart et al. [68] compared MACT with microfracture. MACT had greater improvement in clinical scores and no increased risk of failures. The authors also compared postoperative weight-bearing protocols, reporting that accelerated weight-bearing showed no increased risk of failures and gave higher improvements in subjective clinical scores. This was also confirmed by a specific study by Della Villa et al. [69] showing that athletes treated with on-field rehabilitation and an isokinetic exercise program had faster recovery and an earlier return to competition, thus underlining the importance of intensive rehabilitation for a faster return to sport and to positively influence the clinical outcome. More recently, in a large cohort of 113 patients evaluated at 15 years, Andriolo et al. [64] confirmed the duration of the good results obtained up to this very long-term follow-up.

Hyalofast® (Anika Therapeutics, Inc.—Bedford, MA 01730, USA) is a non-woven biodegradable hyaluronic acid (HA)-based scaffold used for articular cartilage regeneration. This scaffold entraps mesenchymal stem cells (MSCs) to treat chondral lesions and provides structural support for MSCs' attachment, proliferation, and differentiation, allowing for new cartilage deposition and growth and defect filling. The scaffold biodegradation releases hyaluronic acid into the defect, further enhancing cartilage promotion.

Jaramillo Quiceno et al. [70] recently evaluated the use of autologous matrix-induced chondrogenesis (AMIC) with this scaffold in 50 patients with grade IV chondral lesions in a multicenter, non-randomized, retrospective study with a follow-up at 12, 24, and 32 months. Results showed significant improvements in all clinical scores at 32-month follow-up, with patients younger than 45 years presenting better clinical outcomes than older ones. Sofu et al. [71] compared the use of this scaffold applied in combination with microfracture versus microfracture alone in 43 patients with focal osteochondral knee lesions. The authors reported better clinical scores at 1, 12, and 24-month follow-ups for the scaffold-based procedure, and MRI findings were also better in these patients, with complete filling of the defect achieved in 36.8% of the patients vs. 16.6% for microfracture. Finally, Gobbi et al. [72] prospectively evaluated the medium-term effectiveness and regenerative capability of this hyaluronan-based scaffold embedded with autologous adult mesenchymal stem cells, harvested as bone marrow aspirate concentrate (BMAC). The study evaluated 20 patients older than

45 years with ICRS grade 4 chondral lesions of the knee at a 4-year follow-up and compared them with a control group of 20 patients with an age <45 years. According to the authors, treatment of cartilage lesions with BMAC and Hyalofast® is a valid and effective option that is mainly affected by lesion size and number and not by age, showing to be a procedure suitable for older patients with functional results comparable to younger ones.

ChondroTissue® (BioTissue AG, Zurich, Switzerland) is a cell-free polyglycolic acid–hyaluronan (PGA-HA) scaffold immersed in autologous serum. The surgical technique can also be performed arthroscopically. The cartilage defect is first debrided until the subchondral bone is exposed, then the microfracture procedure is performed. The ChondroTissue® implant, after immersion in 3 mL of autologous serum prepared from venous blood pre-operatively, is shaped according to the defect and stabilized using 3 or 4 bioresorbable bone-fixing nails. Fibrin glue can be associated with increasing stability [73].

Siclari et al. [74] evaluated 52 patients with focal chondral defects treated with subchondral drilling and the implantation of this scaffold immersed with autologous PRP. The authors reported significant improvements in clinical scores at a 5-year follow-up, while MRI assessment showed complete defect filling in 20 out of 21 patients at a 4-year follow-up, suggesting this procedure may offer lasting clinical improvements. Similarly, Becher et al. [75] assessed MRI findings of five patients after treatment with microfracture and ChondroTissue® immersed in autologous serum for retropatellar cartilage defects. Results showed good to excellent defect fill with complete integration, although all patients showed subchondral bone alterations. All clinical scores improved, suggesting this procedure represents a safe and feasible solution with improvement at short/medium-term follow-up.

BioCart™ II (ProChon BioTech Ltd, Ness Ziona, Israel) is a fibrin-hyaluronan matrix produced by copolymerization of homologous human fibrinogen and recombinant hyaluronan, subsequently freeze-dried to result in a sponge-like three-dimensional structure. The scaffold, once seeded with chondrocytes, has to be cut according to the defect size and then implanted through an arthrotomy procedure by press-fitting. Fibrin glue is applied at the defect borders to increase stability. Eshed et al. [76] evaluated the use of this scaffold in 31 patients with femoral condyle cartilage defects, demonstrating significant improvements in clinical scores. Clinical scores also showed a significant correlation with the MOCART score for MRI assessment at long-term follow-up.

6.4.3 Chitosan-Based Scaffolds

Cargel Bioscaffold (Smith+Nephew, Watford, UK; formerly BST-CarGel® Piramal, Laval, Quebec, Canada) is a chitosan-based liquid bioscaffold designed to entrap and stabilize the blood clot. The chitosan-based scaffold disperses in uncoagulated autologous blood, strengthening the clot, increasing adhesivity, and thus reducing the risk of clot retraction. This ensures a prolonged effect of the clot and of blood growth and repair factors. The defect is first prepared through accurate debridement and bone marrow stimulation. The Cargel bioscaffold is prepared with 4.5 mL of autologous venous blood in a 3:1 blood to Cargel ratio and then applied via a syringe until the defect is completely covered, avoiding leakage. After delivery, a 15 minutes waiting period is required for polymerization. The use of a tourniquet is recommended. The procedure can also be performed via a dry arthroscopy as long as the defect can be maintained in a horizontal position during the procedure [77].

Shive et al. [78] compared the use of this chitosan-based bioscaffold with microfracture alone in 80 patients at 5-year follow-up in a multicenter RCT. Results showed sustained and significantly superior repair tissue quantity and quality in the CarGel® group over microfracture, but no differences between the treatment groups were seen at 5 years for each WOMAC subscale. Poggi et al. [79] evaluated the use of CarGel® in 14 patients with ICRS grade 3–4 cartilage lesions of the patellar surface at 2-year follow-up. Results showed an improvement in the IKDC subjective score, KOOS Pain, KOOS Sport/Rec, and KOOS QOL from baseline. MRI assessment demonstrated complete defect filling in 70% of the lesions at 2-year follow-up. According to the authors, this chitosan-based bioscaffold may represent a safe surgical treatment in chondral patellar lesions.

6.4.4 Other Scaffolds

Cartipatch® (Tissue Bank of France, Lyon, France) is an agarose-alginate hydrogel scaffold that comes in multiple plug sizes (10, 14, and 18 mm). After debridement, the defect is drilled with a specific instrument until a 4 mm depth is reached. The cell-loaded hydrogel plug has a specific delivery system that transfers it directly onto the defect. The plug can then be squeezed with forceps to adjust its position, and stability is tested with repeated flexion and extension of the knee [80].

A multicenter RCT by Clavé et al. [81] compared the use of Cartipatch® versus mosaicplasty in patients with femoral chondral defects. After 2 years, functional outcomes were significantly worse after Cartipatch® treatment compared to mosaicplasty, and adverse events in the Cartipatch® group were twice as many.

BioSeed® C (BioTissue Technologies, Freiburg im Breisgau, Germany). In this procedure, the cultured chondrocytes are embedded in fibrin and combined with a rectangular resorbable scaffold made of polyglactin 910 and poly-p-dioxanon. Kirschner wires are used to drill transosseous femoral tunnels at each corner of the defect. Resorbable sutures forming loops serve as anchors for the scaffold: the chondrocytes-containing scaffold is shaped according to the defect size and can be fixed at each corner of the defect with an inside-out technique, where the sutures are pulled through the femoral bone using the wires to guide the knots and securely anchor the graft [82]. Erggelet et al. [83] described an arthroscopic approach for this procedure.

Kreuz et al. [84] evaluated patients treated with BioSeed® C for traumatic and degenerative cartilage defects of the knee in 44 patients. Results showed significant improvement in the Lysholm, IKDC, KOOS, and Noyes scores at 48-month follow-up. MRI evaluations showed moderate to complete defect filling in 43 of 44 treated patients. A 4.5% failure was recorded.

6.5 Osteochondral Scaffolds

To date, a small number of multiphasic scaffolds targeting osteochondral lesions have been translated into commercial products, with the most studied being TruFit™, MaioRegen, and CARTIHEAL Agili-C™. All these multilayered scaffolds have been developed as cell-free products, with the aim of exploiting the MSCs coming from the subchondral bone underneath the defect. Various preclinical studies confirmed the rationale of the cell-free use. For example, Kon et al. [85] conducted a study on twelve sheep, where 24 osteochondral lesions were created and randomized in three groups: scaffold alone, scaffold colonized in vitro with autologous chondrocytes, and empty defects. At 6 months of follow-up, significantly better regeneration was observed in the groups receiving the scaffold alone and the scaffold loaded with autologous chondrocytes, without differences between these two groups, when compared with empty defects. The comparable regeneration process observed with or without autologous chondrocytes suggested that the main mode of action of the scaffold is based on the recruitment of local cells, which paved the way to the cell-free use of osteochondral scaffolds.

TRUFIT® (Smith & Nephew, Andover, MA) is a calcium sulfate and polylactic-polyglycolic acid biphasic cylindrical porous scaffold. The surgical technique requires a minimally invasive incision that fully exposes the defect. The use of the tourniquet is required for a bloodless surgical field. The defect is debrided and prepared, then a cylindrical hole (or multiple holes depending on the morphology of the lesion) of 8 to 12 mm in depth is drilled into the defect. A plug of the same height is then introduced into the defect until the surface of the implant is smooth and continuous with the adjacent cartilage. Multiple plugs can be used depending on the lesion size. The implant stability is then tested [86].

Trufit® demonstrated promising preclinical results; however, clinical findings were inconsistent. Some isolated studies showed favorable results after implantation of this scaffold, like Bedi et al. [87], who reported an improvement of the repair tissue at short-term follow-up in 26 patients. Similarly, Bekkers et al. [88] used quantitative MRI analysis to assess 13 patients at 1-year follow-up, demonstrating no damage to the surrounding cartilage and the presence of cartilage-like signal inside the plug. Carmont et al. [89], reporting on a case of an 18-year-old soccer player, showed a delayed incorporation of the scaffold on MRI but positive clinical outcomes at 24 months of follow-up. On the other hand, several authors questioned the results of this scaffold, especially at longer follow-ups. Barber et al. [32] described no signs of maturation, osteoconductivity, or ossification in 9 patients evaluated with CT scans. Dhollander et al. [90] evaluated 15 patients at 12-month follow-up, showing a 20% failure rate, and described fibrous vascularized repair tissue at the histologic assessment. Joshi et al. [91] do not recommend TruFit® implantation for osteochondral patellar defects in active patients after their prospective evaluation of 10 patients showed a 70% revision rate for implant failure at 24-month follow-up. In addition, Hindle et al. [92] retrospectively compared 35 patients who underwent implantation of this osteochondral scaffold with 31 patients who underwent autologous osteochondral mosaicplasty. The results showed significantly lower clinical outcomes and lower return to sport rates in the TruFit® scaffold group. Finally, Shivji et al. [93] demonstrated a high rate of failure of conversion to arthroplasty, no statistically significant improvement, and imaging evidence of absent plug incorporation in 11 patients evaluated at ten years of follow-up. After these controversial clinical findings, this scaffold has currently been withdrawn from the global market.

MaioRegen (Fin-ceramica S.p.A., Faenza, Italy) is an osteochondral nanostructured biomimetic scaffold with a porous three-dimensional tri-layer composite structure that mimics the osteochondral unit biochemical composition. The cartilage layer is made of type I collagen, the intermediate layer (tidemark-like) is made of type I collagen (60%) and hydroxyapatite (HA) (40%), while the lower layer is a mineralized blend of type I collagen (30%) and HA (70%), which mimics the subchondral bone layer. The surgical procedure is performed with a pneumatic tourniquet through a mini-arthrotomic medial or lateral parapatellar approach. The defect is debrided through the removal of the sclerotic subchondral bone with the use of a chisel, until a 7 mm defect depth with stable edges is reached. The scaffold is cut according to the size and the shape of the defect, and the grafts are then implanted by press-fit or with the addition of fibrin glue [94]. Once the tourniquet is released, the implant imbibes blood, and its stability must be tested with repeated knee flexion and extension movements [95]. More recently, a minimally invasive technique with dedicated instrumentation and pre-shaped cylindrical plugs has been introduced [96] (Fig. 6.2).

Promising preliminary results of Kon et al. [29, 97] have been reported in a pilot study on 28 patients affected by complex chondral and osteochondral knee lesions, both at a 2-year follow-up and at a 5-year follow-up, with significant and stable clinical improvements, despite a slow maturation of the scaffold at MRI evaluation. The controversial MRI appearance of the repair tissue at early- to mid-term follow-up has been reported in several studies [98–100], although a slow progression of the graft maturation was shown over time, and MRI alteration showed no correlation with the clinical scores [101]. Moreover, the improvement in clinical scores and the stability at long term were further confirmed by Di Martino et al. [102] at a 10-year follow-up. In 2018 a multicenter RCT by Kon et al. [103] compared MaioRegen and microfracture in 100 patients with knee chondral and osteochondral lesions, reporting significant improvements in all clinical scores at 2-year follow-up in both groups, with no overall statistically significant differences between the two treatments. However, the scaffold group showed better clinical outcomes in sport-active patients

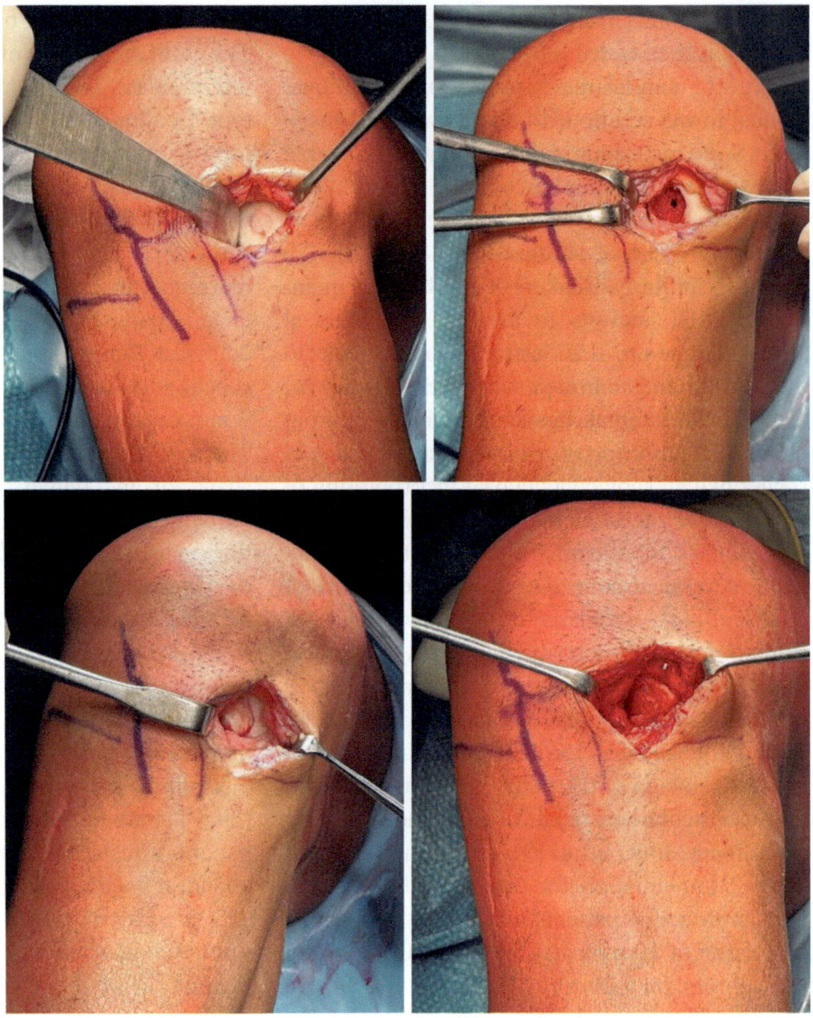

Fig. 6.2 MaioRegen osteochondral scaffold surgical technique. Top left: osteochondral defect; top right: osteochondral defect after debridement; bottom left: implanted scaffold sealed with fibrin glue; bottom right: implanted scaffold after tourniquet release

and in deep osteochondral lesions, i.e., Outerbridge grade IV and OCD. In fact, one of the most validated indications for this scaffold is OCD, with dedicated studies describing positive results at short- and mid-term follow-up both in adult patients [98, 101, 104] and pediatric patients affected by the juvenile form of OCD [105]. On a different note, this scaffold was also applied in more challenging cases. For example, Perdisa et al. [99] treated chondral and osteochondral lesions of the patella in 34 patients, with positive clinical results at short-term follow-up. Kon et al. [106] reported promising clinical results at 2-year follow-up in 11 patients with osteochondral lesions of the tibial plateau. Berruto et al. [42] used this scaffold as a salvage joint-preserving procedure in the treatment of late-stage osteonecrosis of the knee, with significant clinical improvements at 2-year follow-up (with two failures that required total knee replacement out of 11 patients) and at 5-year follow-up [107].

The use of this scaffold offered satisfactory and safe results also in the context of early OA. Di Martino et al. [39] evaluated it in early OA after failure of non-operative treatment in 23 patients. Results showed significant improvements in all clinical scores; however, the activity level was significantly lower than the pre-injury one, with patients younger than 40 years benefitting more from the treatment. Later on, results at 5-year follow-up [40] showed a 16.6% failure rate, suggesting this cell-free osteochondral scaffold can represent a safe and valid alternative in focal articular cartilage defects in the setting of early OA, ensuring significant clinical improvements and stable outcomes with low complication and failure rates. Similarly, Condello et al. [108] evaluated 19 patients with early OA at an average follow-up of 35 months. Clinical scores significantly improved in 69% of the patients, with a complication rate of 11%. Marcacci et al. [109] proposed the use of this scaffold in combination with concurrent knee osteotomy, meniscal allograft transplantation, or meniscal scaffold implantation as an integrated biological and biomechanical approach in 43 patients with unicompartmental OA. Clinical scores at 3-year follow-up significantly improved, with no reported failures or major complications. Higher clinical improvements were observed in patients younger than 40 years, suggesting that this salvage procedure may provide a joint-preserving option in selected young patients who might otherwise be considered for more invasive prosthetic solutions [110].

AGILI-C™ (Smith+Nephew, Watford, UK; formerly CartiHeal Ltd, Israel) is an aragonite-based rigid cell-free scaffold made of two layers: the bone phase, consisting of calcium carbonate in the aragonite crystalline form, and the cartilage phase, consisting of modified aragonite and hyaluronic acid. The technique is a one-step surgical procedure with no cell augmentation. It is performed through a medial or lateral parapatellar arthrotomic approach with a tourniquet to guarantee a bloodless surgical field. After exposure of the defect and size measurement, the lesion is prepared and drilled with specific instrumentation. The scaffold is then implanted by press-fit fixation, leaving the superficial layer 1–2 mm deeper than the adjacent articular surface.

Preclinical analysis revealed promising safety results, a good biodegradability pattern, and adequate cell recruitment from the surrounding tissues, leading to the osteochondral defect healing with both articular hyaline cartilage and subchondral bone regeneration in an animal model [111], which encouraged clinical studies. In 2021, a multicenter prospective study by Kon et al. [112] evaluated a total of 86 patients at 2-year follow-up with mild to moderate knee OA and up to 3 chondral/osteochondral defects (ICRS grades 3 and 4). The results showed significant improvement in all KOOS subscales from baseline. The IKDC subjective score showed a similar trend. In addition, MRI scans demonstrated a significant increase in defect filling over time. More recently a multicenter RCT by Altschuler et al. [41] compared the clinical and radiographic outcomes of this scaffold with a control group that underwent arthroscopic debridement and microfracture in 251 patients affected by knee chondral and osteochondral lesions, including patients with concurrent mild to moderate OA, in a 2:1 ratio. The scaffold group demonstrated a statistically significant superiority in all clinical scores, with a responder rate of 77.8% vs. 33.6% in the control group. An MRI defect fill grade of at least 75% of the defect at a 24-month follow-up was reported in 88.5% of the scaffold-receiving group. The failure rate was 7.2% for the scaffold group as opposed to 21.4% for the control group. These results suggest that this aragonite-based scaffold can be considered a safe and effective solution for chondral and osteochondral knee lesions, including those of patients affected by mild to moderate OA.

6.6 Future Perspectives

Recent advances in biomaterial research and production techniques have offered new opportunities for the development of biomimetic and sophisticated scaffolds. The promotion of minimally manipulated cells techniques (MMCT) favors the shift to a single-step procedure [113]. Moreover, the last generation ACI with three-dimensional bioprinting using computer-aided design (CAD) is currently being developed. Three-dimensional scaffolds bioprinting offers precise control and high flexibility [114, 115]. Gu et al. [116] showed that 3D-printed porous structures allow significantly more cells to infiltrate, with positive results in osteochondral lesion repair in animal models, especially when incorporated with Kartogenin into the upper layer of scaffolds. Similarly, Ding et al. [117] demonstrated that 3D-printed porous scaffolds of hydrogels modified with TGF-β1 binding peptides can promote *in vivo* cartilage regeneration. Three-dimensional composite bioceramic scaffolds for osteochondral regeneration have not only been shown to improve the compressive strength but also the proliferation of both rabbit bone MSCs and chondrocytes, as well as their differentiation, with promising results in the reconstruction of the complex osteochondral interface [118]. New structures are being investigated and are currently undergoing preclinical studies with possible applications in clinical settings in the near future. Among these it is worth mentioning microsphere scaffolds, which can be loaded with drugs, molecules, or genes in order to regulate the local environment [119–121]. Another strategy is the use of decellularized ECM (dECM): dECM scaffolds are biodegradable, present low immunogenicity, and offer a biomimetic microenvironment by providing bioactive molecules and allowing cell growth and proliferation in a native-like structure, making them an attractive research area in tissue engineering [122, 123]. Jiang S et al. [124] applied a dECM scaffold in combination with intra-articular injection of human umbilical cord Wharton's jelly MSC-derived exosomes, promoting osteochondral tissue regeneration in a rabbit model. Despite the promising results, mass industrial implementation and clinical applications are limited by several limitations: narrow range of suitable materials, time-consuming layer-by-layer processing, and high costs [125]. Further exploration is needed to accelerate the clinical translation and fill the gap needed to optimize chondral and osteochondral defect treatments.

6.7 Conclusion

Over the past few decades, biomaterial and tissue engineering studies on scaffolds for the articular surface have seen significant progress. Yet, the anatomical and functional restoration of the chondral layer and of the osteochondral unit is far from perfect: integration with the adjacent tissue, biomechanical and biochemical properties of the repaired tissue, implant survival, and the role of cells still remain key issues to be addressed. The ongoing and future research should work in these directions to offer new insights and provide more effective solutions to treat chondral and osteochondral lesions.

References

1. Sophia Fox AJ, Bedi A, Rodeo SA. The basic science of articular cartilage: structure, composition, and function. Sports Health. 2009;1(6):461–8.
2. Mansfield JC, Winlove CP. A multi-modal multiphoton investigation of microstructure in the deep zone and calcified cartilage. J Anat. 2012;220(4):405–16.
3. Burr DB, Gallant MA. Bone remodelling in osteoarthritis. Nat Rev Rheumatol. 2012;8(11):665–73.
4. Fell NLA, Lawless BM, Cox SC, Cooke ME, Eisenstein NM, Shepherd DET, Espino DM. The role of subchondral bone, and its histomorphology, on the dynamic viscoelasticity of cartilage, bone and osteochondral cores. Osteoarthritis Cartilage. 2019;27(3):535–43.
5. Hu Y, Chen X, Wang S, Jing Y, Su J. Subchondral bone microenvironment in osteoarthritis and pain. Bone Res. 2021;9(1):20.
6. Florencio-Silva R, Sasso GR, Sasso-Cerri E, Simões MJ, Cerri PS. Biology of bone tissue: structure, function, and factors that influence bone cells. Biomed Res Int. 2015;2015:421746.
7. Goldring SR, Goldring MB. Changes in the osteochondral unit during osteoarthritis: structure, function and cartilage-bone crosstalk. Nat Rev Rheumatol. 2016;12(11):632–44.
8. Chau MM, Klimstra MA, Wise KL, Ellermann JM, Tóth F, Carlson CS, Nelson BJ, Tompkins MA. Osteochondritis dissecans: current understanding of epidemiology, etiology, management, and outcomes. J Bone Joint Surg Am. 2021;103(12):1132–51.
9. Ding C, Garnero P, Cicuttini F, Scott F, Cooley H, Jones G. Knee cartilage defects: association with early radiographic osteoarthritis, decreased cartilage volume, increased joint surface area and type II collagen breakdown. Osteoarthritis Cartilage. 2005;13(3):198–205.
10. Morales TI. Chondrocyte moves: clever strategies? Osteoarthritis Cartilage. 2007;15(8):861–71.
11. Shiromoto Y, Niki Y, Kikuchi T, Yoshihara Y, Oguma T, Nemoto K, Chiba K, Kanaji A, Matsumoto M, Nakamura M. Increased migratory activity and cartilage regeneration by superficial-zone chondrocytes in enzymatically treated cartilage explants. BMC Musculoskelet Disord. 2022;23(1):256.
12. Gracitelli GC, Moraes VY, Franciozi CE, Luzo MV, Belloti JC. Surgical interventions (microfrac-

ture, drilling, mosaicplasty, and allograft transplantation) for treating isolated cartilage defects of the knee in adults. Cochrane Database Syst Rev. 2016;9(9):CD010675.
13. Steadman JR, Rodkey WG, Briggs KK. Microfracture to treat full-thickness chondral defects: surgical technique, rehabilitation, and outcomes. J Knee Surg. 2002;15(3):170–6.
14. Brittberg M. Autologous chondrocyte implantation—technique and long-term follow-up. Injury. 2008;39(Suppl 1):S40–9.
15. Orth P, Gao L, Madry H. Microfracture for cartilage repair in the knee: a systematic review of the contemporary literature. Knee Surg Sports Traumatol Arthrosc. 2020;28(3):670–706.
16. Briggs TW, Mahroof S, David LA, Flannelly J, Pringle J, Bayliss M. Histological evaluation of chondral defects after autologous chondrocyte implantation of the knee. J Bone Joint Surg Br. 2003;85(7):1077–83.
17. Harris JD, Siston RA, Brophy RH, Lattermann C, Carey JL, Flanigan DC. Failures, re-operations, and complications after autologous chondrocyte implantation—a systematic review. Osteoarthritis Cartilage. 2011;19(7):779–91.
18. Kon E, Filardo G, Di Matteo B, Perdisa F, Marcacci M. Matrix assisted autologous chondrocyte transplantation for cartilage treatment: a systematic review. Bone Joint Res. 2013;2(2):18–25.
19. Olson A, Graver A, Grande D. Scaffolds for articular cartilage repair. J Long Term Eff Med Implant. 2012;22(3):219–27.
20. Kon E, Filardo G, Di Martino A, Marcacci M. ACI and MACI. J Knee Surg. 2012;25(1):17–22.
21. Rai V, Dilisio MF, Dietz NE, Agrawal DK. Recent strategies in cartilage repair: a systemic review of the scaffold development and tissue engineering. J Biomed Mater Res A. 2017;105(8):2343–54.
22. Frenkel SR, Bradica G, Brekke JH, Goldman SM, Ieska K, Issack P, Bong MR, Tian H, Gokhale J, Coutts RD, Kronengold RT. Regeneration of articular cartilage—evaluation of osteochondral defect repair in the rabbit using multiphasic implants. Osteoarthritis Cartilage. 2005;13(9):798–807.
23. Filardo G, Perdisa F, Gelinsky M, Despang F, Fini M, Marcacci M, Parrilli AP, Roffi A, Salamanna F, Sartori M, Schütz K, Kon E. Novel alginate biphasic scaffold for osteochondral regeneration: an in vivo evaluation in rabbit and sheep models. J Mater Sci Mater Med. 2018;29(6):74.
24. Demoor M, Ollitrault D, Gomez-Leduc T, Bouyoucef M, Hervieu M, Fabre H, Lafont J, Denoix JM, Audigié F, Mallein-Gerin F, Legendre F, Galera P. Cartilage tissue engineering: molecular control of chondrocyte differentiation for proper cartilage matrix reconstruction. Biochim Biophys Acta. 2014;1840(8):2414–40.
25. Wasyłeczko M, Sikorska W, Chwojnowski A. Review of synthetic and hybrid scaffolds in cartilage tissue engineering. Membranes (Basel). 2020;10(11):348.
26. Longley R, Ferreira AM, Gentile P. Recent approaches to the manufacturing of biomimetic multi-phasic scaffolds for osteochondral regeneration. Int J Mol Sci. 2018;19(6):1755.
27. Jeon JE, Vaquette C, Klein TJ, Hutmacher DW. Perspectives in multiphasic osteochondral tissue engineering. Anat Rec. 2014;297(1):26–35.
28. Kon E, Filardo G, Perdisa F, Venieri G, Marcacci M. Clinical results of multilayered biomaterials for osteochondral regeneration. J Exp Orthop. 2014;1(1):10.
29. Kon E, Delcogliano M, Filardo G, Busacca M, Di Martino A, Marcacci M. Novel nano-composite multilayered biomaterial for osteochondral regeneration: a pilot clinical trial. Am J Sports Med. 2011;39(6):1180–90.
30. Xu J, Fahmy-Garcia S, Wesdorp MA, Kops N, Forte L, De Luca C, Misciagna MM, Dolcini L, Filardo G, Labberté M, Vancíková K, Kok J, van Rietbergen B, Nickel J, Farrell E, Brama PAJ, van Osch GJVM. Effectiveness of BMP-2 and PDGF-BB adsorption onto a collagen/collagen-magnesium-hydroxyapatite scaffold in weight-bearing and non-weight-bearing osteochondral defect bone repair: in vitro, ex vivo and in vivo evaluation. J Funct Biomater. 2023;14(2):111.
31. Xu J, Vecstaudza J, Wesdorp MA, Labberté M, Kops N, Salerno M, Kok J, Simon M, Harmand MF, Vancíková K, van Rietbergen B, Misciagna MM, Dolcini L, Filardo G, Farrell E, van Osch GJVM, Locs J, Brama PAJ. Incorporating strontium enriched amorphous calcium phosphate granules in collagen/collagen-magnesium-hydroxyapatite osteochondral scaffolds improves subchondral bone repair. Mater Today Bio. 2024;25:100959.
32. Barber FA, Dockery WD. A computed tomography scan assessment of synthetic multiphase polymer scaffolds used for osteochondral defect repair. Arthroscopy. 2011;27(1):60–4.
33. Gomoll AH, Filardo G, de Girolamo L, Espregueira-Mendes J, Marcacci M, Rodkey WG, Steadman JR, Zaffagnini S, Kon E. Surgical treatment for early osteoarthritis. Part I: cartilage repair procedures. Knee Surg Sports Traumatol Arthrosc. 2012;20(3):450–66.
34. Shao XX, Hutmacher DW, Ho ST, Goh JC, Lee EH. Evaluation of a hybrid scaffold/cell construct in repair of high-load-bearing osteochondral defects in rabbits. Biomaterials. 2006;27(7):1071–80.
35. Zheng P, Hu X, Lou Y, Tang K. A rabbit model of osteochondral regeneration using three-dimensional printed polycaprolactone-hydroxyapatite scaffolds coated with umbilical cord blood mesenchymal stem cells and chondrocytes. Med Sci Monit. 2019;25:7361–9.
36. Filardo G, Andriolo L, Angele P, Berruto M, Brittberg M, Condello V, Chubinskaya S, de Girolamo L, Di Martino A, Di Matteo B, Gille J, Gobbi A,

Lattermann C, Nakamura N, Nehrer S, Peretti GM, Shabshin N, Verdonk P, Zaslav K, Kon E. Scaffolds for knee chondral and osteochondral defects: indications for different clinical scenarios. A Consensus Statement. Cartilage. 2021;13(1_suppl):1036S–46S.
37. Ogura T, Merkely G, Bryant T, Winalski CS, Minas T. Autologous chondrocyte implantation "Segmental-Sandwich" technique for deep osteochondral defects in the knee: clinical outcomes and correlation with magnetic resonance imaging findings. Orthop J Sports Med. 2019;7(5):2325967119847173.
38. Andriolo L, Reale D, Di Martino A, Zaffagnini S, Vannini F, Ferruzzi A, Filardo G. High rate of failure after matrix-assisted autologous chondrocyte transplantation in osteoarthritic knees at 15 years of follow-up. Am J Sports Med. 2019;47(9):2116–22.
39. Di Martino A, Kon E, Perdisa F, Sessa A, Filardo G, Neri MP, Bragonzoni L, Marcacci M. Surgical treatment of early knee osteoarthritis with a cell-free osteochondral scaffold: results at 24 months of follow-up. Injury. 2015;46(Suppl 8):S33–8.
40. Sessa A, Andriolo L, Di Martino A, Romandini I, De Filippis R, Zaffagnini S, Filardo G. Cell-free osteochondral scaffold for the treatment of focal articular cartilage defects in early knee OA: 5 years' follow-up results. J Clin Med. 2019;8(11):1978.
41. Altschuler N, Zaslav KR, Di Matteo B, Sherman SL, Gomoll AH, Hacker SA, Verdonk P, Dulic O, Patrascu JM, Levy AS, Robinson D, Kon E. Aragonite-based scaffold versus microfracture and debridement for the treatment of knee chondral and osteochondral lesions: results of a multicenter randomized controlled trial. Am J Sports Med. 2023;51(4):957–67.
42. Berruto M, Ferrua P, Uboldi F, Pasqualotto S, Ferrara F, Carimati G, Usellini E, Delcogliano M. Can a biomimetic osteochondral scaffold be a reliable alternative to prosthetic surgery in treating late-stage SPONK? Knee. 2016;23(6):936–41.
43. Filardo G, Kon E, Perdisa F, Di Matteo B, Di Martino A, Iacono F, Zaffagnini S, Balboni F, Vaccari V, Marcacci M. Osteochondral scaffold reconstruction for complex knee lesions: a comparative evaluation. Knee. 2013;20(6):570–6.
44. Kon E, Roffi A, Filardo G, Tesei G, Marcacci M. Scaffold-based cartilage treatments: with or without cells? A systematic review of preclinical and clinical evidence. Arthroscopy. 2015;31(4):767–75.
45. Behrens P, Bitter T, Kurz B, Russlies M. Matrix-associated autologous chondrocyte transplantation/implantation (MACT/MACI)—5-year follow-up. Knee. 2006;13(3):194–202.
46. Ebert JR, Fallon M, Ackland TR, Wood DJ, Janes GC. Arthroscopic matrix-induced autologous chondrocyte implantation: 2-year outcomes. Arthroscopy. 2012;28(7):952-64.e1–2.
47. Brittberg M, Recker D, Ilgenfritz J, Saris DBF, SUMMIT Extension Study Group. Matrix-applied characterized autologous cultured chondrocytes versus microfracture: five-year follow-up of a prospective randomized trial. Am J Sports Med. 2018;46(6):1343–51.
48. Basad E, Ishaque B, Bachmann G, Stürz H, Steinmeyer J. Matrix-induced autologous chondrocyte implantation versus microfracture in the treatment of cartilage defects of the knee: a 2-year randomised study. Knee Surg Sports Traumatol Arthrosc. 2010;18(4):519–27.
49. Barié A, Kruck P, Sorbi R, Rehnitz C, Oberle D, Walker T, Zeifang F, Moradi B. Prospective long-term follow-up of autologous chondrocyte implantation with periosteum versus matrix-associated autologous chondrocyte implantation: a randomized clinical trial. Am J Sports Med. 2020;48(9):2230–41.
50. Piontek T, Ciemniewska-Gorzela K, Szulc A, Naczk J, Słomczykowski M. All-arthroscopic AMIC procedure for repair of cartilage defects of the knee. Knee Surg Sports Traumatol Arthrosc. 2012;20(5):922–5.
51. Tradati D, De Luca P, Maione A, Uboldi FM, Volpi P, de Girolamo L, Berruto M. AMIC-autologous matrix-induced chondrogenesis technique in patellar cartilage defects treatment: a retrospective study with a mid-term follow-up. J Clin Med. 2020;9(4):1184.
52. Anders S, Volz M, Frick H, Gellissen J. A randomized, controlled trial comparing autologous matrix-induced chondrogenesis (AMIC®) to microfracture: analysis of 1- and 2-year follow-up data of 2 centers. Open Orthop J. 2013;7:133–43.
53. Volz M, Schaumburger J, Frick H, Grifka J, Anders S. A randomized controlled trial demonstrating sustained benefit of autologous matrix-induced chondrogenesis over microfracture at five years. Int Orthop. 2017;41(4):797–804.
54. Schneider U, Rackwitz L, Andereya S, Siebenlist S, Fensky F, Reichert J, Löer I, Barthel T, Rudert M, Nöth U. A prospective multicenter study on the outcome of type I collagen hydrogel-based autologous chondrocyte implantation (CaReS) for the repair of articular cartilage defects in the knee. Am J Sports Med. 2011;39(12):2558–65.
55. Roessler PP, Pfister B, Gesslein M, Figiel J, Heyse TJ, Colcuc C, Lorbach O, Efe T, Schüttler KF. Short-term follow up after implantation of a cell-free collagen type I matrix for the treatment of large cartilage defects of the knee. Int Orthop. 2015;39(12):2473–9.
56. Schüttler KF, Götschenberg A, Klasan A, Stein T, Pehl A, Roessler PP, Figiel J, Heyse TJ, Efe T. Cell-free cartilage repair in large defects of the knee: increased failure rate 5 years after implantation of a collagen type I scaffold. Arch Orthop Trauma Surg. 2019;139(1):99–106.
57. Müller PE, Gallik D, Hammerschmid F, Baur-Melnyk A, Pietschmann MF, Zhang A, Niethammer TR. Third-generation autologous chondrocyte implantation after failed bone marrow stimulation leads to inferior clinical results. Knee Surg Sports Traumatol Arthrosc. 2020;28(2):470–7.

58. Niethammer TR, Altmann D, Holzgruber M, Goller S, Fischer A, Müller PE. Third generation autologous chondrocyte implantation is a good treatment option for athletic persons. Knee Surg Sports Traumatol Arthrosc. 2021;29(4):1215–23.
59. Tohyama H, Yasuda K, Minami A, Majima T, Iwasaki N, Muneta T, Sekiya I, Yagishita K, Takahashi S, Kurokouchi K, Uchio Y, Iwasa J, Deie M, Adachi N, Sugawara K, Ochi M. Atelocollagen-associated autologous chondrocyte implantation for the repair of chondral defects of the knee: a prospective multicenter clinical trial in Japan. J Orthop Sci. 2009;14(5):579–88.
60. Takazawa K, Adachi N, Deie M, Kamei G, Uchio Y, Iwasa J, Kumahashi N, Tadenuma T, Kuwata S, Yasuda K, Tohyama H, Minami A, Muneta T, Takahashi S, Ochi M. Evaluation of magnetic resonance imaging and clinical outcome after tissue-engineered cartilage implantation: prospective 6-year follow-up study. J Orthop Sci. 2012;17(4):413–24.
61. Kaibara T, Kondo E, Matsuoka M, Iwasaki K, Onodera T, Sakamoto K, Oda Y, Tanei ZI, Momma D, Tanaka S, Iwasaki N. Atelocollagen-associated autologous chondrocyte implantation for the repair of large cartilage defects of the knee: results at three to seven years. J Orthop Sci. 2024;29:207.
62. Marcacci M, Zaffagnini S, Kon E, Visani A, Iacono F, Loreti I. Arthroscopic autologous chondrocyte transplantation: technical note. Knee Surg Sports Traumatol Arthrosc. 2002;10(3):154–9.
63. Marcacci M, Berruto M, Brocchetta D, Delcogliano A, Ghinelli D, Gobbi A, Kon E, Pederzini L, Rosa D, Sacchetti GL, Stefani G, Zanasi S. Articular cartilage engineering with Hyalograft C: 3-year clinical results. Clin Orthop Relat Res. 2005;(435):96–105.
64. Andriolo L, Reale D, Di Martino A, De Filippis R, Sessa A, Zaffagnini S, Filardo G. Long-term results of arthroscopic matrix-assisted autologous chondrocyte transplantation: a prospective follow-up at 15 years. Am J Sports Med. 2020;48(12):2994–3001.
65. Filardo G, Kon E, Di Martino A, Iacono F, Marcacci M. Arthroscopic second-generation autologous chondrocyte implantation: a prospective 7-year follow-up study. Am J Sports Med. 2011;39(10):2153–60.
66. Kon E, Filardo G, Berruto M, Benazzo F, Zanon G, Della Villa S, Marcacci M. Articular cartilage treatment in high-level male soccer players: a prospective comparative study of arthroscopic second-generation autologous chondrocyte implantation versus microfracture. Am J Sports Med. 2011;39(12):2549–57.
67. Brix MO, Stelzeneder D, Chiari C, Koller U, Nehrer S, Dorotka R, Windhager R, Domayer SE. Treatment of full-thickness chondral defects with Hyalograft C in the knee: long-term results. Am J Sports Med. 2014;42(6):1426–32.
68. Everhart JS, Jiang EX, Poland SG, Du A, Flanigan DC. Failures, reoperations, and improvement in knee symptoms following matrix-assisted autologous chondrocyte transplantation: a meta-analysis of prospective comparative trials. Cartilage. 2021;13(1_suppl):1022S–35S.
69. Della Villa S, Kon E, Filardo G, Ricci M, Vincentelli F, Delcogliano M, Marcacci M. Does intensive rehabilitation permit early return to sport without compromising the clinical outcome after arthroscopic autologous chondrocyte implantation in highly competitive athletes? Am J Sports Med. 2010;38(1):68–77.
70. Jaramillo Quiceno GA, Sarmiento Riveros PA, Ochoa Perea GA, Vergara MG, Rodriguez Muñoz LF, Arias Perez RD, Piovesan NO, Muñoz Salamanca JA. Satisfactory clinical outcomes with autologous matrix-induced chondrogenesis in the treatment of grade IV chondral injuries of the knee. J ISAKOS. 2023;8(2):86–93.
71. Sofu H, Kockara N, Oner A, Camurcu Y, Issın A, Sahin V. Results of hyaluronic acid-based cell-free scaffold application in combination with microfracture for the treatment of osteochondral lesions of the knee: 2-year comparative study. Arthroscopy. 2017;33(1):209–16.
72. Gobbi A, Scotti C, Karnatzikos G, Mudhigere A, Castro M, Peretti GM. One-step surgery with multipotent stem cells and Hyaluronan-based scaffold for the treatment of full-thickness chondral defects of the knee in patients older than 45 years. Knee Surg Sports Traumatol Arthrosc. 2017;25(8):2494–501.
73. Siclari A, Mascaro G, Gentili C, Kaps C, Cancedda R, Boux E. Cartilage repair in the knee with subchondral drilling augmented with a platelet-rich plasma-immersed polymer-based implant. Knee Surg Sports Traumatol Arthrosc. 2014;22(6):1225–34.
74. Siclari A, Mascaro G, Kaps C, Boux E. A 5-year follow-up after cartilage repair in the knee using a platelet-rich plasma-immersed polymer-based implant. Open Orthop J. 2014;8:346–54.
75. Becher C, Ettinger M, Ezechieli M, Kaps C, Ewig M, Smith T. Repair of retropatellar cartilage defects in the knee with microfracture and a cell-free polymer-based implant. Arch Orthop Trauma Surg. 2015;135(7):1003–10.
76. Eshed I, Trattnig S, Sharon M, Arbel R, Nierenberg G, Konen E, Yayon A. Assessment of cartilage repair after chondrocyte transplantation with a fibrin-hyaluronan matrix—correlation of morphological MRI, biochemical T2 mapping and clinical outcome. Eur J Radiol. 2012;81(6):1216–23.
77. Steinwachs MR, Waibl B, Mumme M. Arthroscopic treatment of cartilage lesions with microfracture and BST-CarGel. Arthrosc Tech. 2014;3(3):e399–402.
78. Shive MS, Stanish WD, McCormack R, Forriol F, Mohtadi N, Pelet S, Desnoyers J, Méthot S, Vehik K, Restrepo A. BST-CarGel® treatment maintains cartilage repair superiority over microfracture at 5 years in a multicenter randomized controlled trial. Cartilage. 2015;6(2):62–72.
79. Poggi A, Di Martino A, Andriolo L, Reale D, Filardo G, Kon E, Zaffagnini S. Chitosan based scaffold applied in patellar cartilage lesions showed positive clinical and MRI results at minimum 2 years of follow up. Knee Surg Sports Traumatol Arthrosc. 2023;31(5):1714–22.

80. Selmi TA, Verdonk P, Chambat P, Dubrana F, Potel JF, Barnouin L, Neyret P. Autologous chondrocyte implantation in a novel alginate-agarose hydrogel: outcome at two years. J Bone Joint Surg Br. 2008;90(5):597–604.
81. Clavé A, Potel JF, Servien E, Neyret P, Dubrana F, Stindel E. Third-generation autologous chondrocyte implantation versus mosaicplasty for knee cartilage injury: 2-year randomized trial. J Orthop Res. 2016;34(4):658–65.
82. Ossendorf C, Kaps C, Kreuz PC, Burmester GR, Sittinger M, Erggelet C. Treatment of posttraumatic and focal osteoarthritic cartilage defects of the knee with autologous polymer-based three-dimensional chondrocyte grafts: 2-year clinical results. Arthritis Res Ther. 2007;9(2):R41.
83. Erggelet C, Sittinger M, Lahm A. The arthroscopic implantation of autologous chondrocytes for the treatment of full-thickness cartilage defects of the knee joint. Arthroscopy. 2003;19(1):108–10.
84. Kreuz PC, Müller S, Freymann U, Erggelet C, Niemeyer P, Kaps C, Hirschmüller A. Repair of focal cartilage defects with scaffold-assisted autologous chondrocyte grafts: clinical and biomechanical results 48 months after transplantation. Am J Sports Med. 2011;39(8):1697–705.
85. Kon E, Delcogliano M, Filardo G, Fini M, Giavaresi G, Francioli S, Martin I, Pressato D, Arcangeli E, Quarto R, Sandri M, Marcacci M. Orderly osteochondral regeneration in a sheep model using a novel nano-composite multilayered biomaterial. J Orthop Res. 2010;28(1):116–24.
86. Melton JT, Wilson AJ, Chapman-Sheath P, Cossey AJ. TruFit CB bone plug: chondral repair, scaffold design, surgical technique and early experiences. Expert Rev Med Devices. 2010;7(3):333–41.
87. Bedi A, Foo LF, Williams RJ III, Potter HG, Cartilage Study Group. The maturation of synthetic scaffolds for osteochondral donor sites of the knee: an MRI and T2-mapping analysis. Cartilage. 2010;1(1):20–8.
88. Bekkers JE, Bartels LW, Vincken KL, Dhert WJ, Creemers LB, Saris DB. Articular cartilage evaluation after TruFit plug implantation analyzed by delayed gadolinium-enhanced MRI of cartilage (dGEMRIC). Am J Sports Med. 2013;41(6):1290–5.
89. Carmont MR, Carey-Smith R, Saithna A, Dhillon M, Thompson P, Spalding T. Delayed incorporation of a TruFit plug: perseverance is recommended. Arthroscopy. 2009;25(7):810–4.
90. Dhollander AA, Liekens K, Almqvist KF, Verdonk R, Lambrecht S, Elewaut D, Verbruggen G, Verdonk PC. A pilot study of the use of an osteochondral scaffold plug for cartilage repair in the knee and how to deal with early clinical failures. Arthroscopy. 2012;28(2):225–33.
91. Joshi N, Reverte-Vinaixa M, Díaz-Ferreiro EW, Domínguez-Oronoz R. Synthetic resorbable scaffolds for the treatment of isolated patellofemoral cartilage defects in young patients: magnetic resonance imaging and clinical evaluation. Am J Sports Med. 2012;40(6):1289–95.
92. Hindle P, Hendry JL, Keating JF, Biant LC. Autologous osteochondral mosaicplasty or TruFit plugs for cartilage repair. Knee Surg Sports Traumatol Arthrosc. 2014;22(6):1235–40.
93. Shivji FS, Mumith A, Yasen S, Melton JT, Wilson AJ. Treatment of focal chondral lesions in the knee using a synthetic scaffold plug: long-term clinical and radiological results. J Orthop. 2020;20:12–6.
94. Filardo G, Drobnic M, Perdisa F, Kon E, Hribernik M, Marcacci M. Fibrin glue improves osteochondral scaffold fixation: study on the human cadaveric knee exposed to continuous passive motion. Osteoarthritis Cartilage. 2014;22(4):557–65.
95. Kon E, Delcogliano M, Filardo G, Pressato D, Busacca M, Grigolo B, Desando G, Marcacci M. A novel nano-composite multi-layered biomaterial for treatment of osteochondral lesions: technique note and an early stability pilot clinical trial. Injury. 2010;41(7):693–701.
96. Andriolo L, De Marziani L, Di Martino A, Boffa A, Zaffagnini S, Filardo G. Cell-free biomimetic scaffold for chondral and osteochondral lesions: surgical technique for custom and standardized implantation. J Cartilage Joint Preserv. 2024;4(2).
97. Kon E, Filardo G, Di Martino A, Busacca M, Moio A, Perdisa F, Marcacci M. Clinical results and MRI evolution of a nano-composite multilayered biomaterial for osteochondral regeneration at 5 years. Am J Sports Med. 2014;42(1):158–65.
98. Filardo G, Kon E, Di Martino A, Busacca M, Altadonna G, Marcacci M. Treatment of knee osteochondritis dissecans with a cell-free biomimetic osteochondral scaffold: clinical and imaging evaluation at 2-year follow-up. Am J Sports Med. 2013;41(8):1786–93.
99. Perdisa F, Filardo G, Sessa A, Busacca M, Zaffagnini S, Marcacci M, Kon E. One-step treatment for patellar cartilage defects with a cell-free osteochondral scaffold: a prospective clinical and MRI evaluation. Am J Sports Med. 2017;45(7):1581–8.
100. Christensen BB, Foldager CB, Jensen J, Jensen NC, Lind M. Poor osteochondral repair by a biomimetic collagen scaffold: 1- to 3-year clinical and radiological follow-up. Knee Surg Sports Traumatol Arthrosc. 2016;24(7):2380–7.
101. Perdisa F, Kon E, Sessa A, Andriolo L, Busacca M, Marcacci M, Filardo G. Treatment of knee osteochondritis dissecans with a cell-free biomimetic osteochondral scaffold: clinical and imaging findings at midterm follow-up. Am J Sports Med. 2018;46(2):314–21.
102. Di Martino A, Perdisa F, Filardo G, Busacca M, Kon E, Marcacci M, Zaffagnini S. Cell-free biomimetic osteochondral scaffold for the treatment of knee lesions: clinical and imaging results at 10-year follow-up. Am J Sports Med. 2021;49(10):2645–50.

103. Kon E, Filardo G, Brittberg M, Busacca M, Condello V, Engebretsen L, Marlovits S, Niemeyer P, Platzer P, Posthumus M, Verdonk P, Verdonk R, Victor J, van der Merwe W, Widuchowski W, Zorzi C, Marcacci M. A multilayer biomaterial for osteochondral regeneration shows superiority vs microfractures for the treatment of osteochondral lesions in a multicentre randomized trial at 2 years. Knee Surg Sports Traumatol Arthrosc. 2018;26(9):2704–15.
104. Delcogliano M, Menghi A, Placella G, Speziali A, Cerulli G, Carimati G, Pasqualotto S, Berruto M. Treatment of osteochondritis dissecans of the knee with a biomimetic scaffold. A prospective multicenter study. Joints. 2014;2(3):102–8.
105. Sessa A, Romandini I, Andriolo L, Di Martino A, Busacca M, Zaffagnini S, Filardo G. Treatment of juvenile knee osteochondritis dissecans with a cell-free biomimetic osteochondral scaffold: clinical and MRI results at mid-term follow-up. Cartilage. 2021;13(1_suppl):1137S–47S.
106. Kon E, Filardo G, Venieri G, Perdisa F, Marcacci M, Tibial plateau lesions. Surface reconstruction with a biomimetic osteochondral scaffold: results at 2 years of follow-up. Injury. 2014;45(Suppl 6):S121–5.
107. Ricci M, Tradati D, Maione A, Uboldi FM, Usellini E, Berruto M. Cell-free osteochondral scaffolds provide a substantial clinical benefit in the treatment of osteochondral defects at a minimum follow-up of 5 years. J Exp Orthop. 2021;8(1):62.
108. Condello V, Filardo G, Madonna V, Andriolo L, Screpis D, Bonomo M, Zappia M, Dei Giudici L, Zorzi C. Use of a biomimetic scaffold for the treatment of osteochondral lesions in early osteoarthritis. Biomed Res Int. 2018;2018:7937089.
109. Marcacci M, Zaffagnini S, Kon E, Marcheggiani Muccioli GM, Di Martino A, Di Matteo B, Bonanzinga T, Iacono F, Filardo G. Unicompartmental osteoarthritis: an integrated biomechanical and biological approach as alternative to metal resurfacing. Knee Surg Sports Traumatol Arthrosc. 2013;21(11):2509–17.
110. Perdisa F, Bordini B, Salerno M, Traina F, Zaffagnini S, Filardo G. Total knee arthroplasty (TKA): when do the risks of TKA overcome the benefits? Double risk of failure in patients up to 65 years old. Cartilage. 2023;14(3):305–11.
111. Kon E, Filardo G, Robinson D, Eisman JA, Levy A, Zaslav K, Shani J, Altschuler N. Osteochondral regeneration using a novel aragonite-hyaluronate biphasic scaffold in a goat model. Knee Surg Sports Traumatol Arthrosc. 2014;22(6):1452–64.
112. Kon E, Di Matteo B, Verdonk P, Drobnic M, Dulic O, Gavrilovic G, Patrascu JM, Zaslav K, Kwiatkowski G, Altschuler N, Robinson D. Aragonite-based scaffold for the treatment of joint surface lesions in mild to moderate osteoarthritic knees: results of a 2-year multicenter prospective study. Am J Sports Med. 2021;49(3):588–98.
113. Vannini F, Berveglieri L, Boffa A, Filardo G, Viglione V, Buda R, Giannini S, Faldini C. Hyaluronic scaffold transplantation with bone marrow concentrate for the treatment of osteochondral lesions of the talus: durable results up to a minimum of 10 years. Knee Surg Sports Traumatol Arthrosc. 2023;31(10):4551–8.
114. Filardo G, Petretta M, Cavallo C, Roseti L, Durante S, Albisinni U, Grigolo B. Patient-specific meniscus prototype based on 3D bioprinting of human cell-laden scaffold. Bone Joint Res. 2019;8(2):101–6.
115. Zhang H, Wang M, Wu R, Guo J, Sun A, Li Z, Ye R, Xu G, Cheng Y. From materials to clinical use: advances in 3D-printed scaffolds for cartilage tissue engineering. Phys Chem Chem Phys. 2023;25(36):24244–63.
116. Gu Y, Zou Y, Huang Y, Liang R, Wu Y, Hu Y, Hong Y, Zhang X, Toh YC, Ouyang H, Zhang S. 3D-printed biomimetic scaffolds with precisely controlled and tunable structures guide cell migration and promote regeneration of osteochondral defect. Biofabrication. 2023;16(1).
117. Ding X, Gao J, Yu X, Shi J, Chen J, Yu L, Chen S, Ding J. 3D-printed porous scaffolds of hydrogels modified with TGF-β1 binding peptides to promote in vivo cartilage regeneration and animal gait restoration. ACS Appl Mater Interfaces. 2022;14(14):15982–95.
118. Xu N, Lu D, Qiang L, Liu Y, Yin D, Wang Z, Luo Y, Yang C, Ma Z, Ma H, Wang J. 3D-printed composite bioceramic scaffolds for bone and cartilage integrated regeneration. ACS Omega. 2023;8(41):37918–26.
119. Lin L, Wang T, Zhou Q, Qian N. The effects of different amounts of drug microspheres on the vivo and vitro performance of the PLGA/β-TCP scaffold. Des Monomers Polym. 2016;20(1):351–62.
120. Madry H, Venkatesan JK, Carballo-Pedrares N, Rey-Rico A, Cucchiarini M. Scaffold-mediated gene delivery for osteochondral repair. Pharmaceutics. 2020;12(10):930.
121. He J, Hu X, Cao J, Zhang Y, Xiao J, Peng L, Chen D, Xiong C, Zhang L. Chitosan-coated hydroxyapatite and drug-loaded polytrimethylene carbonate/polylactic acid scaffold for enhancing bone regeneration. Carbohydr Polym. 2021;253:117198.
122. Hussey GS, Dziki JL, Badylak SF. Extracellular matrix-based materials for regenerative medicine. Nat Rev Mater. 2018;3:159–73.
123. Zhu W, Cao L, Song C, Pang Z, Jiang H, Guo C. Cell-derived decellularized extracellular matrix scaffolds for articular cartilage repair. Int J Artif Organs. 2021;44(4):269–81.
124. Jiang S, Tian G, Yang Z, Gao X, Wang F, Li J, Tian Z, Huang B, Wei F, Sang X, Shao L, Zhou J, Wang Z, Liu S, Sui X, Guo Q, Guo W, Li X. Enhancement of acellular cartilage matrix scaffold by Wharton's jelly mesenchymal stem cell-derived exosomes to promote osteochondral regeneration. Bioact Mater. 2021;6(9):2711–28.
125. Fu JN, Wang X, Yang M, Chen YR, Zhang JY, Deng RH, Zhang ZN, Yu JK, Yuan FZ. Scaffold-based tissue engineering strategies for osteochondral repair. Front Bioeng Biotechnol. 2022;9:812383.

Microfracture in Cartilage Treatment and Its Effect on Healing

7

Taha Kızılkurt, İsmail Tarık Atasoy, and Mehmet Aşık

7.1 Introduction

Full-thickness cartilage lesions are among the most significant clinical problems despite advances in cartilage repair methods over the years, due to the limited healing capacity of hyaline cartilage [1].

Conservative treatment (non-steroidal anti-inflammatory drugs, activity modification, chondroprotective agents, physical therapy, and rehabilitation), debridement, drilling, microfracture, autologous matrix-induced chondrogenesis, mosaicplasty (osteochondral autologous transplantation), cell-based therapies (autologous chondrocyte implantation and matrix-assisted autologous chondrocyte implantation), osteochondral allograft, and surface replacement arthroplasty are used in the treatment of these lesions [2]. The aim of treating full-thickness cartilage lesions is to fill the defect with mechanically durable hyaline cartilage or hyaline-like cartilage to ensure the integrity of this newly regenerated tissue with the surrounding cartilage and subchondral bone, thus achieving ideal pain-free joint function and minimizing the need for arthroplasty.

T. Kızılkurt (✉) · İ. T. Atasoy · M. Aşık
Istanbul Faculty of Medicine, Department of Orthopedics and Traumatology, Istanbul University, Istanbul, Turkey

No single treatment modality is appropriate for all full-thickness cartilage lesions. The patient's age, the location, size, and depth of the lesion should be taken into consideration when choosing a treatment. Out of these treatments, bone marrow stimulation techniques are a cartilage repair method based on the filling of the defect with fibrocartilage-like regenerative tissue through bleeding, clots, and growth factors formed in the defect area after preparation of the defect bed. Pridie first described it in open surgery in 1959 [3]. Three bone marrow stimulation techniques have been described: abrasion arthroplasty, subchondral drilling, and microfracture. Microfracture is the main surgical approach among bone marrow stimulation techniques for full-thickness cartilage lesions due to its low cost, easy application, and favorable results, especially in young patients.

7.2 Microfracture

Microfracture is a technique described by Steadman in 1994 and popularized by Steadman's clinical studies [4]. It is still the most popular and the most frequently used bone marrow stimulation technique in the world [5–7]. Less damage to the subchondral bone and the absence of the risk of thermal necrosis that may occur during drilling have made microfracture treatment more prominent than other bone marrow stimulation techniques over the years.

M. E. Erdil et al. (eds.), *Current Concept in Cartilage Treatment*,
https://doi.org/10.1007/978-3-032-27099-3_7

The advantages of the microfracture technique are that it is less invasive and less expensive than other cartilage repair methods, it has ease of full arthroscopic application, it is an easily accessible treatment, and it does not preclude subsequent cartilage repair procedures if it fails. Microfracture is still the first-choice repair method used by many surgeons in the treatment of small-to-medium-sized cartilage lesions due to the above-mentioned advantages [8].

7.3 Indications

In the treatment of focal cartilage lesions, accompanying deformity, instability, or meniscal pathology should be evaluated. Treatment of concomitant pathologies should be performed simultaneously or in two stages [2]. Microfracture therapy can be applied in the treatment of symptomatic focal cartilage lesions in young to middle-aged patients with lesions up to 4 cm^2 in size [7, 9, 10]. As a result of clinical experience and publications on microfracture over the years, there has been some controversy in recent years regarding lesion size [10]. Although there are conflicting publications in the literature, treatment is more successful in patients younger than 45 years with lesions smaller than 2 cm^2 [8, 9, 11]. Therefore, some authors report that they recommend this treatment in patients with lesions smaller than 2 or 3 cm^2 [12–14].

7.4 Surgical Technique

In patients with focal cartilage lesions, preoperative anteroposterior (AP) and lateral radiographs of the affected joint, magnetic resonance imaging (MRI), and, in selected patients, computed tomography (CT) imaging of the joint to evaluate the subchondral bone are necessary.

After routine diagnostic arthroscopy, free cartilage fragments in the defect area should be debrided to the subchondral bone using a shaver and open curette. During this process, it is important to obtain stable vertical margins at the edges of the cartilage defect (Fig. 7.1). After preparation of the lesion area, the microfracture procedure is started. Using arthroscopic microfracture awls prepared at different angles depending on the lesion site, 2–4 mm deep holes extending to the subchondral layer are created at 90° to the lesion surface and approximately 3–4 mm apart. Depending on the geometry of the lesion surface, various awl angles ranging from 30° to 90° can be used. 30° and 45° awls are typically used in the tibiofemoral compartment, and 90° awls can be used for the patella, but 90° awls have a high risk of creating larger areas of damage to the subchondral plate because the vector of the force is not favorable. There are also studies in

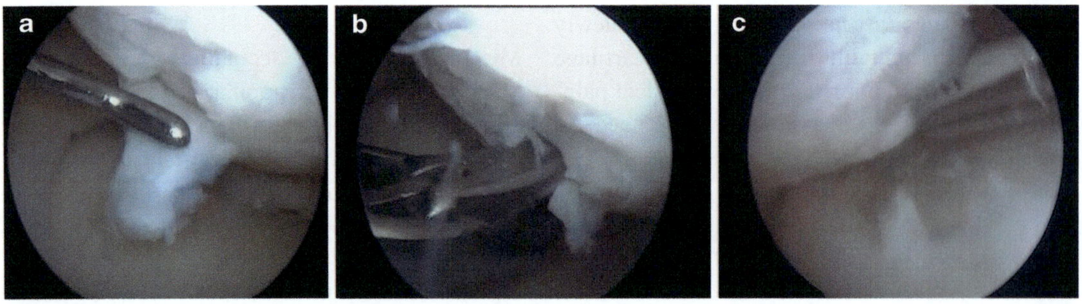

Fig. 7.1 (**a**) Examination and (**b**, **c**) debridement of the osteochondral lesion

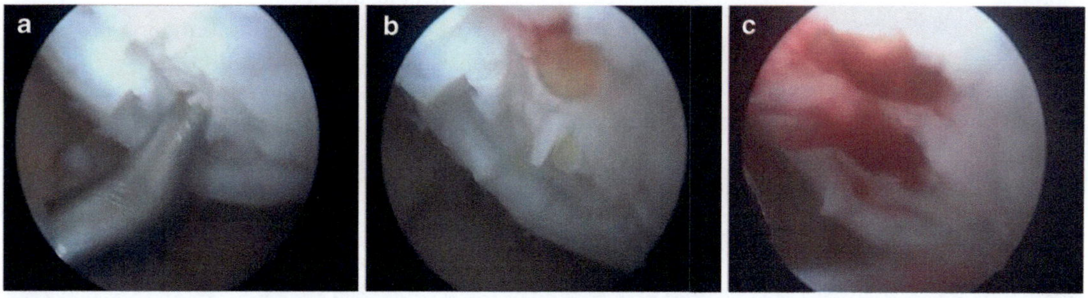

Fig. 7.2 (**a**) Microfracture and (**b**, **c**) bleeding after releasing the tourniquet

the literature that recommend the use of small-diameter wires or nanofracture devices instead of awls because they cause less damage to the subchondral bone [15] (Chap. 21, Fig. 21.6). The microfracture procedure should be started from the periphery of the lesion, and a distance of 3–4 mm should be maintained between the holes to prevent subchondral collapse. After the microfracture procedure, the tourniquet is deflated and inflow pressure is reduced or stopped to confirm adequate marrow bleeding and fat droplets from the holes (Fig. 7.2). It is preferred not to place a drain in the joint for stabilization of the fibrin clot. The procedure is completed with closure of the portals.

7.5 Postoperative Rehabilitation

Postoperative rehabilitation is crucial for the success of microfracture treatment, providing the biological environment necessary for the formation and maturation of regenerative tissue. The location and size of the lesion are decisive in the postoperative rehabilitation of patients. For lesions on the weight-bearing surfaces, walking with toe-touch weight-bearing is allowed for 6 weeks postoperatively. For lesions in the patellofemoral joint, full weight-bearing walking is allowed for 4–6 weeks postoperatively with a hinged knee brace with the flexion setting locked at 20°. Then knee flexion is gradually increased. Quadriceps strengthening and active knee movements are allowed starting from day 1 postoperatively in all patients. In selected patients, a continuous passive motion (CPM) device may be used.

7.6 Discussion

Microfracture is one of the most popular bone marrow stimulation techniques and is still the most commonly used cartilage repair method [5, 6]. Although microfracture treatment is frequently applied in the knee joint, it is also used in cartilage pathologies of the ankle and hip joints [16]. The fibrin clot that fills the defect after the microfracture procedure is a tissue rich in mesenchymal stem cells and growth factors. In the following time period, the mesenchymal stem cells within the existing fibrin plug proliferate and differentiate into chondrocyte-like cells under the influence of local growth factors and environmental factors. This chondrocyte-rich granulation tissue transforms into a fibrocartilage or hyaline-like cartilage structure under appropriate physical and biological stimuli within 6–8 weeks (Fig. 7.3). The newly formed cartilage regenerate tissue has a fibrocartilage structure rich in type 1 collagen or a hyaline-like cartilage structure. However, it is not as durable as hyaline cartilage against mechanical loads such as shear and compression [17, 18].

Clinical experience in the treatment of focal cartilage lesions, especially in the knee joint, with the microfracture technique has increased considerably over the years. In 2001, Steadman published the treatment outcomes of 71 patients with an average follow-up of 11 years. He reported that

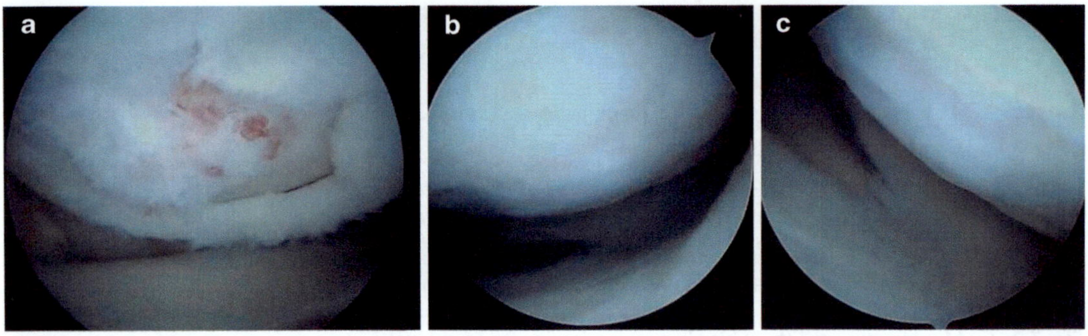

Fig. 7.3 (**a**) Osteochondral lesion and (**b**, **c**) second look arthroscopy image 4 months after microfracture shows healing with fibrocartilage

in these patients who were younger than 45 years of age, the mean Lysholm scores increased from 59 to 89, and the mean Tegner activity scores increased from 3 to 6 after the microfracture procedure [19]. In another study by the same team, which examined the clinical outcomes of 25 athletes treated with the microfracture procedure and followed up for an average of 4.5 years, it was reported that 19 patients (76%) returned to active sports. As a result, the authors reported that the microfracture technique is an appropriate treatment method in cases with full-thickness cartilage lesions that have a high activity expectation [20]. In the literature, there are many studies reporting successful results in the early and mid-term after microfracture treatment [21–23]. In a prospective study reporting the clinical outcomes of 48 patients with a mean follow-up of 41 months, the authors reported 66% good-to-excellent results in the functional evaluation of the patients [23]. In the same study, the fill of the defect area with fibrocartilage during follow-up was evaluated by MRI examinations, and it was reported that functional results were better in patients with more than 66% fill of the defect area [23].

The effect of factors such as patient age, lesion size and location, body mass index (BMI), and lesion depth on treatment outcomes after microfracture treatment has been investigated in numerous studies [9, 23, 24]. Patient age is one of the most important prognostic factors. In the patient group published by Steadman et al. in 2003, patients under 45 years of age had better outcomes [9]. Similarly, Knutsen et al. reported better outcomes in active patients under 30 years of age with lesion sizes less than 4 cm^2 [25]. Kreuz et al. reported a more favorable prognosis in patients under 40 years of age and with femoral condyle lesions [7]. Thomas Neri et al. reported that lesions smaller than 4 cm^2, younger age, a better MOCART score, and a shorter duration of symptoms were associated with a better prognosis in their series of 48 knees [24]. BMI is another important prognostic factor affecting treatment outcomes, and it has been reported in the literature that functional outcomes are worse in patients with a BMI greater than 30 kg/m^2 [23].

In our series of 90 patients (47 male and 43 female patients) who underwent the microfracture procedure in the knee joint, we evaluated the patients with Lysholm, Tegner, and Oxford scores after a mean follow-up of 5.5 years (range, 24–108 months). The mean age of the patients was 34.5 years (range, 20–58). At the last follow-up, there was an increase of 30.4 points in the Lysholm score, 2.6 points in the Tegner score, and 21.7 points in the Oxford score. Our patient series showed that the prognosis was statistically better in patients with lesion sizes less than 2 cm^2, lesions located outside the weight-bearing surface, patients younger than 35 years of age, and patients with a BMI less than 25 [12].

There is no consensus regarding the treatment of cartilage lesions in patients with high activity expectations or athletes [26–29]. In a study evaluating the functional results of 109 athletes after microfracture treatment with an average follow-up of 72 months, the authors reported that the functional and clinical results were generally satisfactory, but they found a decrease in the activity of the athletes over time, and therefore other methods may be required in the knees of athletes [26]. Gobbi et al. published prospective long-term follow-up results of 170 athletes with an average follow-up of 15.1 years [28]. The mean defect size was 4.01 + 0.27 cm^2. It was reported that the functional scores of the patients were the highest in the 2-year follow-up assessments, and a decrease in functional scores was observed after the fifth year. In this study, which reported a total failure rate of 11%, long-term results were found to be more favorable in patients under 30 years of age and with a lesion size of less than 4 cm^2 [28]. In another study comparing microfracture with mosaicplasty as an alternative treatment in athletes, functional outcomes were evaluated in 25 athletes with a mean follow-up of 9.8 years (11 microfractures with a mean defect size of 2.6 cm^2/14 mosaicplasties with a mean defect size of 3.0 cm^2), and no statistical difference was observed between the long-term outcomes of both treatments [29]. In another randomized controlled prospective study on an athlete patient population, after a mean follow-up of 10.4 years in 60 patients with an average age of 24.3 years, it was reported that the treatment outcomes of patients treated with microfracture and mosaicplasty in both groups were successful and there was no statistical difference between the two groups in terms of arthrosis progression at the last follow-up of the patients. However, a 38% failure rate was reported in the microfracture group and a 14% failure rate in the mosaicplasty group during the long-term follow-up, and the authors suggested that mosaicplasty is a more appropriate treatment for athletes regarding faster return to sport and return at the pre-injury level [30]. In addition, in a meta-analysis conducted in 2023 in which 7 randomized prospective studies were examined, it was reported that return to sport after mosaicplasty may be faster and at the pre-injury level [1]. In 2016, Campbell et al. investigated the effectiveness of various cartilage repair techniques in a systemic review and reported that return to sport was lower, especially in microfracture, compared to other treatment methods [31].

There are many studies in the literature comparing microfracture treatment with other cartilage repair methods [29, 30, 32, 33]. In a study by Knutsen et al. comparing autologous chondrocyte implantation (ACI) and microfracture methods, better functional results were reported with microfracture in a 2-year follow-up of 40 patients with a mean lesion size of 4.9 cm^2. However, after 5 years of follow-up, the mean clinical success was 77%, and there was no statistical difference in functional success between the two groups [32]. In another study comparing the 5-year results of ACI and microfracture treatments (51 ACI with a mean defect size of 2.6 cm^2/61 microfractures with a mean defect size of 2.5 cm^2), a 13.7% failure rate in the ACI group and a 16.3% failure rate in the microfracture group were reported. Although both groups reported successful functional results compared to the preoperative status, ACI treatment was found to be more successful in patients with symptoms lasting less than 3 years [33].

Although there are many studies in the literature, the use of different functional scores in the studies and the lack of adequate evaluation of important prognostic criteria such as the weight-bearing surface and location of the lesions make it difficult to compare the studies. In the general evaluation of the literature on full-thickness cartilage lesions, none of the different treatment methods has been proven to be superior to the others [2, 8, 11].

7.7 Conclusion

Microfracture is a successful method in the treatment of full-thickness cartilage lesions in terms of pain and functional results. Its advantages are that it is less invasive, simpler, and less costly than other repair methods while producing comparable postoperative results. Nevertheless, the surgeon should decide on the treatment according to patient characteristics, lesion size, lesion location, and personal experience.

References

1. Han QX, Tong Y, Zhang L, Sun J, Ma J, Liu X, et al. Comparative efficacy of osteochondral autologous transplantation and microfracture in the knee: an updated meta-analysis of randomized controlled trials. Arch Orthop Trauma Surg. 2023;143(1):317–28. https://doi.org/10.1007/s00402-021-04075-9.
2. Hinckel BB, Thomas D, Vellios EE, Hancock KJ, Calcei JG, Sherman SL, et al. Algorithm for treatment of focal cartilage defects of the knee: classic and new procedures. Cartilage. 2021;13(1 Suppl):473s–95s. https://doi.org/10.1177/1947603521993219.
3. Insall J. The Pridie debridement operation for osteoarthritis of the knee. Clin Orthop Relat Res. 1974;101:61–7.
4. Steadman JR, Rodkey WG, Briggs KK, Rodrigo JJ. [The microfracture technic in the management of complete cartilage defects in the knee joint]. Orthopade. 1999;28(1):26–32. https://doi.org/10.1007/s001320050318.
5. Freedman KB, Cole BJ. Microfracture technique in the knee. Textbook of arthoscopy. Amsterdam: Elsevier; 2004. p. 575–9.
6. Marder RA, Hopkins G Jr, Timmerman LA. Arthroscopic microfracture of chondral defects of the knee: a comparison of two postoperative treatments. Arthroscopy. 2005;21(2):152–8. https://doi.org/10.1016/j.arthro.2004.10.009.
7. Kreuz PC, Erggelet C, Steinwachs MR, Krause SJ, Lahm A, Niemeyer P, et al. Is microfracture of chondral defects in the knee associated with different results in patients aged 40 years or younger? Arthroscopy. 2006;22(11):1180–6. https://doi.org/10.1016/j.arthro.2006.06.020.
8. Goyal D, Keyhani S, Lee EH, Hui JH. Evidence--based status of microfracture technique: a systematic review of level I and II studies. Arthroscopy. 2013;29(9):1579–88. https://doi.org/10.1016/j.arthro.2013.05.027.
9. Steadman JR, Briggs KK, Rodrigo JJ, Kocher MS, Gill TJ, Rodkey WG. Outcomes of microfracture for traumatic chondral defects of the knee: average 11-year follow-up. Arthroscopy. 2003;19(5):477–84. https://doi.org/10.1053/jars.2003.50112.
10. Medina J, Garcia-Mansilla I, Fabricant PD, Kremen TJ, Sherman SL, Jones K. Microfracture for the treatment of symptomatic cartilage lesions of the knee: a survey of International Cartilage Regeneration & Joint Preservation Society. Cartilage. 2021;13(1 Suppl):1148s–55s. https://doi.org/10.1177/1947603520954503.
11. Farr J, Cole B, Dhawan A, Kercher J, Sherman S. Clinical cartilage restoration: evolution and overview. Clin Orthop Relat Res. 2011;469(10):2696–705. https://doi.org/10.1007/s11999-010-1764-z.
12. Asik M, Ciftci F, Sen C, Erdil M, Atalar A. The microfracture technique for the treatment of full-thickness articular cartilage lesions of the knee: midterm results. Arthroscopy. 2008;24(11):1214–20. https://doi.org/10.1016/j.arthro.2008.06.015.
13. Jarecki J, Waśko MK, Widuchowski W, Tomczyk--Warunek A, Wójciak M, Sowa I, et al. Knee cartilage lesion management-current trends in clinical practice. J Clin Med. 2023;12(20):6434. https://doi.org/10.3390/jcm12206434.
14. Behery O, Siston RA, Harris JD, Flanigan DC. Treatment of cartilage defects of the knee: expanding on the existing algorithm. Clin J Sport Med. 2014;24(1):21–30. https://doi.org/10.1097/jsm.0000000000000004.
15. Zedde P, Cudoni S, Giachetti G, Manunta ML, Masala G, Brunetti A, et al. Subchondral bone remodeling: comparing nanofracture with microfracture. An ovine in vivo study. Joints. 2016;4(2):87–93. https://doi.org/10.11138/jts/2016.4.2.087.
16. Polat G, Erşen A, Erdil ME, Kızılkurt T, Kılıçoğlu Ö, Aşık M. Long-term results of microfracture in the treatment of talus osteochondral lesions. Knee Surg Sports Traumatol Arthrosc. 2016;24(4):1299–303. https://doi.org/10.1007/s00167-016-3990-8.
17. Goldberg VM, Caplan AI. Biologic restoration of articular surfaces. Instr Course Lect. 1999;48:623–7.
18. Frisbie DD, Oxford JT, Southwood L, Trotter GW, Rodkey WG, Steadman JR, et al. Early events in cartilage repair after subchondral bone microfracture. Clin Orthop Relat Res. 2003;407:215–27. https://doi.org/10.1097/00003086-200302000-00031.
19. Steadman JR, Rodkey WG, Rodrigo JJ. Microfracture: surgical technique and rehabilitation to treat chondral defects. Clin Orthop Relat Res. 2001;(391 Suppl):S362–9. https://doi.org/10.1097/00003086-200110001-00033.
20. Steadman JR, Miller BS, Karas SG, Schlegel TF, Briggs KK, Hawkins RJ. The microfracture technique in the treatment of full-thickness chondral lesions of the knee in National Football League players. J Knee Surg. 2003;16(2):83–6.
21. Solheim E, Hegna J, Strand T, Harlem T, Inderhaug E. Randomized study of long-term (15–17 years) outcome after microfracture versus mosaicplasty in knee articular cartilage defects. Am J Sports Med. 2018;46(4):826–31. https://doi.org/10.1177/0363546517745281.
22. Gill TJ, McCulloch PC, Glasson SS, Blanchet T, Morris EA. Chondral defect repair after the microfracture procedure: a nonhuman primate model. Am J Sports Med. 2005;33(5):680–5. https://doi.org/10.1177/0363546504271744.
23. Mithoefer K, Williams RJ III, Warren RF, Potter HG, Spock CR, Jones EC, et al. The microfracture technique for the treatment of articular cartilage lesions in the knee. A prospective cohort study. J Bone Joint Surg Am. 2005;87(9):1911–20. https://doi.org/10.2106/jbjs.D.02846.
24. Neri T, Dehon M, Klasan A, Putnis SE, Farizon F, Philippot R. Predictors of functional outcome after microfracture treatment of cartilage defects of the knee. Surg Technol Int. 2020;37:341–7.

25. Knutsen G, Engebretsen L, Ludvigsen TC, Drogset JO, Grøntvedt T, Solheim E, et al. Autologous chondrocyte implantation compared with microfracture in the knee. A randomized trial. J Bone Joint Surg Am. 2004;86(3):455–64. https://doi.org/10.2106/00004623-200403000-00001.
26. Gobbi A, Nunag P, Malinowski K. Treatment of full thickness chondral lesions of the knee with microfracture in a group of athletes. Knee Surg Sports Traumatol Arthrosc. 2005;13(3):213–21. https://doi.org/10.1007/s00167-004-0499-3.
27. Solheim E, Hegna J, Inderhaug E, Øyen J, Harlem T, Strand T. Results at 10–14 years after microfracture treatment of articular cartilage defects in the knee. Knee Surg Sports Traumatol Arthrosc. 2016;24(5):1587–93. https://doi.org/10.1007/s00167-014-3443-1.
28. Gobbi A, Karnatzikos G, Kumar A. Long-term results after microfracture treatment for full-thickness knee chondral lesions in athletes. Knee Surg Sports Traumatol Arthrosc. 2014;22(9):1986–96. https://doi.org/10.1007/s00167-013-2676-8.
29. Gudas R, Gudaite A, Pocius A, Gudiene A, Cekanauskas E, Monastyreckiene E, et al. Ten-year follow-up of a prospective, randomized clinical study of mosaic osteochondral autologous transplantation versus microfracture for the treatment of osteochondral defects in the knee joint of athletes. Am J Sports Med. 2012;40(11):2499–508. https://doi.org/10.1177/0363546512458763.
30. Ulstein S, Årøen A, Røtterud JH, Løken S, Engebretsen L, Heir S. Microfracture technique versus osteochondral autologous transplantation mosaicplasty in patients with articular chondral lesions of the knee: a prospective randomized trial with long-term follow-up. Knee Surg Sports Traumatol Arthrosc. 2014;22(6):1207–15. https://doi.org/10.1007/s00167-014-2843-6.
31. Campbell AB, Pineda M, Harris JD, Flanigan DC. Return to sport after articular cartilage repair in athletes' knees: a systematic review. Arthroscopy. 2016;32(4):651–68.e1. https://doi.org/10.1016/j.arthro.2015.08.028.
32. Knutsen G, Drogset JO, Engebretsen L, Grøntvedt T, Isaksen V, Ludvigsen TC, et al. A randomized trial comparing autologous chondrocyte implantation with microfracture. Findings at five years. J Bone Joint Surg Am. 2007;89(10):2105–12. https://doi.org/10.2106/jbjs.G.00003.
33. Vanlauwe J, Saris DB, Victor J, Almqvist KF, Bellemans J, Luyten FP. Five-year outcome of characterized chondrocyte implantation versus microfracture for symptomatic cartilage defects of the knee: early treatment matters. Am J Sports Med. 2011;39(12):2566–74. https://doi.org/10.1177/0363546511422220.

8 Osteochondral Autograft Transfer (OATS and Mosaicplasty) in Cartilage Treatment

Mehmet Emin Şimşek and Rıfat Şahin

8.1 Introduction

Various surgical methods are available for the treatment of partial chondral or osteochondral defects of the articular surfaces. Owing to their poor biomechanical properties and unsatisfactory clinical outcomes, conventional resurfacing procedures can partially and temporarily contribute to lesion healing [1]. Cartilage injuries can lead to persistent pain, stiffness, swelling, and other mechanical symptoms because of the poor healing potential of articular cartilage. Surgical intervention is often required when conservative measures fail to provide significant relief [2].

Currently, the treatment of symptomatic partial articular cartilage defects remains a clinical challenge. Recent advances in treatment options involving osteochondral allografts are focused on promoting the formation of hyaline or hyaline-like cartilage to address articular cartilage injuries [3]. Although previous publications on autogenous osteochondral transplantation have reported long-term hyaline cartilage survival in the transplanted osteochondral block, the clinical use of a single-block large osteochondral autograft plug transfer has been constrained because of limited donor site availability [4]. Additionally, employing large grafts can lead to a mismatch at the recipient site, potentially causing a permanent alteration in the biomechanics of the joint. Preclinical animal studies conducted in the early years of this therapy have indicated that employing multiple small-sized cylindrical grafts rather than a single large block graft not only preserves donor site integrity but also enables a more extensive tissue transplantation with a mosaic-like implantation pattern [5]. The gradual placement of multiple osteochondral autograft plugs enables the shaping of the joint surface. The fundamental concept underlying autogenous osteochondral transplantation is the mosaic-like transplantation of multiple, small-sized, cylindrical osteochondral grafts, which facilitates the creation of a congruent cartilage surface [6]. The grafts are harvested from the relatively low-weight-bearing periphery of the patellofemoral (PF) joint. The transplanted autogenous hyaline cartilage exhibits excellent survival and produces a more durable surface compared to fibrous cartilage repair tissue. The repair at the donor site occurs through natural healing processes, where the tunnels gradually fill with cancellous bone and the surface is lined with reparative fibrocartilage created by bone marrow-derived cells [7].

The mosaicplasty resurfacing technique was developed in the early 1990s. Cadaveric studies

M. E. Şimşek (✉) · R. Şahin
Faculty of Medicine, Department of Orthopedics and Traumatology, Lokman Hekim University, Ankara, Turkey

M. E. Erdil et al. (eds.), *Current Concept in Cartilage Treatment*,
https://doi.org/10.1007/978-3-032-27099-3_8

have aided in the development of surgical equipment capable of providing optimal technical conditions for the harvesting and mosaic-like transplanting of small cylindrical osteochondral grafts. Since 1990, numerous animal experiments have been conducted to assess the mosaicplasty concept and determine the ideal donor site, graft size, optimal filling rate, and compliance with this technique. German Shepherd dogs and horses were the subjects of this experimental study, and subsequently, veterinary clinical trials were conducted on horses to refine the technical details and rehabilitation aspects of mosaicplasty [8].

The most important findings of these experiments were as follows:

- The transplanted hyaline cartilage survives and replaces the hyaline cartilage.
- The implanted grafts demonstrate excellent integration into the host tissue.
- The fibrocartilage tissue forms between the transplanted and intact cartilage.
- Deep matrix integration occurs between the hyaline layer of the grafts and the host cartilage tissue.
- Over time, the donor tunnels were observed to fill with cancellous bone, leading to the creation of an articular surface covered with fibrocartilage tissue that is acceptable for these low-weight-bearing areas [9].

Hjelle et al. found focal chondral lesions in 19% of 1000 consecutive knee arthroscopies. Of these chondral lesions, 58% were located in the medial femoral condyle (MFC), 11% in the patella, 11% in the lateral tibia, 9% in the lateral femoral condyle (LFC), 6% in the LFC, and 5% in the medial tibia. Consequently, 17% of chondral defects in the knee were identified as PF joint lesions, and 67% were medial or FC lesions [10].

During the development phase of mosaicplasty, the first series of instruments for press-fit cartilage transplantation was introduced in 1992. Subsequent research in the following years led to the development of second-generation instruments that enabled the mosaicplasty technique to be performed using an arthroscopic approach. The clinical implementation of the mosaicplasty concept commenced in 1992, owing to its reproducibility and technical ease of application. In subsequent years, based on various clinical data and outcomes obtained from animal experiments, the technique has been employed with similar success in numerous institutions worldwide since 1995 [11].

In this chapter, the current status of osteochondral autograft plug transfer is reviewed, including indications, surgical technique, pitfalls, postoperative complications, and clinical outcomes.

8.2 Indications and Contrandications for Surgery

Small-sized, unifocal lesions of the FCs represent the primary indication for mosaicplasty procedures. However, defects on the tibial, patellar, and trochlear surfaces can also be treated with osteochondral grafting. Mosaicplasty tends to yield less favorable outcomes in cases of multiple defects, particularly in reciprocal lesions. In addition to osteochondral defects in the knee, mosaicplasty can be used to address talus lesions, and in exceptional cases, it can be used to treat lesions of the humeral head and femoral head [12].

The repair of damaged cartilage is restricted to 1–4 cm^2 because of limited donor site availability and certain technical considerations. Typically, the periphery of each PF joint offers suitable graft harvesting for defects of 3–4 cm^2 in size. When all potential donor sites are utilized, this ratio can increase by as much as 8–9 cm^2. Nonetheless, extending resurfacing in this manner may lead to a higher incidence of donor site morbidity [9, 13]. The recommended upper age limit for mosaicplasty is typically set at 50 years because of reduced cartilage repair capacity. Indeed, this limit is derived from clinical experience primarily with single-block osteochondral transfer procedures [14, 15].

Contraindications for mosaicplasty encompass lesions caused by generalized arthritis or rheumatoid arthritis, active infection, or the presence of tumors. At the recipient site, the survival of transplanted hyaline cartilage can be impeded by inadequate intraarticular biochemical conditions [16, 17].

While osteoarthritis is typically considered a contraindication for mosaicplasty, in certain patient groups, it may be contemplated as a salvage procedure for small defects. Matching the contour of the disrupted articular surface to the donor plug can present a technical challenge. Other disadvantages may include donor site morbidity and the risk of cartilage or bone collapse [18].

As with other resurfacing techniques, mosaicplasty is only one part of the treatment of full-thickness chondral and osteochondral defects. It is also essential to address any accompanying joint abnormalities. Treatment of meniscal and ligament tears, joint instabilities, and misalignments should be integrated into the operative and postoperative rehabilitation algorithms. Otherwise, failure to address accompanying joint abnormalities can lead to premature wear of the transplanted cartilage, hinder proper healing, or even contribute to further degeneration. The most common concomitant surgical interventions are anterior cruciate ligament reconstruction, meniscal repair, and femorotibial realignment procedures. Sometimes PF realignment or lateral release may also be required [19–21].

8.3 Surgical Technique

8.3.1 Recommendations for Preoperative Preparation

The patient should be placed in a supine position with the knee flexed at 120°, and the contralateral extremity should be placed on the table to allow movement of the knee to be operated on during the procedure. The use of a tourniquet is recommended under general or regional anesthesia. Preoperative preparations should include antibiotic prophylaxis. The procedure requires standard arthroscopic instruments and the usual mosaicplasty set. In addition to these reusable instruments, disposable chisels, drill bits, and tampons can be utilized to ensure optimal conditions for precise graft harvesting and tunnel preparation [9, 22].

8.3.2 Mosaicplasty Techniques

8.3.2.1 Surgical Approach

Arthroscopic Mosaicplasty

Most femoral condylar defects can be treated arthroscopically. For the majority of these lesions, the anteromedial and anterolateral working portals provide convenient vertical access. A 1.2-mm K-wire or an 18-gauge spinal needle can be used to localize the portal relative to the cartilage defect. These portals tend to be more centralized than standard portals because of the inward curvature of the condyles. Importantly, MFC lesions caused by osteochondritis dissecans may necessitate a lateral approach. In such cases, a central patellar tendon portal can provide good access to the inner regions of both the MFCs and LFCs, as standard portals rarely provide an excessively oblique approach [12, 18] (Chap. 21, Fig. 21.13).

Open Mosaicplasty

Open mosaicplasty may be preferred during the learning curve or when an arthroscopic approach is not appropriate because of the size or location of the lesion. While certain trochlear defects may be accessible via arthroscopic approaches, patellotrochlear and tibial lesions always necessitate an open procedure. The incision can be made in a medial, lateral–anterior–sagittal, or oblique orientation. The most appropriate incision approach can be selected by arthroscopy. Patellotrochlear and tibial implantations may require an extended anteromedial approach. The other steps and techniques of implantation are identical to the arthroscopic procedure [18, 23] (Chap. 21; Figs. 21.12 and 21.14).

8.3.2.2 Preparation of the Defect

Sharp curettes and/or razor blades (shavers) are employed to bring the edges of the defect to right angles with the intact hyaline cartilage. The bony base of the lesion can be cleaned using an arthroscopic burr (such as an abrader or acromionizer) or a half-round file to remove the subchondral sequester layer and freshen the subchondral bone (Fig. 8.1).

Abrasion arthroplasty of the lesion promotes the injection of fibrocartilage from the bone base. A drill guide should be used to determine the required number of grafts and their size in terms of diameter. By gently tapping the cutting edge of the guide on the bone base, a mark can be left on the damaged area. Finally, the depth of the defect should be measured with the ruler of the dilator. Filling the defect with equally sized, contacting cylindrical grafts enables a filling rate of 70%–80%. Additionally, using smaller graft sizes and cutting the grafts into each other can enhance coverage, achieving rates of up to 90%–100% [11] (Fig. 8.2).

8.3.2.3 Graft Harvest

The graft harvesting method plays a crucial role in determining graft quality and preserving the mechanical properties of the osteochondral architecture. The recommended graft harvest sites are the area above the peripheral MFC and the area above the intercondylar notch line of the PF joint. The surface of the LFC above the sulcus terminalis and, in exceptional cases, the notch area may serve as additional donor sites. Grafts harvested from the notch area are considered less suitable because of their concave cartilage heads and reduced elasticity. Recent publications also suggest that the proximal tibiofibular articulation can serve as an exceptional donor site [24–26]. The minimum length of the graft should be at least twice its diameter. However, 15-mm-long grafts for resurfacing chondral lesions and 25-mm-long graft plugs for osteochondral defects can be harvested [13]. The optimal angle of view for graft harvesting from the PF peripheries can be achieved through the standard contralateral portal. Performing full extension of the knee and utilizing the standard ipsilateral portal helps determine whether access to the donor site is perpendicular [11]. A critical concept in graft harvesting is contact steepness. Although this can be achieved with an open or arthroscopic approach, it is crucial to harvest grafts that are orthogonal to the articular surface. This enables a more precise restoration of the condyle inclination and radius of curvature, along with facilitating good joint alignment, which is particularly important in cases with defects requiring multiple plugs. The mini-open arthroscopic technique may be preferred when multiple grafts are required, as it offers a more precise and safer methodology to reduce morbidity at the graft harvest site. With precise planning, this mini-open incision can be used for both graft harvesting and placement, as the knee is positioned between flexion and extension [27]. Gradual flexion of the knee allows additional grafts to be harvested from the lower regions of the PF joint periphery. The graft col-

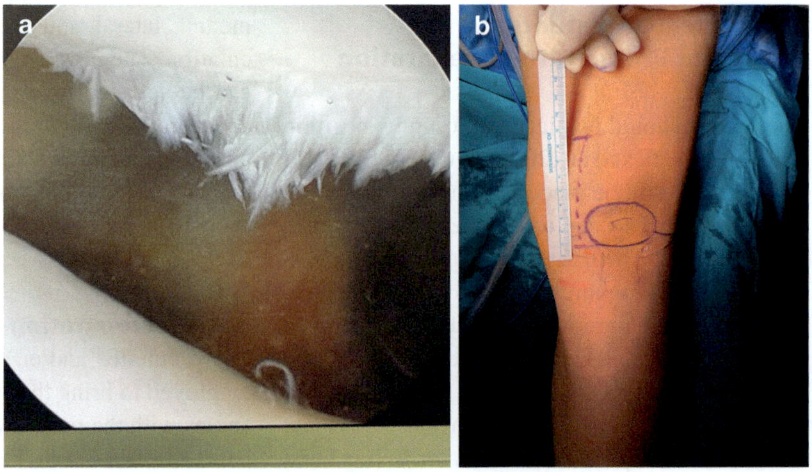

Fig. 8.1 Determination of the chondral damaged area in the patella by arthroscopy (**a**) and determination of the skin incision before osteochondral autograft plug application to the defect (**b**)

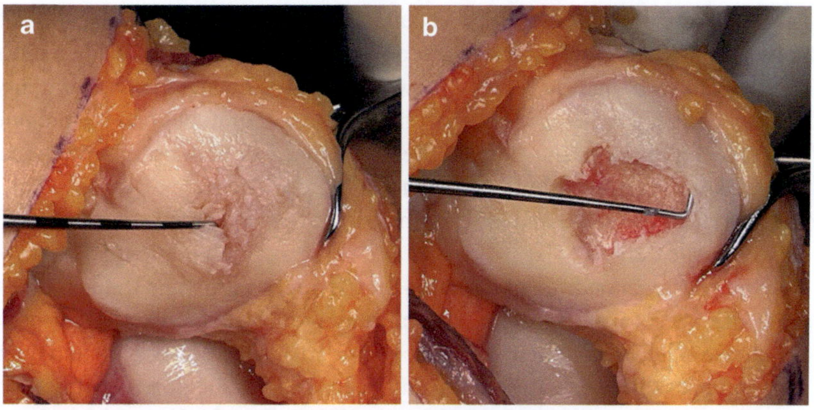

Fig. 8.2 Assessment of the damaged cartilage area (**a**) and a view of the damaged area after debridement with a burr and curette (**b**)

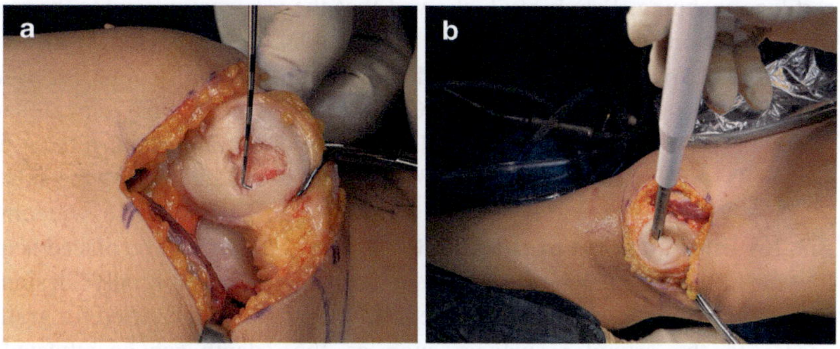

Fig. 8.3 Measurement of defect length (**a**) and preparation of the defect for grafting (**b**)

lection level should not extend above the intercondylar notch (sulcus terminalis). In an arthroscopic approach, accessing the medial PF joint periphery can be more easily achieved through a lateral approach. This is because fluid distension usually moves the patella laterally, facilitating the vertical positioning of the graft harvesting apparatus. If standard portals do not allow vertical access, a spinal needle or a K-wire can be used to locate any additional portals [28, 29] (Fig. 8.3).

Once the portal's location has been determined, the apparatus prepared for graft harvesting should be inserted into the joint. Once the donor site is identified, the chisel should be placed perpendicular to the articular surface. The graft harvesting apparatus should be carefully hammered using a mallet until the appropriate depth is attained. The chisel should be held firmly at the cartilage–bone interface to prevent the apparatus from slipping and creating a curved graft.

The subsequent step involves abruptly rotating the graft-receiving chisel and repeating the movement in the opposite direction. The grafts should be removed from the chisel by sliding the appropriate-sized chisel guard over the insert. Prepared grafts should be placed in isotonic fluid or on a soaked gauze pad. During the learning curve, grafts can also be obtained via mini-arthrotomy (15–20 mm). The incision site is determined using a spinal needle under arthroscopic control [22, 30].

The holes in the donor site should be filled within a few hours with initial repair tissue produced by mesenchymal stem cells, which arrive at the graft harvest site via bleeding. Adequate rehabilitation can promote the transformation of this primary repair tissue into fibrocartilage-covered cancellous bone. Additionally, donor site defects can often be filled using bone grafts from the recipient site. In a canine model reported in 2023, Feczko et al. [31] conducted a comparison of various biodegradable materials for donor site filling, which included hydroxyapatite, carbon fiber, polyglyconate B, compressed collagen, and polycaprolactone. Second-look arthroscopy and histological examination reports show that compressed collagen provides the best fibrocartilage coverage for harvest site defects. Several composite bone graft substitute polymer plugs are commercially available and have been utilized to fill donor site defects [4].

When osteochondral plugs are transferred from the knee to other joints, special attention should be paid to potential differences in cartilage thickness between the donor and recipient sites. Using magnetic resonance imaging (MRI) cartilage mapping, Schub et al. showed that the thinnest region of harvestable knee cartilage is located at the posterior pole of the MFC as well as the distal-most anterior–lateral FC and integrates best with more distal articular receptor sites in the body, such as the elbow [32].

8.3.2.4 Implantation of the Graft

Flexion of the knee helps gain access to the graft placement site. In addition, in areas without access to the articular surface, such as the patella, mosaicplasty may need to be performed with open surgery and rotation of the patella. In arthroscopic mosaicplasty procedures, having a good fluid management system and achieving an appropriate amount of joint distension can ensure excellent visualization. The first step is to place the apparatus perpendicular to the defective surface during the preparation of the area to be grafted [5]. Rotating the arthroscope allows the surgeon to view the surgical site from different angles, enabling proper orientation. The next step involves gently tapping the cutting edge of the guide into the subchondral bone. Depending on the mosaicplasty set used, the appropriately sized graft site preparation apparatus is placed perpendicular to the bone in the area of the defect. Typically, a recipient hole a few millimeters deeper than the graft's length is chosen to reduce the high intraosseous pressure and prevent the prominent graft from being elevated. After removing the defective osteochondral fragment, bone deposits are removed by irrigating the receiving tunnel with an isotonic solution [33].

The fixation of osteochondral autograft plugs is achieved using a press-fit technique. The press-fit technique is employed to enlarge the donor graft beyond the prepared recipient area and to fit it with optimum pressure. Increased stability and better preservation of cartilage thickness were observed when the grafts were 1 mm larger than the recipient site. Accordingly, the donor preparation apparatus is 1 mm larger than the recipient site preparation apparatus. Matching the depth of the donor graft and the recipient site is crucial for achieving an optimal press fit [34] (Fig. 8.4).

Before placing the prepared grafts, the dilator is compressed to the required depth. The depth of the enlargement depends on the stiffness and flexibility of the receiving bone. Hard bone needs further enlargement than normal soft bone. When removing the dilator from the hole, it must be retracted along the axis of the tunnel. In this manner, excessive widening of the area where the graft will be placed is avoided [35].

A specially designed graft-pusher tampon should be used for graft placement. The insertion depth can be adjusted by twisting the handle. Initially, the graft should sit slightly higher than the depth of the defect. It helps minimize the possibility of over-embedding the graft. During arthroscopic procedures, it is recommended to stop the inflow of the fluid at this step, as the continued fluid flow may force the graft out of the tube. The graft must be delivered directly into the receiving tunnel through the guide. The graft can be placed deeper by rotating the handle of the delivery tampon counterclockwise. The graft should align with the original articular surface. If the graft is protruding, the graft should be gently tapped with an appropriately sized dilator or an impactor. Subsequent grafts are placed using a similar technique, with a graft placement guide right next to the previously placed grafts. The edge of the pusher should be placed so that it overhangs the intact cartilage to avoid inadvertent over-insertion of the grafts [36] (Fig. 8.5).

It is recommended to start with the most posterior graft and to place more grafts in less-flexed knee positions. The main advantage of the step-by-step implantation technique is that the next hole allows a secure placement of the surround-

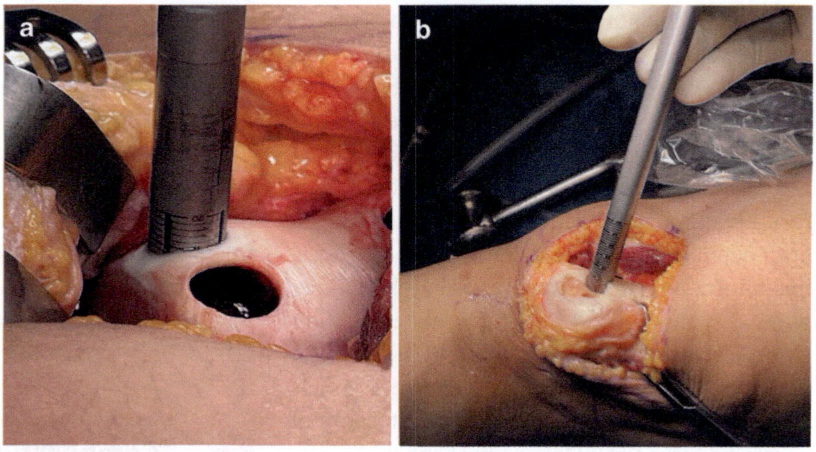

Fig. 8.4 Removal of osteochondral autograft plugs from the lateral trochlear groove according to the slope of the defect (**a**) and the preparation of the defect area according to the size of the prepared graft (**b**)

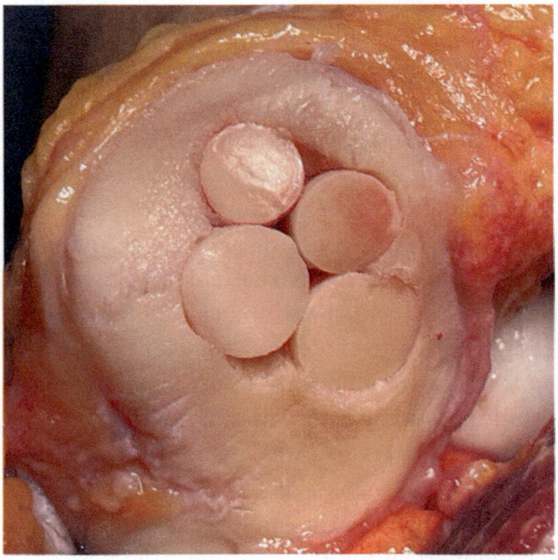

Fig. 8.5 The appearance of osteochondral autograft plugs after placement in the cartilage-damaged area of the patella

ing bone tissue around the previously implanted grafts. Once all grafts are in place, the knee should be moved through the full range of motion, and varus or valgus stress should also be applied depending on the edge of the resurfaced area. Aspiration drainage should be performed from the upper portal, and an elastic bandage should be applied over the dressing after the portals are closed [37].

Although technically more difficult, graft placement through a bone tunnel has also been described, especially for tibial defects. In this technique, an anterior cruciate ligament tibial guide is used to open a tibial bone tunnel, through which a donor graft can be passed in a retrograde manner until it aligns with the articular surface [38].

Manual cutting devices may not be able to cut the retropatellar regions effectively because of the hard subchondral bone characteristic of the retropatellar facets. Alternative surgical techniques involving the use of cutting drills with similar diameters and precise drilling guides to stabilize the process can be employed in regions with hard subchondral bone. Moreover, in cases where manual devices are used, the marked subchondral area can be gradually widened in advance using high-speed reamers [39].

8.4 Surgical Tips

By paying attention to technical considerations and the details of the learning curve, most complications associated with osteochondral autograft plug transfer can be minimized or avoided. Hemarthrosis is perhaps the most common complication, which can be mitigated by filling the donor site and/or utilizing a postoperative drain to prevent bone hemorrhage into the joint [5]. Donor site collapse can occur, often due to placing adjacent donor sites too closely, leading to a loss of structural bone integrity. To prevent collapse, it is recommended to maintain a bone bridge of at least 1–2 mm between harvesting sites [40].

Graft failure at the recipient site can occur for various reasons. The press-fit technique for placing grafts is susceptible to compressive forces. Insufficient impaction force may cause the graft to remain above the articular cartilage level, whereas excessive compression may cause surface chondrocyte cell death [34]. Matching the graft depth to the recipient site depth is crucial, as this allows the surface topography to be aligned without the need for over-embedding. Optimization of the difference between the plug diameter and the receiving seat diameter is essential to allow optimal press fit without applying excessive force [41]. Donor plugs should be handled with caution to prevent damage to the surrounding cartilage at the donor site, minimize microtrauma to the graft articular cartilage, and ensure maximum cellular viability of the graft. In cases where multiple grafts are used, minimizing the distance between the grafts and their proximity to the surrounding cartilage will reduce surface fibrillation and loading on the graft edge. OAPT should be avoided in bipolar lesions as it may result in excessive friction, hindering graft integration and potentially leading to graft failure [42, 43].

8.5 Recommendations for Postoperative Care

Postoperative application of ice packs and elastic bandages may help control excessive bleeding from donor tunnels. The drain should be removed in 24 h. Appropriate pain control, cold therapy, and the use of nonsteroidal anti-inflammatory drugs can help alleviate postoperative complaints. Postoperative thrombosis prophylaxis is also recommended [43].

8.5.1 Rehabilitation

A full range of motion should be allowed immediately after autologous osteochondral plug surgeries. However, it requires a period of non-weight bearing for 2 weeks after surgery and also a period of partial weight bearing for 2–3 weeks afterward. A non-weight-bearing first phase is recommended to prevent graft collapse during bone integration. Patients can return to normal daily activities after 8–10 weeks. High-demand sports activities should be postponed until 5–6 months later. In cases where concurrent procedures, such as ACL reconstruction, high tibial osteotomy, meniscal repair, and meniscal resection, have been performed, it is essential to modify the recommended rehabilitation protocol accordingly [44].

8.6 Complicatıons

Technical difficulties during the osteochondral autograft plug transfer procedure are common and can be avoided by adhering to the main principles of the surgical protocol. Vertical harvesting and graft implantation are crucial for successful transplantation. Graft harvesting and placement at oblique angles can result in a rough joint surface. Comprehensive visual control at different angles with the arthroscope can eliminate such complications [5].

If the grafts are placed deeper than the desired level, the drill guide is placed next to the implanted graft, and the appropriate recipient hole is drilled. The arthroscopic probe can then be used to remove the guide and lift the graft to the required level [40].

Complaints such as pain or swelling following strenuous physical activity are not common complications. However, multiple graft harvesting or graft harvesting without consideration of preexisting PF degeneration may lead to a higher rate of donor site morbidity [34].

Postoperative excessive bleeding from donor tunnels is also a potential postoperative complication and can occur in 7%–8% of cases, according to previous reports. Postoperative drainage, the application of ice packs, and the use of elastic bandages may help reduce the frequency of this complication. Septic or thromboembolic complications can be prevented by adhering to strict aseptic conditions during surgery, administering single-dose antibiotics prophylactically, and implementing thrombosis prophylaxis measures [45].

8.7 Clinical Outcomes

Although the efficacy of treatment for focal cartilage defects needs further investigation, there have been an increasing number of clinical trials published recently that evaluate the short- and long-term clinical outcomes of OAPT compared to alternative therapies. Numerous researchers have used various objective, subjective, and radiologic evaluation criteria to assess clinical outcomes, such as the Knee Injury and Osteoarthritis Outcome Score, International Cartilage Repair Society (ICRS) cartilage repair histological assessment score, International Knee Documentation Committee score, Lysholm scores, modified Hospital for Special Surgery score (HSS score), modified Cincinnati score, subjective activity level assessments using Tegner scores, magnetic resonance observation of cartilage repair tissue score, second-look arthroscopy, and histological analysis of biopsy, and reported positive results about the outcome after OAT in long-term follow-up studies, demonstrating generally successful results.

In a 17-year prospective multicenter study of 354 mosaicplasties using multiple small-diameter graft techniques, Hangody et al. reported autogenous autograft transfers in 187 MFCs, 74 LFCs, 16 tibial plateaus, 18 patellas, and 8 trochleas. Good-to-excellent results were obtained in 91% of FC lesions, 86% of tibial plateau lesions, and 74% of PF lesions. This long-term study showed improvement in overall assessment scores, including HSS, Lysholm, Cincinnati, and ICRS scores [46].

In a 10-year follow-up study comparing OAPT versus microfractures in lesions smaller than 4 cm^2, Gudas et al. reported significantly higher clinical outcome scores on the ICRS scale in both groups [4, 47]. Nevertheless, OAPT achieved significantly higher scores based on the ICRS scales and Tegner scores compared to microfracture. In addition, patients who underwent OAPT showed no evidence of graft loosening at 1- or 10-year follow-up based on MRI [9].

Solheim et al. conducted a study comparing OAPT against microfracture with a minimum follow-up of 15 years. Mean Lysholm scores were found to be significantly higher from baseline in the OAPT group than in the microfracture group at all time points, including 12 months, 5 years, 10 years, and 15 years [48].

In another comparative study, Soleim et al. compared the clinical outcomes of mosaicplasty in the PF joint and tibiofemoral joint in the knee joint. The most remarkable finding of the study was that the survival distribution was not significantly different between the PF joint and tibiofemoral joint groups. For both sites, most OAT repairs remained intact for many years, but in almost half of the cases, they failed after 18 years. Nevertheless, they have reported that regardless of localization (PF or FC), many patients have had remarkably good knee function for many years after the OAT procedure [19].

Jungmann et al. also reported a reduction in the progression of degenerative MRI changes in the OAPT group at an average of 6 years of follow-up on patients with cartilage injuries treated with OAPT versus nonoperatively [49].

Recent studies have investigated the complication rates of cartilage procedures. Gowd et al. reported that both open and arthroscopic OAT procedures resulted in complication rates of less than 2% during a 30-day follow-up, with no significant difference observed between the different cartilage procedures [50]. In a systematic review with a 10-year follow-up, the reported reoperation rate after OAT was 19% and the rate of clinical failure was 29% [14].

Caubère et al. compared the adaptation of the graft diameter to mechanical stresses in the grafted areas. The study found that the differences between the conditions were not statistically significant but showed tendencies. Filling the defect with six 4-mm plugs restores a larger contact surface compared with the other plugs. The use of 8- and 6-mm grafts led to a respective increase of 12% and 52% of the mean pressure compared with the 4-mm grafts. This difference was also found for the maximum pressure (36% and 129%). Regardless of the diameter of the plugs used, filling the lesion reduces the mean pressure exerted on the healthy cartilage by 19% [51].

Kizaki et al. evaluated the results of open and arthroscopic mosaicplasty in a review study. This review aimed to compare clinical outcomes, postoperative complications, defect localization, and defect size between open and arthroscopic OATs. The study evaluated data from 1139 patients (532 in open OAT vs. 607 in arthroscopic OAT). The defect size in open OAT was three times larger than that of arthroscopic OAT (2.96 ± 0.76 vs. 0.97 ± 0.48 cm^2). In terms of defect localization, the MFC was the most common (75.4%), followed by the LFC (12.1%), patella (6.7%), and trochlea (5.7%). All of these defects at these localizations were treated with open OAT, whereas arthroscopic OAT treatments were restricted to the MFC and LFC. The clinical outcomes were overall favorable, with the modified Hospital for Special Surgery knee scores being 89.6 ± 8.0 (36.1-month follow-up) versus 90.4 ± 6.0 (89.5-month follow-up) and the Lysholm scores being 81.6 ± 8.9 (44.2-month follow-up) and 83.3 ± 7.4 (12.0-month follow-up) between open and arthroscopic OATs, respectively. Fifty-three postoperative complications were observed (39/279 vs. 14/594), and the most common complication was hemarthrosis (13/39 in open vs. 1/14 in arthroscopic OAT). The overall clinical outcomes were favorable in open and arthroscopic OATs, with open OAT allowing for the treatment of lesions three times greater in dimension than arthroscopic OAT. Furthermore, defect localization was restricted to MFC and LFC in arthroscopic OAT. The most common complication was hemarthrosis [18].

In the meta-analysis of Matthews et al., where they compared the surgical methods used in the treatment of unstable osteochondritis dissecans (fixation, fragment excision, ACI, MACI, OATs, and scaffold), they concluded that fixation is the most successful treatment method in the treatment of osteochondritis dissecans and that MACI and OAT have similar clinical outcomes with a high success rate [28].

8.8 Conclusion

Osteochondral autograft transplantation is being increasingly used as a treatment option for focal small cartilage and osteochondral defects. This article reviews the surgical technique and indications for this procedure. Clinical trials have demonstrated promising results for OAT, although further randomized controlled trials are required to assess the long-term efficacy of OAT compared to other available techniques.

Take-Home Message

- Injuries to the cartilage of the knee joint are treatable, and there are various treatment options available to address them.
- Autologous osteochondral plug transfer is an excellent procedure for single-stage hyaline cartilage restoration in focal chondral defects of the femur.
- Comprehensive preparation of the defect and subsequent sizing are essential for ensuring a successful surgery.
- As with all cartilage surgeries performed for cartilage damage, it is necessary to consider factors such as age, BMI, the presence of lower extremity malalignment, and the stage of degeneration in the cartilage surrounding the affected area.
- It should be performed together with the treatment of accompanying pathologies such as meniscus tears, ligament damage, and malalignment.
- Defects in the weight-bearing areas of both FCs can typically be addressed arthroscopically, allowing for the possibility of performing a single-plug OATs.
- Larger defects requiring multiple plugs (mosaicplasty) or defects of the posterior FCs are better treated with open surgery.
- Although the success rate of OATs in the PF joint is lower than in the tibiofemoral joint, the outcomes are still satisfactory.
- It should be considered that the success rate is low in "kissing" lesions.
- Strict adherence to the surgical technique for a specific device is crucial to enhancing accuracy and preventing errors.

References

1. Redondo ML, Beer AJ, Yanke AB. Cartilage restoration: microfracture and osteochondral autograft transplantation. J Knee Surg. 2018;31(3):231–8.
2. Armiento AR, Alini M, Stoddart MJ. Articular fibrocartilage—why does hyaline cartilage fail to repair? Adv Drug Deliv Rev. 2019;146:289–305.
3. Wagner KR, et al. Osteochondral allograft transplantation for focal cartilage defects of the femoral condyles. JBJS Essent Surg Tech. 2022;12(3):e21.00037.
4. Krych AJ, et al. Cartilage injury in the knee: assessment and treatment options. J Am Acad Orthop Surg. 2020;28(22):914–22.
5. Rowland R, Colello M, Wyland DJ. Osteochondral autograft transfer procedure: arthroscopic technique and technical pearls. Arthrosc Tech. 2019;8(7):e713–9.
6. Cinti F, Vezzoni L, Vezzoni A. A new generation of osteochondral autograft transfer system for the treatment of osteochondritis dissecans of the femoral condyle: clinical experience in 18 dogs. Vet Comp Orthop Traumatol. 2022;35(3):198–204.
7. Massey PA, et al. Compressibility of osteochondral autograft transfer donor grafts: a comparison of different donor regions and how much shortening occurs of plugs after impaction. Orthop J Sports Med. 2023;11(1):23259671221147329.
8. Pareek A, et al. Osteochondral autograft transfer versus microfracture in the knee: a meta-analysis of prospective comparative studies at midterm. Arthroscopy. 2016;32(10):2118–30.
9. Richter DL, et al. Knee articular cartilage repair and restoration techniques: a review of the literature. Sports Health. 2016;8(2):153–60.
10. Hjelle K, et al. Articular cartilage defects in 1,000 knee arthroscopies. Arthroscopy. 2002;18(7):730–4.
11. Bordes M, et al. Autologous osteochondral transplantation for focal femoral condyle defects: comparison of mosaicplasty by arthrotomy vs. arthroscopy. Orthop Traumatol Surg Res. 2022;108(3):103102.
12. Inderhaug E, Solheim E. Osteochondral autograft transplant (mosaicplasty) for knee articular cartilage defects. JBJS Essent Surg Tech. 2019;9(4):e34.
13. Karmali S, et al. Mosaicplasty technique in the treatment of isolated knee femoral condyle osteochondral lesions—a retrospective study. Rev Bras Ortop (Sao Paulo). 2019;54(3):316–21.
14. Andrade R, et al. Knee donor-site morbidity after mosaicplasty—a systematic review. J Exp Orthop. 2016;3(1):31.
15. Gracitelli GC, et al. Surgical interventions (microfracture, drilling, mosaicplasty, and allograft transplantation) for treating isolated cartilage defects of the knee in adults. Cochrane Database Syst Rev. 2016;9(9):CD010675.
16. De Almeida Lira Neto O, et al. Surgical treatment of osteochondral lesions of the knee by means of mosaicplasty. Rev Bras Ortop. 2010;45(2):166–73.
17. Emre TY, et al. Autologous osteochondral transplantation (mosaicplasty) in articular cartilage defects of the patellofemoral joint: retrospective analysis of 33 cases. Musculoskelet Surg. 2017;101(2):133–8.
18. Kizaki K, et al. Arthroscopic versus open osteochondral autograft transplantation (mosaicplasty) for cartilage damage of the knee: a systematic review. J Knee Surg. 2021;34(1):94–107.
19. Solheim E, Hegna J, Inderhaug E. Clinical outcome after mosaicplasty of knee articular cartilage defects of patellofemoral joint versus tibiofemoral joint. J Orthop. 2020;18:36–40.
20. Banerjee S, Sahanand KS. Managing chondral lesions: a literature review and evidence-based clinical guidelines. Indian J Orthop. 2021;55(2):252–62.
21. Lynch TS, et al. Systematic review of autogenous osteochondral transplant outcomes. Arthroscopy. 2015;31(4):746–54.
22. Bader S, Miniaci A. Mosaicplasty. Orthopedics. 2011;34(9):e491–3.
23. Athanasiou V, et al. Mosaicplasty of the femoral head: a systematic review and meta-analysis of the current literature. Cureus. 2022;14(11):e31874.
24. Evans PJ, Miniaci A, Hurtig MB. Manual punch versus power harvesting of osteochondral grafts. Arthroscopy. 2004;20(3):306–10.
25. Duchow J, Hess T, Kohn D. Primary stability of press-fit-implanted osteochondral grafts. Influence of graft size, repeated insertion, and harvesting technique. Am J Sports Med. 2000;28(1):24–7.
26. Sabaghzadeh A, et al. Osteochondral autograft transfer (mosaicplasty) for treatment of patients with osteochondral lesions of talus. Chin J Traumatol. 2020;23(1):60–2.
27. Nakagawa Y, et al. The effects of alendronate on the suppression of bone resorption and the promotion of cartilage formation in the human mosaicplasty donor site: a randomized, double-blind, placebo-controlled prospective study. J Orthop Sci. 2022;27(4):835–43.
28. Matthews JR, et al. A systematic review of cartilage procedures for unstable osteochondritis dissecans. Phys Sportsmed. 2023;51(6):497–505.
29. Viamont-Guerra MR, et al. Promising outcomes of hip mosaicplasty by minimally invasive anterior approach using osteochondral autografts from the ipsilateral femoral head. Knee Surg Sports Traumatol Arthrosc. 2020;28(3):767–76.
30. Mukai S, et al. Mosaicplasty with high tibial osteotomy for knee subchondral insufficiency fracture had better magnetic resonance observation of cartilage repair tissue scores with less bone marrow edema and better plug union and less plug necrosis compared with mosaicplasty alone. Arthroscopy. 2023;39(2):337–46.
31. Feczko P, et al. Experimental results of donor site filling for autologous osteochondral mosaicplasty. Arthroscopy. 2003;19(7):755–61.
32. Banjar M, et al. Review of quantitative knee articular cartilage MR imaging. Magn Reson Med Sci. 2022;21(1):29–40.

33. Luick L, Steinmetz G, Haleem A. All-arthroscopic osteochondral autograft transfer technique for osteochondritis dissecans of the talus. Arthrosc Tech. 2020;9(4):e499–503.
34. Guzman AJ, et al. Arthroscopic osteochondral autograft transfer system procedure of the lateral femoral condyle with donor-site backfill using osteochondral allograft plug. Arthrosc Tech. 2021;10(12):e2683–9.
35. Kato Y, et al. A large knee osteochondral lesion treated using a combination of osteochondral autograft transfer and second-generation autologous chondrocyte implantation: a case report. Regen Ther. 2019;10:10–6.
36. Yabumoto H, Nakagawa Y, Mukai S. Surgical technique and clinical outcomes of osteochondral autograft transplantation for large osteonecrotic lesions of the femoral condyle with residual normal cartilage: the eyeglass technique. Orthop J Sports Med. 2019;7(10):2325967119872446.
37. Welton KL, et al. Knee cartilage repair and restoration: common problems and solutions. Clin Sports Med. 2018;37(2):307–30.
38. Yabumoto H, et al. Surgical technique and clinical outcomes of retrograde osteochondral autograft transfer for osteochondral lesions of the tibial plateau. Arthroscopy. 2017;33(6):1241–7.
39. Anders S, et al. [Repair of local cartilage defects in the patellofemoral joint]. Orthopade. 2011;40(10):885–8, 890–5.
40. Easley ME, Scranton PE Jr. Osteochondral autologous transfer system. Foot Ankle Clin. 2003;8(2):275–90.
41. Orr JD, et al. Indications for and early complications associated with use of temporary invasive distraction for osteochondral graft transfer procedures for treatment of lateral osteochondral lesions of the talus. Foot Ankle Int. 2014;35(1):50–5.
42. Wetzler MJ. Editorial commentary: is the cure worse than the disease? Harvesting autologous osteochondral transfer plugs for treatment of lesions of the elbow. Arthroscopy. 2018;34(7):2094–5.
43. Burroughs PJ, et al. Subsequent surgery up to 10 years after osteochondral allograft and osteochondral autograft: an analysis of more than 2000 patients. Orthop J Sports Med. 2022;10(12):23259671221139127.
44. Krych AJ, et al. Activity levels are higher after osteochondral autograft transfer mosaicplasty than after microfracture for articular cartilage defects of the knee: a retrospective comparative study. J Bone Joint Surg Am. 2012;94(11):971–8.
45. Anil U, Strauss EJ. Donor-site-related mechanical symptoms following osteochondral autograft transfer: a case report. JBJS Case Connect. 2018;8(4):e84.
46. Hangody L, et al. Autologous osteochondral mosaicplasty. Surgical technique. J Bone Joint Surg Am. 2004;86-A Suppl 1:65–72.
47. Gudas R, et al. Ten-year follow-up of a prospective, randomized clinical study of mosaic osteochondral autologous transplantation versus microfracture for the treatment of osteochondral defects in the knee joint of athletes. Am J Sports Med. 2012;40(11):2499–508.
48. Solheim E, et al. Randomized study of long-term (15-17 years) outcome after microfracture versus mosaicplasty in knee articular cartilage defects. Am J Sports Med. 2018;46(4):826–31.
49. Jungmann PM, et al. Cartilage repair surgery prevents progression of knee degeneration. Knee Surg Sports Traumatol Arthrosc. 2019;27(9):3001–13.
50. Gowd AK, et al. Management of chondral lesions of the knee: analysis of trends and short-term complications using the National Surgical Quality Improvement Program Database. Arthroscopy. 2019;35(1):138–46.
51. Caubere A, et al. Osteochondral autograft transplantation (mosaicplasty): what is the impact of plug diameter in cartilage repair? Int Orthop. 2023;47(3):623–30.

9 Autologous Chondrocyte Implantation and Matrix-Induced Autologous Chondrocyte Implantation

Erkan Alkan and M. Ugur Mermerkaya

9.1 Introduction

Articular cartilage, a critical form of hyaline cartilage, covers the joint surface and facilitates smooth, frictionless movement while absorbing the loads on the joint [1]. Its limited capacity to heal or regenerate itself like native hyaline cartilage often leads to significant movement impairment when damaged. Various treatment methods exist for cartilage lesions, each tailored to the lesion's location, size, and depth. The primary goals of these treatments are to heal the cartilage, mimicking the original hyaline cartilage, prevent permanent damage, restore mobility, impede worsening of the lesion, and alleviate symptoms. The societal cost of cartilage lesions is considerable, stemming from impacts on quality of life, productivity loss, additional medication usage, outpatient procedures, and surgeries, with a notable contribution from those arising as a consequence of untreated cartilage damage leading to osteoarthritis [2]. This chapter explores two such treatment methods, autologous chondrocyte implantation (ACI) and matrix-induced ACI (MACI). Both involve culturing the patient's own cartilage-producing cells in a laboratory, followed by implantation into the chondral defect, promoting healing and regeneration [3].

E. Alkan (✉)
Private Medical Park Ankara Hospital, Ankara, Turkey

Department of Orthopedics and Traumatology, Yuksek Ihtisas University, Ankara, Turkey

M. Ugur Mermerkaya
Department of Orthopedics and Traumatology, Lokman Hekim University, Ankara, Turkey

9.2 Understanding ACI and MACI

ACI is a cartilage restoration technique that was the first cell-based cartilage treatment to be approved by the Food and Drug Administration (FDA) [4], particularly for the knee joint. The procedure involves three stages: the isolation of autologous chondrocytes from surgically harvested articular hyaline cartilage in the non-load-bearing region of the joint, in vitro cultivation of chondrocytes for approximately 6–8 weeks, and implantation of these chondrocytes into the full-thickness articular cartilage lesion.

ACI was first reported clinically in 1994 by Brittberg et al. [5]. This initial study demonstrated satisfactory results for isolated femoral condyle lesions in the midterm. Over time, there have been technological advancements leading to developments in the technique and practice of ACI. With the progression of bioengineering technology, it became possible to embed cultivated chondrocytes into biodegradable matrices, which are used as scaffolds for cell growth and proliferation. This evolved technique is known as MACI, and it was approved by the FDA in 2016 [6] (Chap. 21; Fig. 21.10).

M. E. Erdil et al. (eds.), *Current Concept in Cartilage Treatment*,
https://doi.org/10.1007/978-3-032-27099-3_9

In vitro studies have presented conflicting evidence on the differentiation of cultured cells into fibroblasts and the extent to which the new tissue formed through in vivo chondrocyte implantation resembles native hyaline cartilage [7–10]. Chondrocyte implantation typically results in tissue that is more similar to hyaline cartilage compared to that produced by bone marrow stimulation techniques applied to the cartilage defect area. ACI and MACI do not have some of the disadvantages associated with other techniques such as osteochondral autografts and mosaicplasty, which include a limited amount of obtainable tissue (rendering them unsuitable for large cartilage lesions) and donor site morbidity.

9.3 Indications

- ICRS grade 3 and 4 lesions
- Full-thickness chondral defects with intact subchondral bone (without subchondral cysts and bone edema)
- Deeper, but peripherally contained lesions, which may require simultaneous bone grafting
- Defects larger than 2 cm^2
- Joints without osteoarthritis or with minimal degenerative changes
- Patients with concomitant lesions in the same joint (such as meniscal problems, instability, and malalignment) without treatment, necessitating that such lesions be treated simultaneously with the cartilage lesion or in a staged manner
- Cartilage lesions that have failed previous treatments (such as mosaicplasty and microfracture)
- Patients between the ages of 15 and 55

Contraindications for ACI include severe osteoarthritis, obesity (with a body mass index greater than 35), infection, inflammatory joint disease, and noncompliance [11]. A kissing lesion in the joint is also a contraindication, except for patellofemoral chondral lesions.

9.4 The Technique

Both ACI and MACI have evolved since they were first applied. Initially, the product of chondrocyte culture was a single-layer structure, which supported cell dedifferentiation into fibroblast-like cells. This led to a decrease in the production of proteins specific to articular cartilage by the cells. Consequently, three-dimensional cell cultures have been developed, as they retain chondrogenic potential and have lower dedifferentiation rates compared to single-layer cultures [12].

In ACI, the chondrocyte-implanted lesion is covered with a periosteal flap, which is sutured water-tight to the surrounding healthy cartilage to ensure the liquid chondrocyte layer remains at the graft site; this is known as first-generation ACI. Due to issues with the periosteal flap such as delamination, hypertrophy, and donor site morbidity, a collagen membrane was developed as an alternative covering for the chondrocyte-implanted defect. This technique, known as c-ACI or second-generation ACI, still could not entirely prevent the leakage of implanted chondrocytes (Figs. 9.1, 9.2, 9.3 and 9.4).

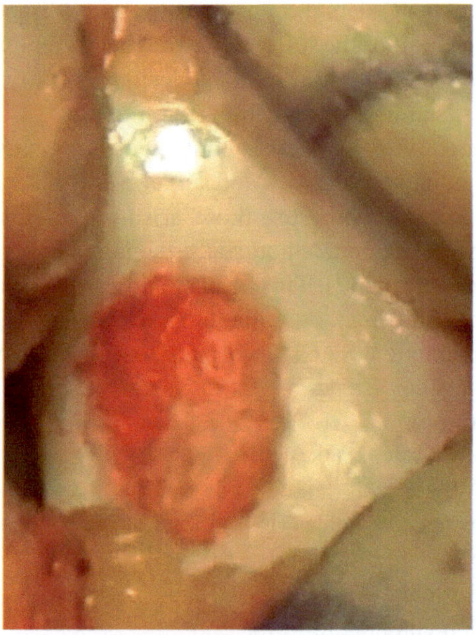

Fig. 9.1 The chondral lesion at the medial femoral condyle is prepared for second-generation ACI application

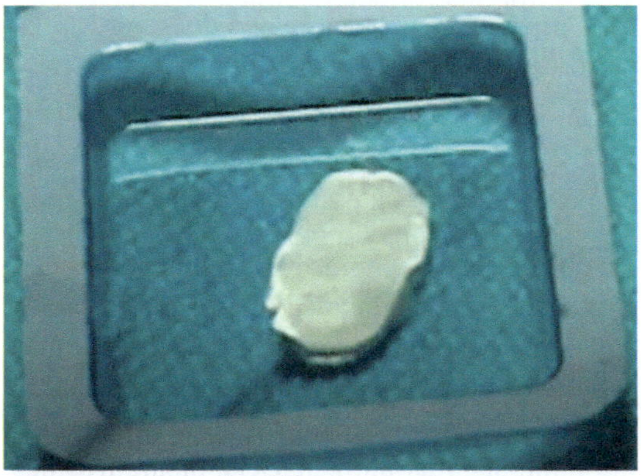

Fig. 9.2 The collagen membrane is adjusted according to the size of the lesion

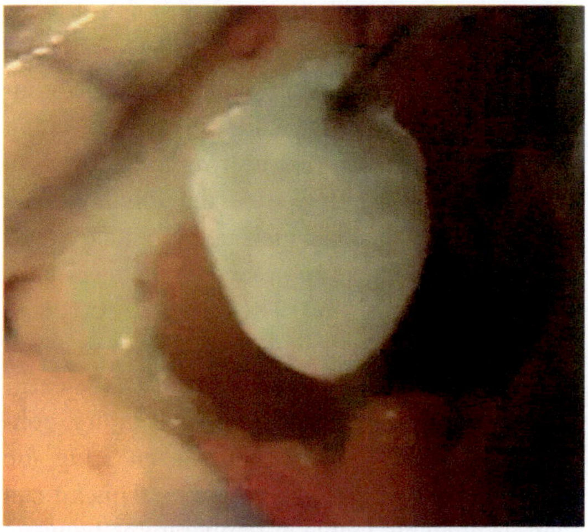

Fig. 9.3 The collagen membrane is placed over the lesion filled with cultivated autologous chondrocytes

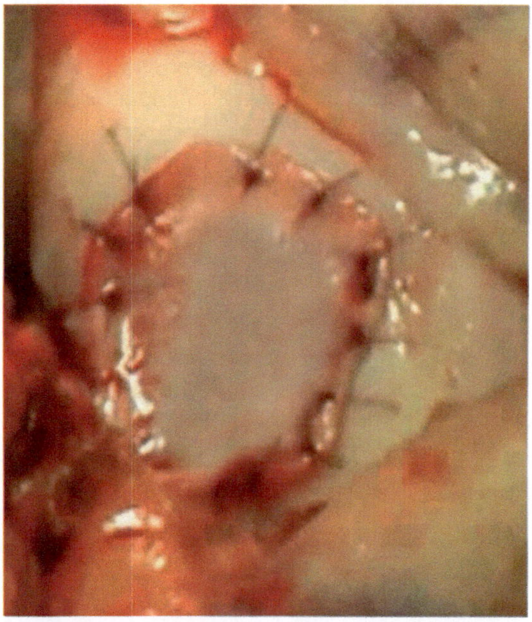

Fig. 9.4 The collagen membrane is secured with absorbable sutures

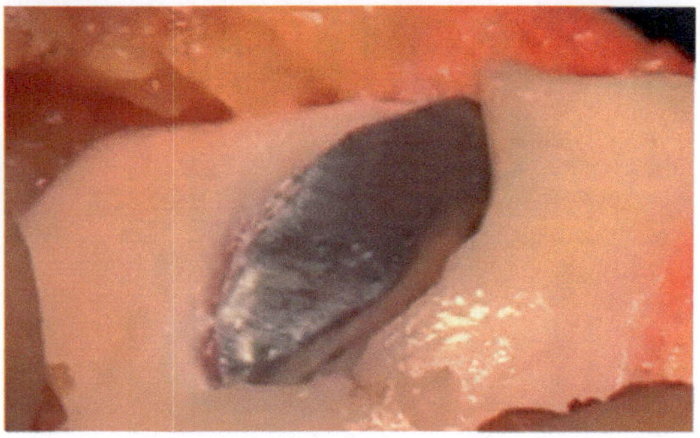

Fig. 9.5 Templating the chondral lesion at the patella is done to determine the dimensions and shape of the scaffold

ACI has certain drawbacks including the need for arthrotomy, donor site morbidity from the periosteal flap, technical difficulties in suturing the periosteum or collagen membrane to surrounding cartilage, and complications such as arthrofibrosis, periosteal hypertrophy, and graft deterioration. To address these issues, third-generation ACI was developed. This approach utilizes biodegradable synthetic membranes or matrices as scaffolds to retain the expanded chondrocytes within the chondral defect. Chondrocytes are seeded into these scaffolds, which can adhere to the chondral lesion without the need for suturing (Figs. 9.5, 9.6 and 9.7). These three-dimensional scaffolds are biodegradable and can be composed of collagen, synthetic polymers, or a demineralized bone matrix with varying mechanical properties. The polymers might include proteins, polyglycolic acid, polylactic acid, or hyaluronic acid. The scaffold is designed with a porous structure to increase the surface area, promoting adhesion and integration with the recipient tissue. It should also have sufficient strength to protect the chondrocytes from mechanical forces until new tissue forms and the scaffold biodegrades [12–14].

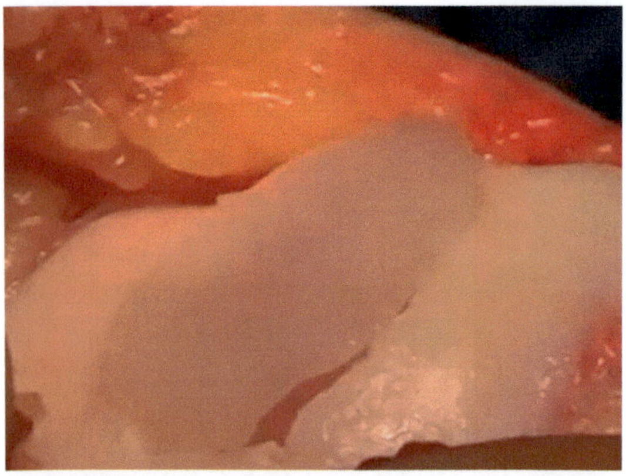

Fig. 9.6 The scaffold containing cultivated autologous chondrocytes is placed into the chondral lesion

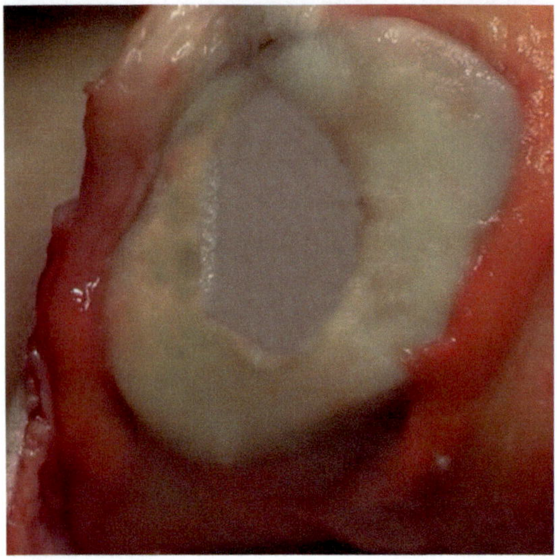

Fig. 9.7 The scaffold is sealed with fibrin glue (no suturing)

MACI, on the other hand, utilizes a resorbable type I/III porcine collagen membrane matrix to deliver the cells, which simplifies surgical implantation [15]. Unlike previous generations of ACI, in MACI the chondrocytes are directly applied to the membrane during manufacturing. Then the membrane can be affixed with fibrin glue or positioned through a press fit. This mitigates problems associated with periosteal hypertrophy and delamination. MACI is associated with lower complication rates than ACI, and it is considered more convenient, less painful, and has a shorter procedure time because it can be performed arthroscopically and does not involve periosteal suturing or donor site morbidity.

9.4.1 Cartilage Harvesting

An arthroscopic technique is employed to secure a full-thickness articular cartilage sample, preferably from the upper and lateral part of the intercondylar notch. However, cartilage can also be harvested from other non-load-bearing regions of the joint, such as the periphery of the trochlea. Typically, around 200 mg articular cartilage tissue is collected [16]. One of the benefits of arthroscopy is that it allows for an assessment of the articular cartilage and other joint structures such as the meniscus and ligaments. This enables comprehensive treatment planning to be conducted in stages. For MACI, cartilage harvesting can occur from non-load-bearing areas or from around the damaged area of the joint with an osteochondral lesion, which helps reduce donor site morbidity. Standard or ring curettes are used for cartilage harvesting. The harvested cartilage is placed into a cartilage biopsy transport kit, a transport container designed to protect the cartilage from physical damage, thermal injury, contamination, and chemical agents, ensuring the vitality and durability of the biopsy. This kit can keep its contents viable at temperatures between 2 and 37 °C for up to 3 days, following cold chain rules until it reaches the lab for further processing. Blood samples taken at the time of biopsy are also included in the kit and tested for infectious agents such as HIV-1, HIV-2, hepatitis B, hepatitis C, and *Treponema palladium*.

9.4.2 Cell Cultivation

The harvested cartilage is processed in a lab to isolate autologous chondrocytes. The process of chondrocyte separation involves the use of special enzymes to degrade the extracellular matrix, releasing the cells, which are then cultivated in a medium containing growth factors. The number of cultured chondrocytes should reach a certain threshold before the chondrocyte implantation surgery can take place. If the initial expansion does not produce a sufficient cell count for the matrix scaffold, a second expansion culture is pursued. If the chondrocyte implantation is planned for a later date, the cultured cells are cryopreserved. This is also done to control the number of population doublings during the production of MACI. The number of membranes needed and the required cell passage cycles for inoculation are determined by the size of the defect. After the final passage, the cells are counted and condensed by centrifugation. The recommended cell concentration for a MACI implant is 0.5–1 million cells/cm^2 of the defect, a dosage that remains the same for all patients, regardless of age [17]. Then the membrane is rinsed with a serum-free, antibiotic-free transport medium. A strip is cut from the membrane for release testing. Once the final product is confirmed to be intact, it is aseptically transferred, cell-side up, into the primary transport container, where it is covered with transport medium. Then the final product is sent to the hospital for implantation. The final MACI product requires no thawing, reconstitution, dilution, resuspension, or rinsing steps before use.

9.4.3 Chondrocyte Implantation

A surgical plan is formulated by integrating radiological findings obtained prior to surgery with arthroscopic observations made during the cartilage harvesting stage. This plan includes the incision, chondrocyte implantation, and any supplementary surgical interventions, such as realignment procedures or ligament and meniscal treatments. During the procedure, the lesion is meticulously inspected, and its boundaries are identified. It is imperative to ensure that the cartilage lesion has clearly defined borders. Any damaged cartilage within these boundaries is carefully excised down to the subchondral bone using ring curettes. While performing this, it is critical not to inflict any damage to the subchondral bone. However, if the subchondral bone is already marginally compromised, debridement is required to expose healthy bone, which may necessitate support through an autologous bone graft.

The dimensions of the borders of the cartilage defect are assessed using aluminum foil to create a template. In first- and second-generation ACI, a periosteal flap or collagen membrane is tailored according to this template. Then it is sutured to the area of the defect where cultured chondrocytes are introduced, followed by the application of fibrin sealant. By contrast, for MACI, a scaffold matrix impregnated with chondrocytes is fashioned based on the template, positioned within the defect, and secured with fibrin sealant. In addition, MACI affords the flexibility of employing a mini-open or arthroscopic technique at this juncture, which is considered an advantage over ACI.

In MACI, the membrane matrix includes a conducive biological milieu that allows chondrocytes to adhere and integrate into the collagen fibers. The implanted chondrocytes synthesize proteoglycans and type II collagen, indicative of active cellular function. In this setting, chondrocytes within the matrix demonstrate the capacity to redifferentiate and progressively migrate from the fibrin adhesive to the healthy subchondral bone in the host. Moreover, chondrocytes are capable of maturing and migrating from the matrix to the subchondral bone, fostering a setting that is favorable for the proliferation and development of immature mesenchymal and chondral cells, ultimately culminating in the formation of healthy hyaline cartilage [18].

9.5 Rehabilitation

The rehabilitation process plays a crucial role in ensuring the regeneration of healthy cartilage and the restoration of normal joint function. The objectives of the rehabilitation program include mitigating postoperative pain, reducing swelling, preserving range of motion in the joint, and maintaining the vitality and endurance of the implanted chondrocytes.

For 6 weeks following the surgery, the joint is immobilized using a splint or brace while the patient is in a standing position or at rest. During this time, patients are encouraged to move around with the assistance of crutches or a walker, initially non-weight-bearing for 2 weeks, followed by partial weight-bearing (approximately 10–20 kg) for the subsequent 4 weeks. Concurrently, patients are guided through a regimen of early range-of-motion exercises, as well as isotonic and isometric exercises. The application of a continuous passive motion (CPM) device is also incorporated, with the range of motion incrementally increased; initially from 0° to 60° for the first 4 weeks and subsequently from 0° to 90° over the next 2 weeks.

Post the 6-week mark, patients are permitted to progressively bear weight as per their tolerance levels. Full weight-bearing should be initiated within this 2-week window. At the same time, progression into strengthening exercises, closed-chain exercises, and proprioceptive exercises is recommended. Notably, for chondral lesions of the patella, immediate weight-bearing is allowed [19].

For athletes, training and aerobic exercises can be cautiously reintroduced at 12 weeks post-surgery, with a gradual increase in intensity. Jogging can commence at 16 weeks, and the training load can be escalated over a period extending up to 24 weeks. Thereafter, slalom movements and high-intensity running can be gradually integrated into the training regimen. Although the general timeline for return to sports activities is estimated at 1 year, this period may vary based on individual healing characteristics, as well as the quality of bioengineering products and chondrocyte culture [20].

9.6 Discussion

Treatment options for articular cartilage lesions include microfractures, mosaicplasty, ACI, and MACI. The selection of a suitable treatment approach is influenced by various factors such as the location, size, and extent of a lesion; the patient's activity level; as well as the availability of resources and technology. ACI, as a regenerative technique, has evolved over time, giving rise to MACI. It is anticipated that MACI will continue to progress, establishing a foundation for more reliable and efficacious tissue engineering-based regenerative therapies.

First-generation ACI is associated with satisfactory clinical outcomes in terms of patient contentment, alleviation of pain, and enhancement in knee functionality. However, it is noteworthy that complete restoration of knee function remains elusive [21].

Ogura et al. [22] presented long-term findings of patients who underwent ACI. They reported a 20-year survival rate of 63% in a sample of 24 knees. Among the 15 knees with preserved grafts, significant improvements were observed in all clinical scores, except the WOMAC subscore for stiffness and the SF-36 mental component summary score, and these improvements were sustained up to 20 years post-surgery. A striking 93% of these patients rated the knee-specific outcomes as good or excellent. Among the 24 knees, outcomes for 9 were deemed failures, including 5 that underwent revision ACI and 4 that were converted into arthroplasty at an average of 1.7 and 5.9 years, respectively. Overall, 79% of patients retained their native knee at the 20-year mark, expressing satisfaction with the results [22].

An issue that emerged among patients undergoing p-ACI was the occurrence of hypertrophied grafts. Gooding et al. [23] revealed that a significant proportion of the patients in their study required shaving of a hypertrophied graft. Consequently, the study concluded that employing periosteum as a covering for retaining chondrocytes within an osteochondral defect does not confer any advantage. This finding advocates for the utilization of alternative covers, such as a manufactured type I/III collagen membrane [23].

Bartlett et al. [24] published a randomized controlled trial that compared the short-term outcomes of patients treated with c-ACI and MACI for knee cartilage lesions. Both treatments led to improvements in clinical scores 1 year post-treatment. Arthroscopic evaluations conducted after 1 year indicated good to excellent International Cartilage Repair Society scores in 79.2% of ACI-C patients and 66.6% of MACI patients. Hyaline-like cartilage or a combination of hyaline-like cartilage with fibrocartilage was observed in 43.9% of ACI-C biopsies and 36.4% of MACI biopsies after 1 year. The incidence of graft hypertrophy was 9% in the ACI-C group and 6% in the MACI group. The reoperation rate stood at 9% for both groups [24].

Another notable study was a single-center prospective evaluation that compared the long-term results of first-generation ACI with the second-generation c-ACI technique. One of the key findings was the long-term reliability of the ACI technique, which exhibited excellent clinical outcomes. Interestingly, no significant differences were observed between the first and second generations of the technique. The study also revealed that clinical outcomes were notably better for defects in the femoral condyles, but these outcomes were influenced by age, with less favorable results in patients over 30 years old. The study concluded that ACI is a robust technique for treating chondral and osteochondral lesions in the knee across a diverse population with respect to age, sex, and activity levels, exhibiting promising results even in the long term [25]. In contrast, another investigation reported superior clinical long-term outcomes for second-generation ACI, which utilizes a collagen membrane in conjunction with autologous chondrocytes, compared to first-generation ACI. This led to the recommendation of favoring second-generation ACI [26].

In a 10-year study that evaluated the outcomes of MACI treatment in 16 patients with knee chondral injuries, significant improvements were observed in three outcome measures. This suggested that MACI could be a viable treatment option for localized cartilage defects in the knee [27]. Supporting these findings, Gille et al. [28] reported significantly improved results on three functional scores 15 years after MACI treatment, which further validates MACI as a suitable treatment for localized cartilage defects in the knee [28].

Long-term results were published in a study by Lenz et al. [29] on talus chondral lesions undergoing MACI surgery. They found a significant improvement in mean AOFAS score from 60 preoperatively to a mean of 84 at 12 years postoperatively [29].

In a randomized controlled study by Barié et al. [30], long-term results of patients who underwent ACI and MACI were compared. The long-term results suggested that first- and third-generation ACI methods were equally effective treatments for isolated full-thickness cartilage defects of the knee. With the number of participants available, no significant difference was noted between MACI and ACI at any time point [30].

A systematic review that focused on randomized controlled trials found that, at short-term follow-up, third-generation ACI demonstrated a lower failure rate and greater improvement in patient-reported outcomes than microfracture treatment for focal cartilage defects in the knee joint [31].

Conversely, another study, based on long-term follow-up evaluations, compared ACI and microfracture techniques and found no significant differences in clinical scoring systems. At the 15-year evaluation, there were 17 failures in the ACI group compared to 13 in the microfracture group. Interestingly, more total knee replacements were needed in the ACI group than in the microfracture group (6 compared to 3). However, patients who did not experience failure, in both groups, showed significant improvements in clinical scores relative to baseline across short, medium, and long-term evaluations. This study raised concerns regarding the efficacy of these procedures in delaying the progression of osteoarthritis and preventing subsequent surgeries [32].

A systematic review that evaluated various treatment modalities concluded that restorative cartilage procedures, such as c-ACI or MACI and osteochondral autograft transplantation (OAT), are associated with superior long-term clinical outcomes, including lower complication and failure rates, compared to reparative techniques such as microfracture. Furthermore, among the restorative procedures, OAT appeared to be less effective than ACI, particularly for larger defects over extended follow-up periods [33].

Migliorini et al. [34] conducted an extensive systematic review involving data from 184 published articles, including 8905 procedures concerning reparative and regenerative treatment techniques for chondral lesions. The review found that female sex exhibited a moderate positive association with the visual analog scale at the final follow-up. Patient age showed a negative association with the American Orthopaedic Foot and Ankle Score and Lysholm Knee Scoring Scale. Body mass index had a strong association with graft hypertrophy. Intriguingly, the study concluded that clinical outcomes were primarily associated with patients' performance status before surgery, while cartilage defect size did not show any association with surgical outcomes. Furthermore, lesion size and duration of symptoms did not present any correlation with surgical outcomes [34].

Beck et al. [35] investigated the histological and immunohistochemical characteristics of repair tissue in chondral lesions of patients who underwent MACI surgery. They found that the predominant tissue in biopsies taken at the time of revision surgery or total joint arthroplasty was of a fibrocartilaginous nature. The repair tissue in MACI grafts was predominantly fibrocartilage and was histologically different from healthy cartilage. Notably, tissue morphology and overall assessment scores were highest for ankle grafts and lowest for patellar grafts, with significant differences between them. Furthermore, the repair tissue from ankle specimens predominantly consisted of hyaline-like cartilage and fibrocartilage, whereas all patellar grafts mainly contained fibrous tissue. The study emphasized the variation in repair tissue composition and characteristics depending on the anatomical location [35].

9.7 Future Directions

Moving forward, research efforts can focus on the production of chondrocytes from mesenchymal or multipotent stem cells (sourced from blood, adipose tissue, and so forth) through the utilization of suitable growth factors in appropriate culture media.

Moreover, current techniques predominantly rely on cell culture, which poses challenges in terms of cost-effectiveness and necessitates two-step surgeries. The ideal surgical treatment should aim for a single-stage procedure, preferably via an arthroscopic approach.

In the pursuit to circumvent the challenges associated with ex vivo chondrocyte culture and expansion in scaffolds, there is an evolving interest in cell-free implants capable of inducing orderly and durable tissue regeneration. Such implants are being extensively investigated in animal studies and are gradually garnering attention in clinical practice. These novel and emerging technologies signify an exhilarating frontier in regenerative treatments, the development and progress of which will be captivating to monitor in the future.

References

1. Mansour JM. Biomechanics of cartilage (Chapter 5). In: Oatis C, editor. Kinesiology: the mechanics and pathomechanics of human movement. Philadelphia, PA: Lippincott Williams and Wilkins; 2003. p. 66–79.
2. Glyn-Jones S, Palmer AJR, Agricola R, Price AJ, Vincent TL, Weinans H, Carr AJ. Seminar "osteoarthritis". Lancet. 2015;386(9991):25–31, pages 376–387.
3. Kon E, Filardo G, Di Martino A, Marcacci M. ACI and MACI. Review. J Knee Surg. 2012;25(1):17–22. https://doi.org/10.1055/s-0031-1299651.
4. https://www.fda.gov/media/165428/download.
5. Brittberg M, Lindahl A, Nilsson A, Ohlsson C, Isaksson O, Peterson L. Treatment of deep cartilage defects in the knee with autologous chondrocyte transplantation. N Engl J Med. 1994;331(14):889–95. https://doi.org/10.1056/NEJM199410063311401.
6. https://www.fda.gov/news-events/press-announcements/fda-approves-first-autologous-cellularized-scaffold-repair-cartilage-defects-knee#:~:text=Press%20Announcements-,FDA%20approves%20first%20autologous%20cellularized%20scaffold%20for%20the,cartilage%20defects%20of%20the%20knee&text=The%20U.S.%20Food%20and%20Drug,the%20knee%20in%20adult%20patients.
7. Ghosh S, Scott AK, Seelbinder B, Barthold JE, St. Martin BM, Kaonis S, Schneider SE, Henderson JT, Neu CP. Dedifferentiation alters chondrocyte nuclear mechanics during in vitro culture and expansion. Biophys J. 2022;121(1):131–41. https://doi.org/10.1016/j.bpj.2021.11.018.
8. Chen Y, Yu Y, Wen Y, Chen J, Lin J, Sheng Z, Zhou W, Sun H, An C, Chen J, Wu W, Teng C, Wei W, Ouyang H. A high-resolution route map reveals distinct stages of chondrocyte dedifferentiation

for cartilage regeneration. Bone Res. 2022;10:38. https://doi.org/10.1038/s41413-022-00209-w.
9. Yu L, Lin Y, Yan M, Li T, Wu EY, Zimmel K, Qureshi O, Falck A, Sherman KM, Huggins SS, Hurtado DO, Suva LJ, Gaddy D, Cai J, Brunauer R. Hyaline cartilage differentiation of fibroblasts in regeneration and regenerative medicine. Development. 2022;149(2):dev200249. https://doi.org/10.1242/dev.200249.
10. Chen J-L, Duan L, Zhu W, Xiong J, Wang D. Extracellular matrix production in vitro in cartilage tissue engineering. J Transl Med. 2014;12:88. https://doi.org/10.1186/1479-5876-12-88.
11. Wood D, Janes GC. Chapter 9E—Autologous chondrocyte implantation: matrix-induced autologous chondrocyte implantation (MACI). In: Cartilage surgery; 2011. P. 161–73. https://doi.org/10.1016/B978-1-4377-0878-3.10016-6.
12. Thorp H, Kim K, Kondo M, Maak T, Grainger DW, Okano T. Trends in articular cartilage tissue engineering: 3D mesenchymal stem cell sheets as candidates for engineered hyaline-like cartilage. Cells. 2021;10(3):643. https://doi.org/10.3390/cells10030643.
13. Li YY, Choy TH, Ho FC, Chan PB. Scaffold composition affects cytoskeleton organization, cell-matrix interaction and the cellular fate of human mesenchymal stem cells upon chondrogenic differentiation. Biomaterials. 2015;52:208–20. https://doi.org/10.1016/j.biomaterials.2015.02.037.
14. Benders KEM, van Weeren PR, Badylak SF, Saris DBF, Dhert W, Malda J. Extracellular matrix scaffolds for cartilage and bone regeneration. Trends Biotechnol. 2013;31(3):169–76. https://doi.org/10.1016/j.tibtech.2012.12.004.
15. Huang BJ, Hu JC, Athanasiou KA. Cell-based tissue engineering strategies used in the clinical repair of articular cartilage. Biomaterials. 2016;98:1–22. https://doi.org/10.1016/j.biomaterials.2016.04.018.
16. Hinckel BB, Thomas D, Vellios EE, Hancock KJ, Calcei JG, Sherman SL, Eliasberg CD, Fernandes TL, Farr J, Lattermann C, Gomoll AH. Algorithm for treatment of focal cartilage defects of the knee: classic and new procedures. Cartilage. 2021;13(1 Suppl):473S–95S. https://doi.org/10.1177/1947603521993219.
17. https://www.ema.europa.eu/en/documents/assessment-report/maci-epar-public-assessment-report_en.pdf.
18. Guo X, Xi L, Yu M, Fan Z, Wang W, Ju A, Liang Z, Zhou G, Ren W. Regeneration of articular cartilage defects: therapeutic strategies and perspectives. J Tissue Eng. 2023;14:20417314231164765. https://doi.org/10.1177/20417314231164765.
19. Flanigan DC, Sherman SL, Chilelli B, Gersoff W, Jones D, Lee CA, Toth A, Cramer C, Zaporojan V, Carey J. Consensus on rehabilitation guidelines among orthopedic surgeons in the United States following use of third-generation articular cartilage repair (MACI) for treatment of knee cartilage lesions. Cartilage. 2021;13(1 Suppl):1782S–90S. https://doi.org/10.1177/1947603520968876.
20. Toyooka S, Moatshe G, Persson A, Engebretsen L. Return to pivoting sports after cartilage repair surgery of the knee: a scoping review. Cartilage. 2023;14(1):17–25. https://doi.org/10.1177/19476035221141416.
21. Niemeyer P, Porichis S, Steinwachs M, Christoph E, Kreuz PC, Schmal H, Uhl M, Ghanem N, Südkamp NP, Salzmann G. Long-term outcomes after first-generation autologous chondrocyte implantation for cartilage defects of the knee. Am J Sports Med. 2014;42(1):150–7. https://doi.org/10.1177/0363546513506593.
22. Ogura T, Mosier BA, Bryant T, Minas T. A 20-year follow-up after first-generation autologous chondrocyte implantation. Am J Sports Med. 2017;45(12):2751–61. https://doi.org/10.1177/0363546517716631.
23. Gooding CR, Bartlett W, Bentley G, Skinner JA, Carrington R, Flanagan A. A prospective, randomised study comparing two techniques of autologous chondrocyte implantation for osteochondral defects in the knee: periosteum covered versus type I/III collagen covered. Knee. 2006;13(3):203–10. https://doi.org/10.1016/j.knee.2006.02.011.
24. Bartlett W, Skinner JA, Gooding CR, Carrington RWJ, Flanagan AM, Briggs TWR, Bentley G. Autologous chondrocyte implantation versus matrix-induced autologous chondrocyte implantation for osteochondral defects of the knee: a prospective, randomised study. Clinical trial. J Bone Joint Surg Br. 2005;87(5):640–5. https://doi.org/10.1302/0301-620X.87B5.15905.
25. Berruto M, Ferrua P, Pasqualotto S, Uboldi F, Maione A, Tradati D, Usellini E. Long-term follow-up evaluation of autologous chondrocyte implantation for symptomatic cartilage lesions of the knee: a single-centre prospective study. Injury. 2017;48(10):2230–4. https://doi.org/10.1016/j.injury.2017.08.005.
26. Niemeyer P, Salzmann G, Feucht M, Pestka J, Porichis S, Ogon P, Südkamp N, Schmal H. First-generation versus second-generation autologous chondrocyte implantation for treatment of cartilage defects of the knee: a matched-pair analysis on long-term clinical outcome. Int Orthop. 2014;38(10):2065–70. https://doi.org/10.1007/s00264-014-2368-0.
27. Aldrian S, Zak L, Wondrasch B, Albrecht C, Stelzeneder B, Binder H, Kovar F, Trattnig S, Marlovits S. Clinical and radiological long-term outcomes after matrix-induced autologous chondrocyte transplantation: a prospective follow-up at a minimum of 10 years. Am J Sports Med. 2014;42(11):2680–8. https://doi.org/10.1177/0363546514548160.
28. Gille J, Behrens P, Schulz AP, Oheim R, Kienast B. Matrix-associated autologous chondrocyte implantation: a clinical follow-up at 15 years. Cartilage. 2016;7(4):309–15. https://doi.org/10.1177/1947603516638901.

29. Lenz CG, Tan S, Carey AL, Ang K, Schneider T. Matrix-induced autologous chondrocyte implantation (MACI) grafting for osteochondral lesions of the talus. Foot Ankle Int. 2020;41(9):1099–105. https://doi.org/10.1177/1071100720935110.
30. Barié A, Kruck P, Sorbi R, Rehnitz C, Oberle D, Walker T, Zeifang F, Moradi B. Prospective long-term follow-up of autologous chondrocyte implantation with periosteum versus matrix-associated autologous chondrocyte implantation. Am J Sports Med. 2020;48(9):2230–41. https://doi.org/10.1177/0363546520928337.
31. Dhillon J, Decilveo AP, Kraeutler MJ, Belk JW, McCulloch PC, Scillia AJ. Third-generation autologous chondrocyte implantation (cells cultured within collagen membrane) is superior to microfracture for focal chondral defects of the knee joint: systematic review and meta-analysis. Arthroscopy. 2022;38(8):2579–86. https://doi.org/10.1016/j.arthro.2022.02.011.
32. Knutsen G, Drogset JO, Engebretsen L, Grøntvedt T, Ludvigsen TC, Løken S, Solheim E, Strand T, Johansen O. A randomized multicenter trial comparing autologous chondrocyte implantation with microfracture: long-term follow-up at 14 to 15 years. J Bone Joint Surg Am. 2016;98(16):1332–9. https://doi.org/10.2106/JBJS.15.01208.
33. Angele P, Zellner J, Schröter S, Flechtenmacher J, Fritz J, Niemeyer P. Biological reconstruction of localized full-thickness cartilage defects of the knee: a systematic review of level 1 studies with a minimum follow-up of 5 years. Cartilage. 2022;13(4):5–18. https://doi.org/10.1177/19476035221129571.
34. Migliorini F, Maffulli N, Eschweiler J, Götze C, Hildebrand F, Betsch M. Prognostic factors for the management of chondral defects of the knee and ankle joint: a systematic review. Eur J Trauma Emerg Surg. 2023;49(2):723–45. https://doi.org/10.1007/s00068-022-02155-y.
35. Beck A, Wood D, Vertullo CJ, Ebert J, Janes G, Sullivan M, Zheng M-H. Morphological assessment of MACI grafts in patients with revision surgery and total joint arthroplasty. Cartilage. 2021;13(1 Suppl):526S–39S. https://doi.org/10.1177/1947603519890754.

Third-Generation GACI (Gel-Based Autologous Chondrocyte Implantation)

10

Niyazi Ercan, Sancar Alp Ovalı, and Ramazan Akmeşe

10.1 Introduction

Chondral defects of the knee are common and can significantly affect quality of life. Cartilage tissues that are damaged have a limited inherent ability to self-repair [1]. Research indicates that up to 61%–66% of patients undergoing knee arthroscopy have chondral or osteochondral lesions [2, 3]. Determining the true incidence and prevalence is challenging, as many defects are asymptomatic, but if untreated, these defects can progress to osteoarthritis [4, 5].

Various approaches have been developed to address lesions, including abrasion arthroplasty and microfracture, which promote healing by activating the subchondral bone. However, despite these techniques' simplicity, their long-term outcomes have been unsatisfactory because the regenerated fibrocartilage tissue possesses inferior mechanical properties [6, 7]. Autologous chondrocyte implantation (ACI) has proven to be an effective treatment for significant knee articular cartilage lesions, facilitating hyaline-rich cartilage repair [8–12]. This procedure involves collecting chondrocytes from a non-weight-bearing region of the knee's articular cartilage and expanding them ex vivo. ACI has demonstrated advantages in pain reduction, quality of life enhancement, and improved functional scores for patients with symptomatic chondral defects sized 2–9 cm^2, with benefits lasting up to 10–13 years [13, 14].

The evolution of ACI has seen significant advancements from the first-generation to the third-generation procedures, addressing several technical limitations and improving clinical outcomes [15, 16]. First-generation ACI utilized a periosteal patch to create a chondrogenic chamber over the cartilage defect, within which cultured chondrocytes were implanted [17]. This method encountered numerous issues such as the complexity of periosteal suturing and periosteal hypertrophy. These challenges prompted the development of second-generation techniques, which replaced the periosteum with a collagen membrane [18, 19]. While this approach resolved some of the first-generation issues, it remained difficult to suture the collagen membrane, particularly in less accessible lesion locations. Additionally, the meticulous attention required for watertight sealing to prevent leakage of the implanted chondrocytes and the need for an extended surgical incision for better visualization further complicated the procedure and prolonged

N. Ercan
Department of Orthopedics and Traumatology, Yüksek İhtisas University, Ankara, Turkey

S. A. Ovalı
Department of Orthopedics and Traumatology, Zonguldak Bülent Ecevit University, Zonguldak, Turkey

R. Akmeşe (✉)
Department of Orthopedics and Traumatology, Private Çankaya Hospital, Ankara, Turkey

M. E. Erdil et al. (eds.), *Current Concept in Cartilage Treatment*,
https://doi.org/10.1007/978-3-032-27099-3_10

operative time. To overcome these hurdles, third-generation ACI techniques introduced the use of matrices as scaffolds for chondrocyte implantation [17, 20, 21]. Among these, Gel-type ACI (GACI) and matrix-induced ACI (MACI) are notable advancements. GACI employs a fibrin gel scaffold that solidifies within minutes, facilitating easier application in three-dimensional spaces regardless of lesion size, depth, or shape [22–24]. This method eliminates the need for suturing, as the membrane-seeded cultured chondrocytes are prepared in the laboratory and directly implanted during surgery. The solidification of the glue into a gel ensures that the application is efficient and adaptable, addressing issues related to the complexity and time-consuming nature of earlier techniques.

This section aims to discuss the indications, contraindications, decision-making, surgical techniques, and post-operative management of gel-based ACI.

10.2 Indications and Contraindications

ACI is the preferred treatment option when certain conditions are met. Ideal candidates are symptomatic patients typically aged between 14 and 55 years. However, in physiologically active patients with localized lesions and healthy margins, consideration can be given to those slightly older, while younger patients are not strictly excluded. The presence of a full-thickness cartilage defect, classified as ICRS grade III or IV, or osteochondritis dissecans (OCD) stage III or IV, is necessary. The defect should preferably be larger than 2 cm^2 since smaller lesions may be treated effectively with less invasive techniques. Though there is no upper limit to defect size, larger lesions generally yield poorer outcomes compared to mid-sized ones. Suitable defects may be purely chondral or osteochondral with reconstructed subchondral bone. In the knee joint, defects localized to the femoral condyles, patella, trochlea, or tibial articular surfaces are considered, with the best results typically observed in the femoral condyles. It is essential that the joint has normal or corrected biomechanics, and the patient must be cooperative and committed to the post-operative rehabilitation program. Conversely, ACI should not be attempted if certain contraindications are present. These include altered or untreated abnormal joint biomechanics, such as tibia vara, degenerative joint diseases, inflammatory joint diseases like rheumatoid arthritis, septic joint diseases such as infective arthritis, and metabolic disorders like uric acid crystallopathy. Smoking is a contraindication due to its negative impact on healing. Obesity, defined as a body mass index (BMI) greater than 30, is a relative contraindication unless all other conditions are ideal. Non-cooperative patients are also not suitable candidates. While age over 55 years is generally a contraindication, ACI may still be performed in physiologically active patients with stable and healthy cartilage margins in a single localized chondral defect [25, 26].

10.3 Surgical Technique

ACI is a two-stage procedure that includes culturing chondrocytes in a certified laboratory after the initial surgery. During the first stage, the key steps involve validating clinical findings, addressing any associated injuries or biomechanical issues, and obtaining a cartilage biopsy for chondrocyte culture. Cartilage damage is evaluated thoroughly using ICRS or Outerbridge classifications. For gel-based ACI, a hexagonal osteochondral cylinder is harvested, ensuring it includes full-thickness cartilage. Preferred sites for biopsy are the non-weight-bearing areas of the medial or lateral trochlea above the sulcus terminalis. Hyperextending the knee helps in covering all weight-bearing areas of the femoral condyles with the tibial articular surface. The biopsy sample is then dispatched to the cartilage lab for culturing. The second stage of ACI generally involves an open procedure performed via a mini-arthrotomy. However, experienced surgeons may choose an arthroscopic approach for specific sites, such as the tibial plateau. For medial femoral condyle lesions, a mini medial parapatellar approach parallel to the patellar tendon is recommended, while a mini lateral parapatellar approach is suggested for lateral femoral condyle lesions. For patellofemoral lesions, a limited medial parapatellar approach, starting from the inferior patella, circling the medial patellar margin, and ending near the superior patella, is advised. These approaches can be extended if necessary during surgery. To prepare the lesion, retractors are placed around the soft tissues to fully expose the cartilage defect. The lesion base is cleared of all fibrous tissue and fibrocartilage to reveal raw subchondral bone. Any internal osteophytes or subchondral bone thickening is removed to align with the surrounding subchondral bone plate. If subchondral bone cysts are present, they are cleaned and filled with autogenous bone grafts, converting the procedure to the overlay ACI technique. The margins of the cartilage lesion are shaped using a blade and a sharp ring curette to create beveled edges, which provide stability for the gel-based ACI implant. Any remaining irregular or damaged cartilage is carefully removed with a ring curette or periosteum elevator to ensure that only healthy cartilage surrounds the defect. The size of the prepared defect is documented for future reference and follow-up. Tiny holes may be made in the lesion base to help anchor the ACI implant. For the implantation phase, two 1 mL syringes are used with a "Y" mixing connector. One syringe contains 1 mL of fibrinogen, and the other holds 0.9 mL of cultured chondrocytes mixed with 0.1 mL of thrombin. Each drop from these syringes combines chondrocytes with the fibrinogen-thrombin mixture to form fibrin, creating a three-dimensional, layer-by-layer scaffold on the cartilage defect. The cultured chondrocytes populate this scaffold, creating a multi-layered ACI implant. To ensure the gel remains contained within the defect, it is essential to keep the base level. Any gel that spills out should be promptly removed with a dry gauze sponge. The gel takes 8–10 min to solidify completely [27]. After this period, a thorough inspection is conducted to confirm that the ACI graft completely fills the defect, leaving no gaps or bubbles. A slight elevation of the graft above the surrounding cartilage surface is permissible but should be kept to a minimum. Gentle movements of the knee through flexion and extension are performed three to five times, followed by another inspection to ensure the implant remains securely in place. The area is then washed, and the surgical site is meticulously closed in layers. MRI images of a chondral lesion and the application of the MACI procedure are shown in Figs. 10.1 and 10.2.

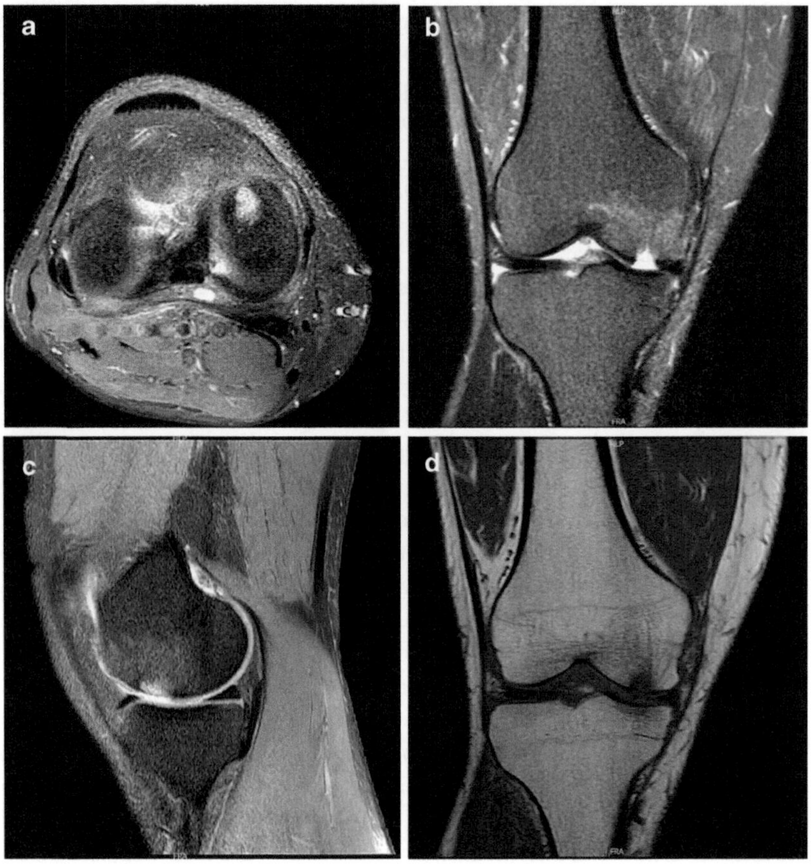

Fig. 10.1 MRI images of the chondral lesion in the medial condyle of the left knee are shown in axial, sagittal, and coronal views, respectively (**a**–**d**)

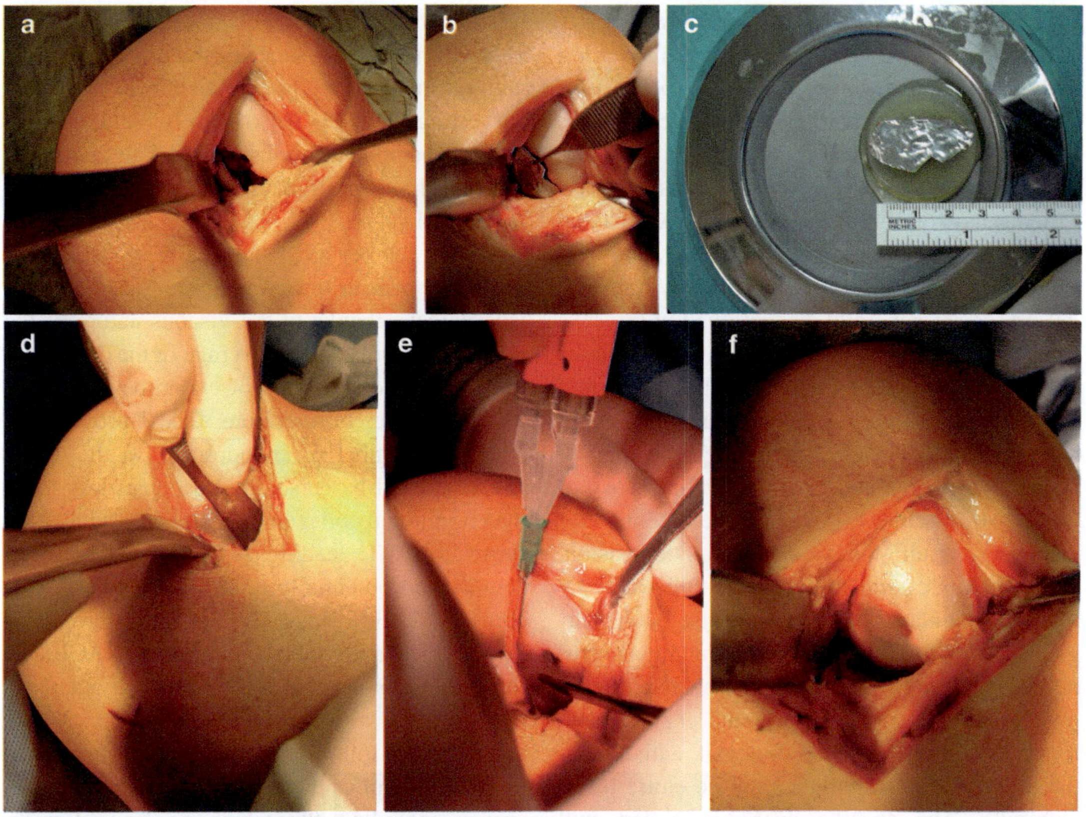

Fig. 10.2 After arthrotomy of the left knee, the cartilage lesion in the medial condyle was revealed after debriding (**a**); the area of the cartilage lesion is measured with a suitable aluminum foil template (**b**); the prepared MACI graft is cut according to the defect size (**c**). The graft is placed in the defective area and fixation is supported with fibrin glue (**d**, **e**). Final image after the graft is placed in the cartilage defect and fixed with fibrin (**f**)

10.4 Postoperative Management

Effective management of pain and inflammation is crucial in the immediate postoperative period following ACI [28]. Key strategies include ice application, compression bandages, and elevation of the limb. These measures help alleviate pain and reduce inflammation, which are essential for a successful recovery. A well-structured rehabilitation program is vital for the long-term success of the ACI procedure. The primary goal is to facilitate the gradual maturation of the repair tissue. Prematurely overloading the graft increases the risk of failure. Therefore, the initial phase of rehabilitation emphasizes achieving a full range of motion (ROM), protecting the graft from mechanical overload, and performing strengthening exercises to support functional gait. Early controlled ROM and weight-bearing exercises are critical for stimulating cellular orientation and chondrocyte development. However, it is important to avoid shear forces, particularly during activities like stair climbing, where maintaining full extension is necessary. Active and active-assisted flexion exercises should begin early to achieve a full ROM by 3–6 weeks unless contraindicated by the surgeon for specific reasons. Once the pain subsides, patients are encouraged to walk. The use of a full-length leg brace is important initially to prevent undue shear forces on the knee. For ACI performed in the tibiofemoral region, non-weight-bearing walking with crutches is recommended, whereas partial weight-bearing with a full-length leg brace locked in full extension is advised for ACI in the patellofemoral region. Smaller defects may permit early weight-bearing within 1–2 weeks, while larger or deeper lesions typically require partial weight-bearing at 2–4 weeks, depending on the surgeon's evaluation. Approximately 2–3 weeks post-surgery, patients may transition to a ROM brace with a dial lock function, increasing the ROM by about 40° per week until full ROM is achieved by 6 weeks. All braces are generally discontinued at 6 weeks if quadriceps strength is sufficient. Continuous passive motion (CPM) machines should be used 6–12 h after surgery and continued for up to 8 weeks. CPM encourages cartilage healing by signaling cells to regenerate into hyaline-like cartilage, while active movements are essential for achieving full flexion and extension. Physiotherapists aim to achieve a full ROM by 3–6 weeks, unless specified otherwise by the surgeon. Both CPM and active movements are crucial, each playing a distinct role in the rehabilitation process. Early static strengthening exercises are introduced to support functional gait, with a gradual progression to strengthening the entire lower extremity. The specific exercises added will depend on the size, location, and containment of the lesion by the surrounding cartilage. The graft site generally becomes firm within 6–9 months, and any sudden shear or extreme loading forces should be avoided until that time [29]. Low-impact activities such as swimming and biking can begin after 12 weeks. Moderate activities like jogging and dancing should be deferred for at least 9 months, and high-impact activities should be postponed until after 1 year to ensure the durability of the repair tissue [30].

10.5 Discussion

GACI has demonstrated its effectiveness in treating large focal cartilage defects in the knee, particularly due to its simplified and less invasive surgical technique. In contrast to conventional ACI, which involves periosteal grafting—a process that requires an additional procedure to harvest the periosteum and meticulous suturing to create a watertight seal—GACI eliminates these complexities. The use of a fibrin-based gel scaffold allows for faster application, as the gel solidifies within minutes, securing the implant in place without the need for large incisions or periosteal harvesting [31, 32]. This not only reduces surgical time but also minimizes the risk of complications such as graft detachment and periosteal hypertrophy.

One of the key advantages of GACI is its ability to conform to the irregular contours of cartilage defects, thanks to the viscous nature of the gel. This ensures better coverage of the defect and a more even distribution of chondrocytes within the lesion site. Furthermore, GACI provides an increased number of chondrocytes at the defect site, as the gel-based scaffold occupies less space than traditional collagen membranes used in other forms of ACI, leading to higher biosynthetic activity and potentially improved long-term outcomes [33, 34]. Short-term studies have confirmed the safety and efficacy of GACI. For instance, Choi et al. [27] analyzed the outcomes of 98 patients with a mean lesion size of 5.23 cm^2 and a mean follow-up of 24.35 months. They observed significant improvements in functional scores, including the telephone Knee Society Score (tKSS), with no major postoperative complications. Similarly, Goyal et al. [35] performed a systematic review of second- and third-generation ACI techniques, concluding that third-generation ACI, including GACI, provides comparable results to first-generation ACI, but with fewer complications and a more straightforward surgical approach. Additionally, Peterson et al. [36] presented long-term data on first-generation ACI, showing that 92% of patients were willing to undergo the procedure again if necessary. However, despite the substantial evidence supporting the long-term benefits of first-generation ACI, there is limited data on the long-term outcomes of third-generation techniques such as GACI. Most studies, including those by Goyal et al. [35] and Pareek et al. [14], have focused on short- to mid-term results, showing that third-generation ACI provides favorable outcomes in terms of cartilage regeneration and functional improvement. Recent studies have further confirmed these outcomes. For instance, a retrospective multicenter study with a mean follow-up of 9.8 years demonstrated significant improvements in both the Lysholm Knee Scoring Scale and the Knee Outcome Sports Activity Scale, along with high MOCART scores indicating successful cartilage repair. The study also reported a low complication and revision rate, with 56.7% of patients returning to sports at the same or higher level [37]. Additionally, a prospective observational study of 25 patients treated with GACI reported substantial functional gains, with significant improvements in both Lysholm and IKDC scores at 24 months. MRI evaluations also showed successful cartilage repair, with no major complications reported, further reinforcing the safety and effectiveness of GACI in the medium term [23]. Moreover, studies such as those by Siebold et al. [38] and Enea et al. [39] have reported promising histological outcomes, with many cases showing the regeneration of hyaline or mixed hyaline-fibrocartilage tissue. These findings suggest that GACI can provide similar cartilage quality to earlier ACI generations, but with fewer complications and a simpler surgical process. Nonetheless, limitations still exist. For example, arthroscopic GACI requires meticulous bleeding control for clear visualization during the application of chondrocytes, which can be challenging in certain areas of the knee, such as the posterior condyle. In these cases, a mini-open arthrotomy may be necessary to achieve the desired results [13]. Despite these limitations, GACI offers significant advantages in terms of surgical ease and patient outcomes. Studies such as those by Kim et al. [40] and Choi et al. [27] have shown that GACI can achieve significant improvements in functional scores and cartilage quality with minimal complications. Furthermore, the use of a fibrin scaffold in GACI provides a 3D construct that promotes effective cell distribution and regeneration, making it an appealing option for patients with large cartilage defects.

10.6 Conclusion

While GACI represents a significant improvement over earlier generations of ACI, particularly in terms of reducing surgical complexity and complications, further research is needed to confirm its long-term effectiveness. The procedure has demonstrated favorable short- and mid-term outcomes, with studies showing improvements in functional scores and cartilage regeneration. However, as the field continues to evolve, long-term studies will be crucial in determining whether GACI can deliver sustained benefits comparable to those seen with first-generation ACI [14, 27, 36].

References

1. Ossendorf C, Kaps C, Kreuz PC, Burmester GR, Sittinger M, Erggelet C. Treatment of posttraumatic and focal osteoarthritic cartilage defects of the knee with autologous polymer-based three-dimensional chondrocyte grafts: 2-year clinical results. Arthritis Res Ther. 2007;9:1–11.
2. Årøen A, Løken S, Heir S, Alvik E, Ekeland A, Granlund OG, et al. Articular cartilage lesions in 993 consecutive knee arthroscopies. Am J Sports Med. 2004;32:211–5.
3. Hjelle K, Solheim E, Strand T, Muri R, Brittberg M. Articular cartilage defects in 1,000 knee arthroscopies. Arthroscopy. 2002;18:730–4.
4. Lefkoe TP, Trafton PG, Ehrlich MG, Walsh WR, Dennehy DT, Barrach H-J, et al. An experimental model of femoral condylar defect leading to osteoarthrosis. J Orthop Trauma. 1993;7:458–67.
5. Messner K, Maletius W. The long-term prognosis for severe damage to weight-bearing cartilage in the knee: a 14-year clinical and radiographic follow-up in 28 young athletes. Acta Orthop Scand. 1996;67:165–8.
6. Oussedik S, Tsitskaris K, Parker D. Treatment of articular cartilage lesions of the knee by microfracture or autologous chondrocyte implantation: a systematic review. Arthroscopy. 2015;31:732–44.
7. Saris DBF, Vanlauwe J, Victor J, Haspl M, Bohnsack M, Fortems Y, et al. Characterized chondrocyte implantation results in better structural repair when treating symptomatic cartilage defects of the knee in a randomized controlled trial versus microfracture. Am J Sports Med. 2009;36:235–46.
8. Wei W, Dai H. Articular cartilage and osteochondral tissue engineering techniques: recent advances and challenges. Bioact Mater. 2021;6:4830–55.
9. Paatela T, Vasara A, Nurmi H, Kautiainen H, Jurvelin JS, Kiviranta I. Biomechanical changes of repair tissue after autologous chondrocyte implantation at long-term follow-up. Cartilage. 2021;13:1085S–91S.
10. Niethammer TR, Altmann D, Holzgruber M, Goller S, Fischer A, Müller PE. Third generation autologous chondrocyte implantation is a good treatment option for athletic persons. Knee Surg Sports Traumatol Arthrosc. 2021;29:1215–23.

11. Kreuz PC, Kalkreuth RH, Niemeyer P, Uhl M, Erggelet C. Long-term clinical and MRI results of matrix-assisted autologous chondrocyte implantation for articular cartilage defects of the knee. Cartilage. 2019;10:305–13.
12. Na Y, Shi Y, Liu W, Jia Y, Kong L, Zhang T, et al. Is implantation of autologous chondrocytes superior to microfracture for articular-cartilage defects of the knee? A systematic review of 5-year follow-up data. Int J Surg. 2019;68:56–62.
13. Beck JJ, Sugimoto D, Micheli L. Sustained results in long-term follow-up of autologous chondrocyte implantation (ACI) for distal femur juvenile osteochondritis dissecans (JOCD). Adv Orthop. 2018;2018:7912975.
14. Pareek A, Carey JL, Reardon PJ, Peterson L, Stuart MJ, Krych AJ. Long-term outcomes after autologous chondrocyte implantation: a systematic review at mean follow-up of 11.4 years. Cartilage. 2016;7:298–308.
15. Goyal D, Keyhani S, Lee EH, Hui JHP. Evidence-based status of microfracture technique: a systematic review of level I and II studies. Arthroscopy. 2013;29:1579–88.
16. Minas T, Ogura T, Bryant T. Autologous chondrocyte implantation. JBJS Essent Surg Tech. 2016;6:e24.
17. Basad E, Ishaque B, Bachmann G, Stürz H, Steinmeyer J. Matrix-induced autologous chondrocyte implantation versus microfracture in the treatment of cartilage defects of the knee: a 2-year randomised study. Knee Surg Sports Traumatol Arthrosc. 2010;18:519–27.
18. Nixon AJ, Sparks HD, Begum L, McDonough S, Scimeca MS, Moran N, et al. Matrix-induced autologous chondrocyte implantation (MACI) using a cell-seeded collagen membrane improves cartilage healing in the equine model. JBJS. 2017;99:1987–98.
19. Haddo O, Mahroof S, Higgs D, David L, Pringle J, Bayliss M, et al. The use of chondrogide membrane in autologous chondrocyte implantation. Knee. 2004;11:51–5.
20. Ebert JR, Schneider A, Fallon M, Wood DJ, Janes GC. A comparison of 2-year outcomes in patients undergoing tibiofemoral or patellofemoral matrix-induced autologous chondrocyte implantation. Am J Sports Med. 2017;45:3243–53.
21. Gille J, Behrens P, Schulz AP, Oheim R, Kienast B. Matrix-associated autologous chondrocyte implantation: a clinical follow-up at 15 years. Cartilage. 2016;7:309–15.
22. Samsudin EZ, Kamarul T. The comparison between the different generations of autologous chondrocyte implantation with other treatment modalities: a systematic review of clinical trials. Knee Surg Sports Traumatol Arthrosc. 2016;24:3912–26.
23. Shankar AN, Jeyaraman M, Jayakumar T, Jeyaraman N, Nallakumarasamy A, Pranav NG. Gel-based autologous chondrocyte implantation (GACI) in the chondral defects of the knee: an observational study. Indian J Orthop. 2023;57:1809–18.
24. Yoon T-H, Jung M, Choi C-H, Kim H-S, Lee Y-H, Choi Y-S, et al. Arthroscopic gel-type autologous chondrocyte implantation presents histologic evidence of regenerating hyaline-like cartilage in the knee with articular cartilage defect. Knee Surg Sports Traumatol Arthrosc. 2020;28:941–51.
25. Cole BJ, Corpus KT, Bajaj S, Daley EL, Karas V, Kercher JS, et al. Prospective evaluation of autologous chondrocyte implantation procedure: minimum seven-year follow-up (SS-26). Arthroscopy. 2011;27:e43–4.
26. Niemeyer P, Albrecht D, Andereya S, Angele P, Ateschrang A, Aurich M, et al. Autologous chondrocyte implantation (ACI) for cartilage defects of the knee: a guideline by the working group "Clinical Tissue Regeneration" of the German Society of Orthopaedics and Trauma (DGOU). Knee. 2016;23:426–35.
27. Choi N-Y, Kim B-W, Yeo W-J, Kim H-B, Suh D-S, Kim J-S, et al. Gel-type autologous chondrocyte (ChondronTM) implantation for treatment of articular cartilage defects of the knee. BMC Musculoskelet Disord. 2010;11:1–8.
28. Goyal D, Modi V. Gel based autologous chondrocyte implantation: the surgical technique. Asian J Arthrosc. 2019;4:27–33.
29. Peterson L, Minas T, Brittberg M, Nilsson A, Sjögren-Jansson E, Lindahl A. Two-to 9-year outcome after autologous chondrocyte transplantation of the knee. Clin Orthop Relat Res. 2000;374:212–34.
30. Goyal DR. The illustrative third generation autologous chondrocyte implantation for cartilage repair: the gel based ACI technique. In: The illustrative book of cartilage repair. Cham: Springer; 2021. p. 157–66.
31. Brittberg M. Autologous chondrocyte implantation—technique and long-term follow-up. Injury. 2008;39:40–9.
32. Gooding CR, Bartlett W, Bentley G, Skinner JA, Carrington R, Flanagan A. A prospective, randomized study comparing two techniques of autologous chondrocyte implantation for osteochondral defects in the knee: periosteum covered versus type I/III collagen covered. Knee. 2006;13:203–10.
33. Chen AC, Nagrampa JP, Schinagl RM, Lottman LM, Sah RL. Chondrocyte transplantation to articular cartilage explants in vitro. J Orthop Res. 1997;15:791–802.
34. Ho W, Tawil B, Dunn JCY, Wu BM. The behavior of human mesenchymal stem cells in 3D fibrin clots: dependence on fibrinogen concentration and clot structure. Tissue Eng. 2006;12:1587–95.
35. Goyal D, Goyal A, Keyhani S, Lee EH, Hui JHP. Evidence-based status of second- and third-

generation autologous chondrocyte implantation over first generation: a systematic review of level I and II studies. Arthroscopy. 2013;29:1872–8.
36. Peterson L, Vasiliadis HS, Brittberg M, Lindahl A. Autologous chondrocyte implantation: a long-term follow-up. Am J Sports Med. 2010;38:1117–24.
37. Pardiwala DN, Tapasvi S, Chaudhary D, Babhulkar A, Varghese J, Rajan D, et al. Outcomes following gel-based autologous chondrocyte implantation for articular cartilage defects of the knee. Knee. 2024;49:70–8.
38. Siebold R, Suezer F, Schmitt B, Trattnig S, Essig M. Good clinical and MRI outcome after arthroscopic autologous chondrocyte implantation for cartilage repair in the knee. Knee Surg Sports Traumatol Arthrosc. 2018;26:831–9.
39. Enea D, Cecconi S, Busilacchi A, Manzotti S, Gesuita R, Gigante A. Matrix-induced autologous chondrocyte implantation (MACI) in the knee. Knee Surg Sports Traumatol Arthrosc. 2012;20:862–9.
40. Kim MK, Choi SW, Kim SR, Oh IS, Won MH. Autologous chondrocyte implantation in the knee using fibrin. Knee Surg Sports Traumatol Arthrosc. 2010;18:528–34.

Particulated Cartilage Applications in Cartilage Treatment

11

Andriolo Luca, Grassi Alberto, Zanasi Lorenzo, Filardo Giuseppe, and Zaffagnini Stefano

11.1 Introduction

Articular cartilage can be damaged by trauma, repetitive mechanical overload, or degenerative joint disease, resulting in pain and functional impairment. The limited ability of cartilage to heal spontaneously is mainly related to its avascular structure, low cellular density, and restricted chondrocyte proliferation and migration [1, 2]. As a consequence, focal cartilage defects may persist, enlarge, and contribute over time to joint degeneration and symptomatic osteoarthritis (OA) [3]. This led to the development of several cartilage restoration surgical procedures in the context of joint-preserving surgery. The main therapeutic goal is to reduce pain, restore function, and delay or avoid arthroplasty, particularly in young and active patients, in whom joint replacement may be associated with relevant morbidity and a higher lifetime risk of revision [4]. Numerous treatments have been developed since the 1990s, and each approach, with its advantages and disadvantages, must be tailored to the patient's own clinical features and functional demands. The damaged cartilage may be repaired or replaced using cell-based or cell-free strategies. Treatment with microfracture has been proven effective for small and intermediate-size cartilage defects, offering satisfactory clinical short- to mid-term improvement in most patients [5]. However, the repair tissue is predominantly fibrocartilaginous rather than hyaline cartilage, and clinical benefits generally decline at longer follow-ups [6, 7]. Autologous chondrocyte implantation (ACI) has been implemented in larger lesions and offered promising results both at short- and long-term follow-up [8]. Nevertheless, the high cost of cell cultures and two-step surgeries severely limited their use, with healthcare providers in many countries not adopting or abandoning their use in favor of other options with a more favorable cost/reimbursement profile [9]. This led to the widespread use of procedures based on minimally manipulated cell techniques or cell-free scaffolds, which have considerably lower costs and offer positive results at short- and mid-term follow-up [10, 11]. However, their long-term outcomes and the repaired tissue quality showed controversial results, and no high-level study provided definitive answers. Fresh osteochondral allografts represent another option which has high versatility and showed satisfactory results even at long-term, especially in lesions >2 cm^2 [12–14],

A. Luca · G. Alberto (✉) · Z. Lorenzo · Z. Stefano
Clinica Ortopedica e Traumatologica 2, IRCCS Istituto Ortopedico Rizzoli, Bologna, Italy
e-mail: luca.andriolo@ior.it; alberto.grassi@ior.it; lorenzo.zanasi@ior.it; stefano.zaffagnini@unibo.it

F. Giuseppe
Service of Orthopaedics and Traumatology, Department of Surgery, EOC, Lugano, Switzerland

Faculty of Biomedical Sciences, Università della Svizzera Italiana, Lugano, Switzerland
e-mail: giuseppe.filardo@usi.ch

M. E. Erdil et al. (eds.), *Current Concept in Cartilage Treatment*,
https://doi.org/10.1007/978-3-032-27099-3_11

but the limited graft availability, logistical issues, cost, and regulatory constraints make it a treatment not always feasible on a large scale in many countries.

In this context, particulated (or minced) cartilage implantation represents an interesting alternative, as it is a single-step surgical procedure in which autologous articular cartilage is harvested from the defect edge (or, alternatively, from non-weight bearing or low-weight bearing articular surface), mechanically fragmented into millimetric or sub-millimetric cartilage pieces, and then re-implanted to cover the defect [15, 16]. Graft fixation can be done with fibrin glue, scaffolds, autologous platelet-rich plasma (PRP), or a combination of these. The biological rationale is that fragmentation increases the exposed cartilage surface and may facilitate chondrocyte migration from the native extracellular matrix, allowing the fragments to serve as a local source of viable cells and matrix components. The increase in the use of this technique in articular cartilage regeneration has been driven by its single-stage nature, its good regulatory and cost profiles and by the promising in vitro and in vivo results both for chondral and osteochondral lesions [58]. The following paragraphs will review the preclinical rationale, clinical indications, and specific application methods of particulated cartilage.

11.2 Preclinical Evidence and Rationale

The biological rationale for particulated cartilage implantation was first supported by early experimental work from 1983 showing that cartilage fragmentation could contribute to osteochondral defect repair. In a rabbit model, Albrecht et al. [17] treated osteochondral defects with cartilage fragments fixed with fibrin glue and observed histological evidence of hyaline cartilage formation and defect closure, whereas untreated or differently sealed control defects did not show comparable repair at 40 weeks. More recently, other preclinical studies further supported the concept that mechanically fragmented cartilage may serve as an intraoperative source of viable chondrocytes and extracellular matrix components. Lu et al. [18] showed that chondrocytes released from minced cartilage could migrate into three-dimensional scaffolds and generate cartilage-like tissue, with additional evidence of hyaline-like repair in full-thickness chondral defects in a goat model. Similarly, Tsuyuguchi et al. [19], reported that minced cartilage placed within an atelocollagen gel scaffold promoted greater cell migration, proliferation, and glycosaminoglycan production than isolated enzymatically treated chondrocytes. The way cartilage is fragmented also appears to be biologically relevant. Experimental evidence suggests that sharp mechanical injury preserves a more favorable cellular response than blunt trauma.

Redman et al. [20] showed that sharp cartilage wounds were associated with limited cell death at the cut edge and signs of chondrocyte proliferation and matrix synthesis, whereas blunt injury produced a wider zone of cell death and little reparative activity. However, when different mincing methods were directly compared, Levinson et al. [21] found similar cell viability, outgrowth, and matrix deposition between hand-mincing and device-assisted mincing, although device-assisted preparation was faster and produced smaller fragments. Fragment size may also influence the reparative potential of minced cartilage. Smaller particles have been associated with greater extracellular matrix production and enhanced chondrocyte outgrowth compared with larger fragments [22, 23], supporting the concept that increasing the exposed cartilage surface may facilitate cell migration from the native matrix.

Other factors may influence the regenerative potential of particulated cartilage, including the harvest site and the age of the cartilage donor. Cartilage collected from the peripheral area of a lesion appears to preserve better tissue quality, viability, and chondrogenic capacity than cartilage obtained from more central degenerative areas [24, 25]. Donor age is also relevant: younger cartilage has been associated with greater chondrocyte migration and stronger chondrogenic activity than adult cartilage in a study by Marmotti et al. [26]. Similarly, Adkisson et al. [27] reported a marked age-related decline in cartilage biological potential, with juvenile cartilage showing higher proteoglycan content and increased collagen type II and IX expression, together with limited immunogenicity.

These findings have supported the development of particulated juvenile allograft cartilage (PJAC), which aims to exploit the enhanced biological activity of immature cartilage. *In vitro* studies suggest that juvenile cartilage fragments may stimulate matrix production when combined with adult cartilage [28], while animal data have shown higher expression of proliferative markers after PJAC compared with autologous cartilage chips [29]. Overall, the available evidence supports the biological rationale of both autologous minced cartilage and PJAC, while indicating that fragment size, preparation method, harvest location, and donor age may all affect regenerative performance.

11.3 Indications

There is no official consensus on the use of particulated cartilage in chondral and osteochondral defects, although in the literature the most accepted indications are the following:

- Symptomatic ICRS grade III-IV chondral or osteochondral defects.
- Etiology: traumatic injuries, degenerative lesions, osteochondritis dissecans (OCD).
- Defect size: depending on the procedure performed (suggested 1–3 cm^2).
- Age: younger than 50 years of age is recommended.
- Body mass index (BMI): up to 30 kg/m^2.

On the other hand, commonly accepted contraindications are the following:

- Moderate or advanced OA.
- Uncorrected mechanical malalignment.
- Joint instability.
- Active joint infection.
- Patients suffering from rheumatic diseases, Reiter syndrome, psoriatic arthritis, gout, ankylosing spondylitis, or arthritis secondary to other inflammatory diseases.
- Patients with active malignant neoplasms or uncontrolled systemic diseases (e.g., diabetes, thyroid disorders).

11.4 Particulated Cartilage Applications

Particulated cartilage can essentially be divided into two major categories: autologous minced cartilage and allograft minced cartilage implantation. The following paragraphs will provide a brief review of these procedures and the most relevant literature investigating their clinical use.

11.4.1 Autologous Particulated Cartilage

11.4.1.1 Cartilage Autograft Implantation System

The Cartilage Autograft Implantation System (CAIS; DePuy Mitek, Raynham, MA, USA) was developed as a one-stage technique for the treatment of knee articular cartilage defects and osteochondritis dissecans. The procedure combined autologous minced cartilage with a biodegradable scaffold composed of 35% polycaprolactone and 65% polyglycolic acid, reinforced with a polydioxanone mesh. The scaffold was designed to provide mechanical support, retain the cartilage fragments within the defect, and facilitate matrix formation. During the procedure, cartilage was first harvested from a non-load- or low-load-bearing area of the joint and processed with a specific mincing device to obtain small fragments, generally measuring approximately 1–2 mm. These fragments were distributed onto the scaffold and secured with fibrin sealant. After preparation of the defect, the cartilage–scaffold construct was trimmed to match the lesion and implanted with the cartilage surface oriented toward the subchondral bone. Fixation was achieved using biodegradable staple anchors. Clinical evidence for CAIS remains limited. Cole et al. [30] performed the only randomized trial on this technique, comparing CAIS with microfracture in 29 patients. Outcomes included SF-36, International Knee

Documentation Committee (IKDC) score, and Knee injury and Osteoarthritis Outcome Score (KOOS) assessed up to 24 months, together with serial MRI evaluations. Both groups improved clinically, but the CAIS group showed greater improvement in IKDC and most KOOS subscales at 24 months. MRI findings were broadly comparable, although intralesional osteophytes were more frequently observed after microfracture. Despite encouraging early results, further development of CAIS was discontinued and the procedure is no longer commercially available.

11.4.1.2 Minced Cartilage Implantation and Autologous Dual Tissue Transplantation

Minced cartilage implantation (MCI), previously referred to as autologous cartilage chip implantation, is a single-stage surgical technique in which autologous cartilage is harvested, usually from the intercondylar notch or from the defect margins, mechanically fragmented with a scalpel, and implanted into the prepared lesion with fibrin glue fixation. In osteochondral defects, this approach may be combined with autologous bone grafting, as in Autologous Dual Tissue Transplantation (ADTT), where cancellous bone is used to restore the subchondral component before the cartilage fragments are applied. Initial clinical evidence for MCI was mainly based on small case series. Christensen et al. [31] reported improved clinical scores, better MOCART findings, and substantial bone defect filling at 1 year in patients with knee osteochondritis dissecans treated with combined autologous bone and cartilage chips. Massen et al. [32] described significant pain reduction, functional improvement, and improved MRI repair scores at 2 years after single-stage autologous MCI for chondral and osteochondral knee lesions in 27 patients, with the authors suggesting it as a possible alternative to standard ACI. Wodzig et al. [33] reported similar short-term clinical and radiological improvements, using cartilage obtained from the lesion periphery or loose bodies and adding cancellous bone grafting in deeper defects. Runer et al. [34] reported favourable 5-year outcomes after MCI in 34 patients with knee chondral and osteochondral lesions, with good patient-reported results, low complication rates, and sustained graft survival. In a subsequent matched-pair analysis, the same group found comparable short-term outcomes and revision rates between MCI and ACI, further supporting MCI as a promising single-stage alternative to more complex cell-based procedures [49]. Finally, Shim et al. [50] extended the concept to osteochondral lesions of the talus, suggesting that particulated autologous cartilage transplantation may also be feasible in the ankle and that lesion-derived cartilage could be reused as a biological source in selected cases.

11.4.1.3 Augmented Minced Cartilage Implantation

The same procedure can also be performed with autologous platelet-rich plasma (PRP) or autologous conditioned plasma (ACP) augmentation. Cugat et al. [35] treated 15 patients affected by full-thickness knee chondral or osteochondral lesions with autologous cartilage chips embedded in a mixture of platelet-poor plasma and PRP. Results showed significant improvements in all clinical scores (IKDC, WOMAC, Lysholm, VAS) and in the MOCART score at 15-month follow-up. Gebhardt et al. [36] studied the viability and proliferation of cartilage tissue that was harvested and minced with an arthroscopic shaver. Results showed that chondrocytes retained proliferation capability and cell viability. The addition of PRP did not modify these characteristics and demonstrated an enhanced proteoglycan production, suggesting the ability to produce cartilage-specific extracellular matrix. According to the authors, shaver mincing and augmentation with PRP can be considered a safe technique for MCI. On the other hand, in 2021 Olesen et al. [37] assessed histological and macroscopic changes in cartilage repair tissue in an animal model with and without repeated injections of PRP, showing no difference in the content of hyaline cartilage, fibrocartilage, or fibrous tissue between the two groups.

11.4.1.4 AutoCart™

AutoCart™ (Arthrex Inc., Naples, FL) is an all-arthroscopic procedure that allows treatment of cartilage lesions with only autologous material, augmenting MCI with ACP and autologous fibrin. Cartilage is cut with a SabreTooth™ shaver blade into 3 or 4 mm particulates, collected in a specific device (GraftNet™) and then transferred into a 1 ml application syringe. The collected cartilage fragments are then augmented with PRP and placed into the defect with the use of a specific cannula, as shown in figure 11.1 (Fig. 11.1). Fixation is done through an autologous thrombin solution produced by a specific device (Thrombinator™). A final sealing is done with an additional layer of an ACP/thrombin mix. This procedure has been increasingly investigated across different anatomical sites and lesion patterns. Schneider et al. [51] reported satisfactory 2-year outcomes in an arthroscopic series of 62 patients with knee cartilage defects of the femoral condyles, showing significant improvements in patient-reported outcomes, moderate MRI repair tissue quality, and a low revision rate, mainly related to graft hypertrophy. Gebhardt et al. [38] evaluated clinical outcomes and safety of arthroscopic, autologous MCI for acetabular cartilage lesions to treat femoroacetabular impingement syndrome in 11 male patients at short-term follow-up. Harvesting was done from the loose cartilage flap at the chondrolabral lesion, and mincing was performed with a shaver. The tissue was then augmented with ACP, implanted, and then stabilized into the lesion by autologous thrombin. Results showed a significant increase in all clinical scores at 2-year follow-up, with 10 out of 11 patients reaching the minimal clinically important difference (MCID) in terms of functional outcome and pain.

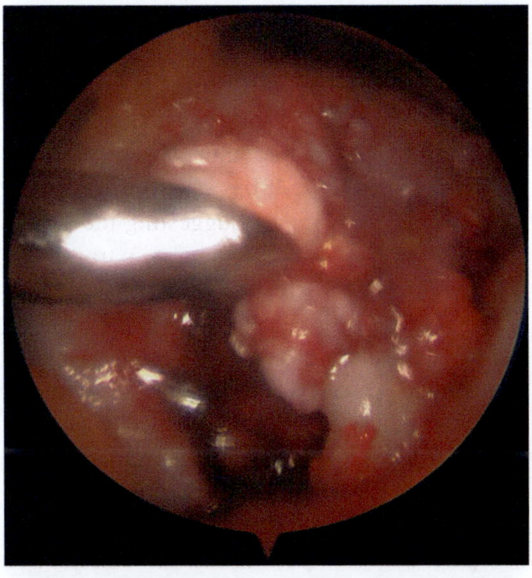

Fig. 11.1 Autocart™ procedure: Arthroscopic positioning of cartilage fragments

Roth et al. [39] treated five patients with circumscribed cartilage defects in the first metatarsophalangeal joint in combination with hallux rigidus using autologous cartilage fragments harvested from the dorsal rim portion. Mincing was done with a 3.0 mm shaver, and cartilage fragments were then augmented with ACP. Results were satisfactory for all five patients, with no relevant surgery-associated complications. Finally, a further experience investigated the use of this approach for a shoulder cartilage lesion. Karkosch et al. [40] presented a case report on arthroscopic minced cartilage repair with the AutoCart™ procedure in the glenohumeral joint, underlying the short-term positive clinical outcome obtained in a 33-year-old man and suggesting the possibility to apply this approach also outside of the more common knee applications.

11.4.2 Allograft Particulated Cartilage

As previously mentioned, several in vitro studies demonstrated the benefits of allograft juvenile cartilage. The first clinical studies for PJAC were published in the early 2010s [41], with literature reports on the treatment of chondral and osteochondral defects of the knee (including the patellofemoral joint) and of the talus [58].

11.4.2.1 DeNovo NT Natural Tissue Graft

DeNovo NT® Natural Tissue Graft (ISTO Technologies, St. Louis, MO, USA; distributed by Zimmer, Warsaw, IN, USA) is an

FDA-listed listed particulated juvenile articular cartilage allograft used as a single-stage treatment option for focal chondral and osteochondral defects. Its rationale is based on the higher proliferative and matrix-producing potential of juvenile cartilage, while avoiding autologous cartilage harvest, cell expansion, and staged surgery. Donors are younger than 13 years of age, although most grafts are obtained from approximately 2-year-old donors, without the use of stillborn or fetal tissue. Each package remains viable for up to 49 days and contains enough particulated cartilage to treat a defect of approximately 2.5 cm^2. The graft consists of viable juvenile chondrocytes embedded within their native extracellular matrix. After defect preparation, the cartilage fragments are implanted without completely filling the lesion, and the remaining defect depth is sealed with fibrin glue to stabilize the graft.

Most available evidence concerns knee cartilage defects, particularly patellar and patellofemoral lesions. Early studies reported significant improvements in clinical scores, satisfactory MRI defect fill, and, in some cases, repair tissue with both hyaline-like and fibrocartilaginous features. Farr et al. showed improved IKDC and KOOS scores in 25 patients at 2 years [42], while Tompkins et al. and Grawe et al. reported favourable MRI findings in patellar defects [43, 44]. Wang et al. [45] also found clinical improvement in patellofemoral lesions at mid-term follow-up, although clinical scores had no correlation with MRI scores, with defect fill > 67% being reached in 69% of the defects. More recent studies have further supported the role of PJAC in selected patellofemoral indications. Marmor et al. [52] reported significant clinical improvement after PJAC implantation for full-thickness patellar lesions, again showing that MRI defect fill was not strongly associated with patient-reported outcomes. Davie et al. [53] found comparable short-term clinical and imaging results between shouldered and unshouldered patellar defects treated with PJAC and concomitant stabilization, highlighting the importance of correcting associated biomechanical factors such as instability or maltracking. Dawkins et al. [46] treated 34 young patients with patellofemoral cartilage defects using DeNovo NT®, reporting satisfactory short-term clinical and MRI outcomes, a 100% return-to-sport rate, and low complication and graft failure rates. Pearsall et al. [54] also reported favourable return-to-sport rates and patient-reported outcomes after PJAC transplantation for patellofemoral defects. On the other hand, comparative evidence remains limited. Marom et al. [57] found similar postoperative patient-reported outcomes between PJAC and osteochondral allograft transplantation for patellar defects, but lower reoperation and graft failure rates in the osteochondral allograft group.

Outside the patellofemoral joint, Walker et al. [55] described a technique combining PJAC with autogenous bone grafting for symptomatic osteochondral defects of the tibial plateau, highlighting a possible role in challenging osteochondral lesions. In contrast, results in the ankle appear less predictable. A recent systematic review by Butler et al. [56] evaluated PJAC for osteochondral lesions of the talus across 12 studies and 241 patients. Although the procedure was associated with some short-term symptomatic improvement, the radiological quality of the repair tissue was limited, and relatively high complication rate (25.2%) and failure rate (12.4%) were reported. These findings led the authors to question the reliability of PJAC in this setting, particularly for large talar osteochondral lesions, and to advise caution until stronger evidence is available. DeNovo NT® has also been applied in other joints, with preliminary reports describing its use for wrist cartilage lesions and osteochondral defects of the first metatarsal head, with encouraging clinical outcomes in small case series [47, 48].

11.5 Conclusions

Particulated cartilage techniques and their related commercial products have attracted renewed interest because of their biological rationale, technical simplicity, logistical advantages, and encouraging early results. Although preclinical studies provide strong support for their regenerative potential, clinical evidence remains limited and heterogeneous. Further high-level clinical studies are required to better define indications, optimize implantation techniques, clarify repair tissue quality, and determine the role of minced cartilage implantation relative to other cartilage restoration procedures for chondral and osteochondral lesions.

References

1. Sophia Fox AJ, Bedi A, Rodeo SA. The basic science of articular cartilage: structure, composition, and function. Sports Health. 2009;1(6):461–8. https://doi.org/10.1177/1941738109350438.
2. Shiromoto Y, Niki Y, Kikuchi T, Yoshihara Y, Oguma T, Nemoto K, Chiba K, Kanaji A, Matsumoto M, Nakamura M. Increased migratory activity and cartilage regeneration by superficial-zone chondrocytes in enzymatically treated cartilage explants. BMC Musculoskelet Disord. 2022;23(1):256. https://doi.org/10.1186/s12891-022-05210-2.
3. Ding C, Garnero P, Cicuttini F, Scott F, Cooley H, Jones G. Knee cartilage defects: association with early radiographic osteoarthritis, decreased cartilage volume, increased joint surface area and type II collagen breakdown. Osteoarthr Cartil. 2005;13(3):198–205. https://doi.org/10.1016/j.joca.2004.11.007.
4. Perdisa F, Bordini B, Salerno M, Traina F, Zaffagnini S, Filardo G. Total knee arthroplasty (TKA): when do the risks of TKA overcome the benefits? Double risk of failure in patients up to 65 years old. Cartilage. 2023;14(3):305–11. https://doi.org/10.1177/19476035231164733. Epub 2023 Apr 19.
5. Steadman JR, Rodkey WG, Briggs KK. Microfracture to treat full-thickness chondral defects: surgical technique, rehabilitation, and outcomes. J Knee Surg. 2002;15(3):170–6.
6. Mithoefer K, Williams RJ 3rd, Warren RF, Potter HG, Spock CR, Jones EC, Wickiewicz TL, Marx RG. Chondral resurfacing of articular cartilage defects in the knee with the microfracture technique. Surgical technique. J Bone Joint Surg Am. 2006;88(Suppl 1 Pt 2):294–304. https://doi.org/10.2106/JBJS.F.00292.
7. Solheim E, Hegna J, Strand T, Harlem T, Inderhaug E. Randomized study of long-term (15-17 years) outcome after microfracture versus mosaicplasty in knee articular cartilage defects. Am J Sports Med. 2018;46(4):826–31. https://doi.org/10.1177/0363546517745281. Epub 2017 Dec 18
8. Brittberg M. Autologous chondrocyte implantation—technique and long-term follow-up. Injury. 2008;39(Suppl 1):S40–9. https://doi.org/10.1016/j.injury.2008.01.040.
9. De Marziani L, Boffa A, Di Martino A, Andriolo L, Reale D, Bernasconi A, Corbo VR, de Caro F, Delcogliano M, di Laura Frattura G, Di Vico G, Manunta AF, Russo A, Filardo G. The reimbursement system can influence the treatment choice and favor joint replacement versus other less invasive solutions in patients affected by osteoarthritis. J Exp Orthop. 2023;10(1):146. https://doi.org/10.1186/s40634-023-00699-5.
10. Filardo G, Andriolo L, Angele P, Berruto M, Brittberg M, Condello V, Chubinskaya S, de Girolamo L, Di Martino A, Di Matteo B, Gille J, Gobbi A, Lattermann C, Nakamura N, Nehrer S, Peretti GM, Shabshin N, Verdonk P, Zaslav K, Kon E. Scaffolds for knee chondral and osteochondral defects: indications for different clinical scenarios. A consensus statement. Cartilage. 2021;13(1_suppl):1036S–46S. https://doi.org/10.1177/1947603519894729. Epub 2020 Jan 15.
11. Andriolo L, Reale D, Di Martino A, Boffa A, Zaffagnini S, Filardo G. Cell-free scaffolds in cartilage knee surgery: a systematic review and meta-analysis of clinical evidence. Cartilage. 2021;12(3):277–92. https://doi.org/10.1177/1947603519852406. Epub 2019 Jun 5.
12. Assenmacher AT, Pareek A, Reardon PJ, Macalena JA, Stuart MJ, Krych AJ. Long-term outcomes after osteochondral allograft: a systematic review at long-term follow-up of 12.3 years. Arthroscopy. 2016;32(10):2160–8. https://doi.org/10.1016/j.arthro.2016.04.020. Epub 2016 Jun 15
13. Campbell AB, Pineda M, Harris JD, Flanigan DC. Return to sport after articular cartilage repair in athletes' knees: a systematic review. Arthroscopy. 2016;32(4):651–68.e1. https://doi.org/10.1016/j.arthro.2015.08.028. Epub 2015 Oct 30
14. Crawford ZT, Schumaier AP, Glogovac G, Grawe BM. Return to sport and sports-specific outcomes after osteochondral allograft transplantation in the knee: a systematic review of studies with at least 2 years' mean follow-up. Arthroscopy. 2019;35(6):1880–9. https://doi.org/10.1016/j.arthro.2018.11.064. Epub 2019 Apr 30
15. Ossendorff R, Walter SG, Schildberg FA, Spang J, Obudzinski S, Preiss S, Schneider S, Salzmann GM. Biologic principles of minced cartilage implantation: a narrative review. Arch Orthop Trauma Surg. 2023;143(6):3259–69. https://doi.org/10.1007/s00402-022-04692-y. Epub 2022 Nov 16.
16. Salzmann GM, Ossendorff R, Gilat R, Cole BJ. Autologous minced cartilage implantation for treatment of chondral and osteochondral lesions in the knee joint: an overview. Cartilage. 2021;13(1_suppl):1124S–36S. https://doi.org/10.1177/1947603520942952. Epub 2020 Jul 25.
17. Albrecht F, Roessner A, Zimmermann E. Closure of osteochondral lesions using chondral fragments and fibrin adhesive. Arch Orthop Trauma Surg (1978). 1983;101(3):213–7. https://doi.org/10.1007/BF00436773.
18. Lu Y, Dhanaraj S, Wang Z, Bradley DM, Bowman SM, Cole BJ, Binette F. Minced cartilage without cell culture serves as an effective intraoperative cell source for cartilage repair. J Orthop Res.

2006;24(6):1261–70. https://doi.org/10.1002/jor.20135.
19. Tsuyuguchi Y, Nakasa T, Ishikawa M, Miyaki S, Matsushita R, Kanemitsu M, Adachi N. The benefit of minced cartilage over isolated chondrocytes in atelocollagen gel on chondrocyte proliferation and migration. Cartilage. 2021;12(1):93–101. https://doi.org/10.1177/1947603518805205. Epub 2018 Oct 12.
20. Redman SN, Dowthwaite GP, Thomson BM, Archer CW. The cellular responses of articular cartilage to sharp and blunt trauma. Osteoarthr Cartil. 2004;12(2):106–16. https://doi.org/10.1016/j.joca.2002.12.001.
21. Levinson C, Cavalli E, Sindi DM, Kessel B, Zenobi-Wong M, Preiss S, Salzmann G, Neidenbach P. Chondrocytes from device-minced articular cartilage show potent outgrowth into fibrin and collagen hydrogels. Orthop J Sports Med. 2019;7(9):2325967119867618. https://doi.org/10.1177/2325967119867618.
22. Bonasia DE, Marmotti A, Mattia S, Cosentino A, Spolaore S, Governale G, Castoldi F, Rossi R. The degree of chondral fragmentation affects extracellular matrix production in cartilage autograft implantation: an in vitro study. Arthroscopy. 2015;31(12):2335–41. https://doi.org/10.1016/j.arthro.2015.06.025. Epub 2015 Aug 28
23. Lei Y, Peng J, Dai Z, Liao Y, Liu Q, Li J, Jiang Y. Articular cartilage fragmentation improves chondrocyte migration by upregulating membrane type 1 matrix metalloprotease. Cartilage. 2021;13(2_suppl):1054S–63S. https://doi.org/10.1177/19476035211035435. Epub 2021 Oct 15.
24. Acevedo L, Iselin L, Berkelaar MHM, Salzmann GM, Wolf F, Feliciano S, Vogel N, Pagenstert G, Martin I, Pelttari K, Barbero A, Arnold MP. Comparison of human articular cartilage tissue and chondrocytes isolated from peripheral versus central regions of traumatic lesions. Cartilage. 2021;13(2_suppl):68S–81S. https://doi.org/10.1177/1947603520958154. Epub 2020 Sep 22.
25. Aurich M, Hofmann GO, Best N, Rolauffs B. Induced redifferentiation of human chondrocytes from articular cartilage lesion in alginate bead culture after monolayer dedifferentiation: an alternative cell source for cell-based therapies? Tissue Eng Part A. 2018;24(3-4):275–86. https://doi.org/10.1089/ten.TEA.2016.0505. Epub 2017 Jul 19
26. Marmotti A, Bonasia DE, Bruzzone M, Rossi R, Castoldi F, Collo G, Realmuto C, Tarella C, Peretti GM. Human cartilage fragments in a composite scaffold for single-stage cartilage repair: an in vitro study of the chondrocyte migration and the influence of TGF-β1 and G-CSF. Knee Surg Sports Traumatol Arthrosc. 2013;21(8):1819–33. https://doi.org/10.1007/s00167-012-2244-7. Epub 2012 Nov 10
27. Adkisson HD 4th, Martin JA, Amendola RL, Milliman C, Mauch KA, Katwal AB, Seyedin M, Amendola A, Streeter PR, Buckwalter JA. The potential of human allogeneic juvenile chondrocytes for restoration of articular cartilage. Am J Sports Med. 2010;38(7):1324–33. https://doi.org/10.1177/0363546510361950. Epub 2010 Apr 27.
28. Bonasia DE, Martin JA, Marmotti A, Amendola RL, Buckwalter JA, Rossi R, Blonna D, Adkisson HD 4th, Amendola A. Cocultures of adult and juvenile chondrocytes compared with adult and juvenile chondral fragments: in vitro matrix production. Am J Sports Med. 2011;39(11):2355–61. https://doi.org/10.1177/0363546511417172. Epub 2011 Aug 9.
29. Zhang C, Zhao X, Ao Y, Cao J, Yang L, Duan X. Proliferation ability of particulated juvenile allograft cartilage. J Orthop Surg Res. 2021;16(1):56. https://doi.org/10.1186/s13018-020-02199-z.
30. Cole BJ, Farr J, Winalski CS, Hosea T, Richmond J, Mandelbaum B, De Deyne PG. Outcomes after a single-stage procedure for cell-based cartilage repair: a prospective clinical safety trial with 2-year follow-up. Am J Sports Med. 2011;39(6):1170–9. https://doi.org/10.1177/0363546511399382. Epub 2011 Apr 1
31. Christensen BB, Foldager CB, Jensen J, Lind M. Autologous dual-tissue transplantation for osteochondral repair: early clinical and radiological results. Cartilage. 2015;6(3):166–73. https://doi.org/10.1177/1947603515580983.
32. Massen FK, Inauen CR, Harder LP, Runer A, Preiss S, Salzmann GM. One-step autologous minced cartilage procedure for the treatment of knee joint chondral and osteochondral lesions: a series of 27 patients with 2-year follow-up. Orthop J Sports Med. 2019;7(6):2325967119853773. https://doi.org/10.1177/2325967119853773.
33. Wodzig MHH, Peters MJM, Emanuel KS, Van Hugten PPW, Wijnen W, Jutten LM, Boymans TA, Loeffen DV, Emans PJ. Minced autologous chondral fragments with fibrin glue as a simple promising one-step cartilage repair procedure: a clinical and MRI study at 12-month follow-up. Cartilage. 2022;13(4):19–31. https://doi.org/10.1177/19476035221126343. Epub 2022 Oct 28.
34. Runer A, Ossendorff R, Öttl F, Stadelmann VA, Schneider S, Preiss S, Salzmann GM, Hax J. Autologous minced cartilage repair for chondral and osteochondral lesions of the knee joint demonstrates good postoperative outcomes and low reoperation rates at minimum five-year follow-up. Knee Surg Sports Traumatol Arthrosc. 2023;31(11):4977–87. https://doi.org/10.1007/s00167-023-07546-1. Epub 2023 Aug 27.
35. Cugat R, Alentorn-Geli E, Navarro J, Cuscó X, Steinbacher G, Seijas R, Álvarez-Díaz P, Barastegui D, Laiz P, Samitier G, García-Balletbó M. A novel autologous-made matrix using hyaline cartilage chips and platelet-rich growth factors for the

treatment of full-thickness cartilage or osteochondral defects: preliminary results. J Orthop Surg (Hong Kong). 2020;28(1):2309499019887547. https://doi.org/10.1177/2309499019887547.
36. Gebhardt S, Zimmerer A, Balcarek P, Wassilew GI, Schoon J. The influence of arthroscopic shaver mincing and platelet-rich plasma on chondrocytes of intraoperatively harvested human cartilage. Am J Sports Med. 2023;51(10):2679–87. https://doi.org/10.1177/03635465231181633. Epub 2023 Jul 14.
37. Olesen ML, Christensen BB, Foldager CB, Hede KC, Jørgensen NL, Lind M. No effect of platelet-rich plasma injections as an adjuvant to autologous cartilage chips implantation for the treatment of chondral defects. Cartilage. 2021 Dec;13(2_suppl):277S-284S. https://doi.org/10.1177/1947603519865318. Epub 2019 Jul 22.
38. Gebhardt S, Hofer A, Wassilew GI, Sobau C, Zimmerer A. Minced cartilage implantation in acetabular cartilage defects: case series with 2-year results. Cartilage. 2023;14(4):393–9. https://doi.org/10.1177/19476035231189840. Epub 2023 Aug 3
39. Roth KE, Klos K, Simons P, Ossendorff R, Drees P, Maier GS, Salzmann GM. Minced cartilage bei Knorpeldefekten am Großzehengrundgelenk [cartilage chip transplantation for cartilage defects of the first metatarsophalangeal joint]. Oper Orthop Traumatol. 2021;33(6):480–6. https://doi.org/10.1007/s00064-021-00745-4. German. Epub 2021 Nov 1
40. Karkosch RF, Smith T, Jensen G, Tuecking LR, Horstmann H. Arthroscopic minced cartilage repair in the Glenohumeral joint—short term clinical outcome in a 33-year-old handyman: a case report. Orthop Res Rev. 2023;15:245–51. https://doi.org/10.2147/ORR.S418032.
41. Bonner KF, Daner W, Yao JQ. 2-year postoperative evaluation of a patient with a symptomatic full-thickness patellar cartilage defect repaired with particulated juvenile cartilage tissue. J Knee Surg. 2010;23(2):109–14. https://doi.org/10.1055/s-0030-1267465.
42. Farr J, Tabet SK, Margerrison E, Cole BJ. Clinical, radiographic, and histological outcomes after cartilage repair with particulated juvenile articular cartilage: a 2-year prospective study. Am J Sports Med. 2014;42(6):1417–25. https://doi.org/10.1177/0363546514528671. Epub 2014 Apr 9. Erratum in: Am J Sports Med. 2014 Oct;42(10):NP50
43. Tompkins M, Hamann JC, Diduch DR, Bonner KF, Hart JM, Gwathmey FW, Milewski MD, Gaskin CM. Preliminary results of a novel single-stage cartilage restoration technique: particulated juvenile articular cartilage allograft for chondral defects of the patella. Arthroscopy. 2013;29(10):1661–70. https://doi.org/10.1016/j.arthro.2013.05.021. Epub 2013 Jul 20
44. Grawe B, Burge A, Nguyen J, Strickland S, Warren R, Rodeo S, Shubin SB. Cartilage regeneration in full-thickness patellar chondral defects treated with particulated juvenile articular allograft cartilage: an MRI analysis. Cartilage. 2017;8(4):374–83. https://doi.org/10.1177/1947603517710308. Epub 2017 Jun 12.
45. Wang T, Belkin NS, Burge AJ, Chang B, Pais M, Mahony G, Williams RJ. Patellofemoral cartilage lesions treated with particulated juvenile allograft cartilage: a prospective study with minimum 2-year clinical and magnetic resonance imaging outcomes. Arthroscopy. 2018;34(5):1498–505. https://doi.org/10.1016/j.arthro.2017.11.021. Epub 2018 Feb 1
46. Dawkins BJ, Shubin Stein BE, Mintz DN, Fabricant PD, Gomoll AH, Strickland SM, Aitchison AH, Hidalgo Perea S, Green DW. Patellofemoral joint cartilage restoration with particulated juvenile allograft in patients under 21 years old. Knee. 2022;36:120–9. https://doi.org/10.1016/j.knee.2021.07.006. Epub 2021 Aug 8
47. Hess DE, Werner BC, Deal DN. Use of particulated juvenile articular cartilage allograft for osteochondral lesions of the wrist. Hand (N Y). 2017;12(5):NP62–7. https://doi.org/10.1177/1558944716673047. Epub 2016 Oct 11.
48. Van Dyke B, Berlet GC, Daigre JL, Hyer CF, Philbin TM. First metatarsal head osteochondral defect treatment with particulated juvenile cartilage allograft transplantation: a case series. Foot Ankle Int. 2018;39(2):236–41. https://doi.org/10.1177/1071100717737482. Epub 2017 Nov 7
49. Runer A, Leuthard L, Hoheisel L, Stadelmann VA, Preiss S, Salzmann GM, Hax J. Minced cartilage implantation provides comparable outcomes to autologous chondrocyte implantation (ACI) for knee cartilage lesions: A matched-pair analysis. Knee Surg Sports Traumatol Arthrosc. 2025. https://doi.org/10.1002/ksa.70210. Epub ahead of print.
50. Shim DW, Hong H, Lee JW, Kim BS. Particulated autologous cartilage transplantation for the treatment of osteochondral lesion of the talus: can the lesion cartilage be recycled? Bone Jt Open. 2023;4(12):942–947. https://doi.org/10.1302/2633-1462.412.BJO-2023-0097.R1.
51. Schneider S, Ossendorff R, Walter SG, Berger M, Endler C, Kaiser R, Ilg A, Salzmann GM, Holz J. Arthroscopic Autologous Minced Cartilage Implantation of Cartilage Defects in the Knee: A 2-Year Follow-up of 62 Patients. Orthop J Sports Med. 2024;12(12):23259671241297970. https://doi.org/10.1177/23259671241297970.
52. Marmor WA, Dennis ER, Buza SS, Gruber S, Propp BE, Burge AJ, Nguyen JT, Shubin Stein BE. Outcomes of Particulated Juvenile Articular Cartilage and Association With Defect Fill in Patients With Full-Thickness Patellar Chondral Lesions. Orthop J Sports Med. 2024;12(6):23259671241249121. https://doi.org/10.1177/23259671241249121.
53. Davie R, Ammerman B, Propp B, Marigi E, Marmor W, Pahapill N, Kingston K, Gruber S, Burge A, Wimberly A, Nguyen J, Dennis E, Stein

BES. Comparative Clinical and Imaging Outcomes of Particulated Juvenile Articular Cartilage Implantation in Shouldered and Unshouldered Patellar Cartilage Lesions With Concomitant Stabilization at 2-Year Follow-up. Orthop J Sports Med. 2025;13(9):23259671251369018. https://doi.org/10.1177/23259671251369018.

54. Pearsall C, Chen AZ, Reynolds AW, Saltzman BM, Ahmad CS, Popkin CA, Redler LH, Trofa DP. Particulated Juvenile Articular Cartilage Allograft Transplantation for Patellofemoral Defects Shows Favorable Return-to-Sport Rates and Patient-Reported Outcomes. Arthroscopy. 2024;40(12):2875–83. https://doi.org/10.1016/j.arthro.2024.02.018. Epub 2024 Feb 22.
55. Walker PB, Cope S, Trikha R, Kremen TJ, Jones KJ. Combined Particulated Juvenile Articular Cartilage Allograft Transplantation With Autogenous Bone Graft for Symptomatic Osteochondral Defects in the Tibial Plateau. Arthrosc Tech. 2025;14(8):103689. https://doi.org/10.1016/j.eats.2025.103689.
56. Butler JJ, Rizla MRM, Egol AJ, Campbell H, Schoof L, Dahmen J, Azam MT, Kerkhoffs GMMJ, Kennedy JG. Particulated juvenile cartilage allograft for the treatment of osteochondral lesions of the talus is associated with a high complication rate and a high failure rate at short-term follow-up: A systematic review. Knee Surg Sports Traumatol Arthrosc. 2024;32(3):529–41. https://doi.org/10.1002/ksa.12069. Epub 2024 Feb 6.
57. Marom N, Coxe F, Wang D, Williams R, Ode G. Particulate juvenile articular cartilage vs osteochondral allograft for patellar cartilage defects: a matched cohort analysis. Orthop J Sports Med. 2020;8(7 suppl6):2325967120S00510. https://doi.org/10.1177/2325967120S00510.
58. Christensen BB, Olesen ML, Hede KTC, Bergholt NL, Foldager CB, Lind M. Particulated cartilage for chondral and osteochondral repair: a review. Cartilage. 2021;13(1_suppl):1047S–57S. https://doi.org/10.1177/1947603520904757. Epub 2020 Feb 13.

12 Bone Marrow Aspirate Concentrate and Hyaluronic Acid-Based Scaffold Applications and the Healing Cycle

Zirvecan Güneş and Gazi Huri

12.1 Introduction

Bone marrow aspirate concentrate (BMAC) and hyaluronic acid (HA)-based porous scaffolds are a newly defined and efficient treatment in the field of regenerative medicine. All of these treatment options combine the values of BMAC with the structural and biochemical properties of HA scaffolds to build up the extracellular matrix that may solve the low healing potential of cartilage. BMAC consists of mesenchymal stem cells (MSCs), growth factors, and cytokines that play important roles in inflammation regulation, cell growth, and new tissue formation. HA-based scaffolds, on the other hand, provide an extracellular matrix-like scaffold to aid in the process of cell adhesion, proliferation, and integration during the healing process. All of these elements come together in harmony during the stages of healing and formation of a new and durable cartilage. Moreover, due to the evolution of the disciplines of BMAC and HA scaffolds, there are emerging strategies for enhancing the outcomes of current therapies for cartilage injuries that are less invasive, personalized for the patient, and that harness the natural resources of the body to regenerate the cartilage.

12.1.1 Overview and Importance of Regenerative Medicine

The twenty-first century has seen an exponential growth in the field of regenerative medicine [1, 2]. This is a relatively new field of research that focuses on the surgical procedures and the most recent biotechnological developments, which can transform the conventional approach to medicine [3]. Advanced cellular therapies, tissue engineering, novel gene manipulations, artificial organic tissues, and new disease phenotyping have already started to change the face of medicine and have a potential to do more in the future [4, 5].

Regenerative medicine is a branch of medicine that relies on the body's self-heal ability. While the conventional therapies only attempt to suppress the symptoms or replace the affected joints with artificial implants, regenerative medicine aims to create new native tissue that has the same form and function as the lost one. Based on stem cell biology, biomaterials, tissue engineering, and molecular medicine, regenerative medicine offers new strategies for diseases of tissues that have limited or no healing ability, such as cartilage tissue [6, 7]. Cartilage has been a hot

Z. Güneş (✉)
Orthopaedics and traumatology, Hacettepe University, Ankara, Türkiye

G. Huri
Orthopaedics and Traumatology, Hacettepe University, Ankara, Türkiye

Orthopaedics and Traumatology, Aspetar, FIFA Medical Center of Excellence, Doha, Qatar

M. E. Erdil et al. (eds.), *Current Concept in Cartilage Treatment*,
https://doi.org/10.1007/978-3-032-27099-3_12

topic in musculoskeletal medicine because of its avascular nature and low cell density, and therefore it has been a challenge in the field with conventional treatments offering only a transient improvement or a partial restoration of the damaged structure [8].

Regenerative medicine offers revolutionary approaches to overcome these limitations by developing therapies that target the underlying biological mechanisms of tissue healing. Some of the major players include the mesenchymal stem cells (MSCs), growth factors, cytokines, and extracellular vesicles that together regulate inflammation, cell number, and the synthesis of extracellular matrix (ECM) [9]. Advanced biomaterials like HA-based scaffolds can deliver the necessary elements on-site of the injury while reproducing native ECM and offering support in a bioactive microenvironment at the site of tissue regeneration [10, 11]. HA has excellent biodegradability, biocompatibility, and local retention ability of bioactive molecules and stem cells at the injury sites. These scaffolds facilitate the retention and proliferation of cells and provide growth factors in a time-dependent fashion throughout the repair process [12, 13].

The incorporation of biologics into biomaterials is one of the most outstanding progressions made in the field of regenerative medicine. The combination of BMAC and HA-based scaffolds is a good example of how regenerative medicine can be developed. It combines cellular and molecular therapy to deal with the complex nature of cartilage repair [14, 15].

12.1.1.1 Current Challenges in Tissue Repair and Healing

The first challenge is the matter of acquiring and managing stem cells, which are crucial to the field of regenerative medicine. The problem is how to get and grow enough of them and how to keep them in good condition [15]. The second challenge raises ethical questions, especially when it comes to embryonic stem cells (e.g., induced pluripotent stem cells). Pluripotent stem cells also have technical safety problems, such as a risk of inducing tumor formation. The immune response also complicates healing; inflammation or immune reactions can impede the repair of tissue, particularly for allogeneic therapies, which carry risks of rejection requiring immunosuppressive therapies [16]. Creating scaffolds and biomaterials is another challenge. These materials should be biocompatible, biodegradable, and mimic the natural extracellular matrix (ECM) to promote cell adhesion, differentiation, and vascularization. Moreover, the expense and lengthy development timeline of these therapies limit their accessibility. These therapies also require extensive clinical trials for evaluating their safety and efficacy [16, 17].

12.1.2 What Is BMAC

BMAC has been receiving attention in the field of regenerative medicine because of its ability to harness the body's natural healing capability. Resulting from the collection of a patient's iliac crest, BMAC is concentrated into high-density mesenchymal stem cells (MSCs), growth factors, and bioactive molecules that are critical for tissue repair [18]. BMAC contains MSCs that can differentiate into specific tissues and secrete growth factors and cytokines that promote local cell regeneration and proliferation. Furthermore, since BMAC is autologous, it has a low risk of immunological reactions [19].

12.1.2.1 Mechanism of Action

The bone marrow plays a crucial role in tissue repair, as it is the source of MSCs, hematopoietic stem cells, and bioactive factors that participate in healing. Regenerative treatments are applied in the field of orthopedics to promote healing, especially in cartilage defects, osteoarthritis, tendon pathologies, and fracture nonunions [20]. BMAC is a treatment method that concentrates MSCs, growth factors, and cytokines for use in local delivery to the injury site. In cartilage repair, BMAC is frequently used in combination with biomaterials, such as HA-based scaffolds, to increase the retention of cells and ECM production [21]. MSCs are derived from the stroma of the bone marrow and are important for the regeneration of cartilage, as they have the potential to become chondrocytes and produce ECM components (e.g., collagen type II, proteoglycans) and secrete paracrine factors that modulate inflammation and promote matrix remodeling [22]. They further induce angiogenesis and recruit reparative cells to the injury site for tissue healing [22].

The most important mechanism of this regenerative effect of BMAC is attributed to the presence of multipotent MSCs, which can differentiate into various types of tissues such as bone, cartilage, fat, or muscle and provide a major contribution during normal orthopedic healing such as cartilage defects and bone fractures [21]. Moreover, MSCs confer a "trophic effect" through secretion of molecules and cytokines that are involved in modulating inflammation, stimulating progenitor cells, and augmenting vascularization to promote healing [22]. Hematopoietic stem cells promote hematopoiesis and cytokine production in order to stimulate angiogenesis and immune modulation [23]. Endothelial progenitor cell activation is vital for neovascularization and thus to supply nutrients and oxygen to the regenerating tissue [24]. BMAC also has important growth factors that trigger and maintain tissue repair. Vascular endothelial growth factor (VEGF) induces angiogenesis, providing oxygen delivery and nutrients to the damaged tissue during the healing process. Whereas transforming growth factor-beta (TGF-β) induces chondrogenesis and extracellular matrix (ECM) production [18]. Platelet-derived growth factor (PDGF) stimulates cell proliferation and migration, while fibroblast growth factor (FGF) promotes progenitor cell expansion and differentiation [25, 26]. These growth factors work synergistically with stem cells to enhance their healing properties [27, 28].

BMAC's interaction with immune cells is necessary for coordinating inflammation during healing. By modulating immune cells, including macrophages and T cells, MSCs drive excessive inflammation suppression toward the reparative M2 phenotype, which secretes anti-inflammatory cytokines, such as interleukin-10 (IL-10), and growth factors, such as transforming growth factor-beta (TGF-β) [29]. Anti-inflammatory cytokines such as interleukin-10 (IL-10) and prostaglandin E2 (PGE2) support an immune context that counteracts overwhelming inflammatory responses and aids in tissue remodeling. Collectively, these factors work together to orchestrate the three phases of the healing cycle: inflammation, proliferation, and remodeling [30].

In osteoarthritis and cartilage damage, BMAC reduces inflammation, decreases pain, and regenerates cartilage. In tendon and ligament injuries, the bioactive factors found in BMAC stimulate fibroblast proliferation and collagen production, facilitating soft tissue repair [18]. BMAC also promotes bone healing by promoting the differentiation of MSCs into osteoblasts and stimulating vascularization through factors like VEGF [31, 32]. Therefore, BMAC is an important method in the treatment of complex orthopedic conditions and provides cellular repair, matrix production, vascular integration, and modulation of inflammation. BMAC is becoming more important as orthopedic research continues to provide biologically mediated strategies for an array of musculoskeletal injuries and degenerative diseases [33, 34].

BMAC treatments are minimally invasive and usually performed on an outpatient basis, resulting in shorter recovery times and reduced hospital costs. However, BMAC suffers from the same challenges as bone marrow due to variability in stem cell quality based on patient age, health, and harvesting technique [35]. Developing better techniques for BMAC preparation may produce optimal cell counts and quality to achieve the best outcomes. BMAC is a promising step forward in the field of regenerative therapies, as it promotes healing using the patient's own cells and may help minimize the need for surgeries in the future. BMAC represents the potential future of the field as it demonstrates harnessing the body's own reparative capability, which can lead to novel treatments. Future work will focus on improving harvesting, characterizing the isolation at the cellular and molecular levels, and sequential usage of BMAC with biomaterial scaffolds to maximize the therapeutic impact.

12.1.2.2 Composition and Cellular Components of Bone Marrow

Bone marrow is a highly dynamic tissue critical for hematopoiesis and tissue regeneration, which consists of a microenvironment formed by the stroma, hematopoietic cells, ECM, cytokines, and growth factors. Mesenchymal stem cells (MSCs), which are responsible for chondrogenesis, osteogenesis, and adipogenesis, are located in the stromal compartment and play an important role in cartilage repair. MSCs also secrete substances that counteract inflammation and promote tissue repair. Hematopoietic stem cells (HSCs) include the generation of blood cells and enable tissue repair/recovery through reciprocal interactions with stromal cells. Furthermore, bone marrow contains supportive cells such as fibroblasts, which synthesize ECM. Endothelial cells stimulate angiogenesis. Macrophages, in particular the M2 subtype, produce and release anti-inflammatory cytokines and growth factors such as VEGF and PDGF to promote tissue reconstruction and vascularization [18].

Bone marrow contains diverse cellular components, classified into hematopoietic and stromal cells. The components include approximately 40% red blood cells, 15% granulocytes, 2% nucleated erythroid precursors, 2–5% platelets, 40% lymphocytes, and less than 1% progenitor cells. These progenitor cells include hematopoietic stem and progenitor cells and mesenchymal stromal cells and can be therapeutically applicable after selection [36].

12.1.2.3 The Significance of Mesenchymal Stem Cells (MSCs) in Tissue Repair

MSCs are critical to tissue repair, as they can differentiate into chondrocytes, osteoblasts, and adipocytes. These cells, which reside in tissues such as bone marrow and adipose tissue, are particularly useful for repairing cartilage, which has low regenerative capacity. In addition to differentiation potentials, MSCs also have various secretory functions. It releases bioactive molecules that include growth factors, like transforming growth factor-beta and vascular endothelial growth factor, and cytokines, which may modulate inflammation and enhance cellular proliferation. This generally induces a pro-regenerative microenvironment by recruiting reparative cells, suppressing inflammation, and stimulating angiogenesis and ECM reorganization [37, 38]. Their immunomodulatory effects also reduce secondary damage caused by inflammation, thus speeding up healing [39].

12.1.3 Hyaluronic Acid (HA) as a Scaffold

HA is one of the most promising biomaterials for cartilage tissue engineering because of its distinctive physical and chemical characteristics. HA, a naturally occurring glycosaminoglycan, is among the principal components of the extracellular matrix (ECM) and is important in maintaining the structure, hydration, and signaling. HA scaffolds can mimic the native ECM, facilitating cell adhesion, migration, and proliferation. Their inherent hydrophilicity permits nutrient and oxygen diffusion, while their biocompatibility and biodegradability render HA appropriate for clinical application. Chemical modifications, such as cross-linking, strengthen mechanical properties and modulate degradation rates, enabling adjustable tissue engineering applications [14, 40].

12.1.3.1 Properties of Hyaluronic Acid (HA) and its Role in Tissue Engineering

HA is an important glycosaminoglycan and has significance in tissue engineering. Because of its high water retention, viscoelasticity, and biocompatibility, HA enhances adhesion, proliferation, and migration [39]. Compared to other polymers, HA shows better hydrophilic properties and provides mechanical cushioning, essential in load-bearing tissues, like cartilage. HA can bind to cell surface receptors such as CD44 and RHAMM, activating the signaling pathways that modulate tissue growth and remodeling [41]. The scaffolds mimic the native extracellular environment and are unique signaling molecules that can act as autocrine, paracrine, or endocrine agents with chemoattractant and mitogenic properties [13].

HA scaffolds can be chemically modified to improve mechanical properties, porosity, and degradation rates, rendering these scaffolds ideal for wound healing, cartilage repair, and soft tissue engineering [13]. The HA-based scaffolds serve as structural supports and can also be used to deliver bioactive molecules or cells to damaged tissues. As a carrier for growth factors and stem cells, it enhances tissue regeneration. In cartilage, HA-based scaffolds induce chondrogenesis and differentiate MSCs into chondrocytes. HA, therefore, is crucial in regenerative medicine, providing both structure and biology for advanced therapeutic approaches for tissue repair [39, 42].

When combined with BMAC, HA-based scaffolds enhance the viability and action of BMAC while limiting its escape from the injury site. HA has anti-inflammatory effects and promotes immune tolerance, thus enhancing its regenerative potential [43]. Systematic research, however, is needed to optimize the clinical use of the HA and BMAC solutions, with a focus not only on material performance but also on tissue interaction, cell infiltration, and ECM synthesis. HA-based scaffold with BMAC has great potential to treat joint arthritis and cartilage injuries, but more studies need to be performed to optimize its clinical use. Long-term validation and robust outcome measures are key to translating HA scaffolds from preclinical research to clinical applications, particularly for regenerative procedures.

12.1.3.2 Advantages of HA-Based Scaffolds over Traditional Methods

Traditionally used scaffolding materials, including synthetic polymers and decellularized tissues, has restrictiveness due to immunogenic responses, poor biocompatibility, and mechanical characteristics [44]. Compared with other biopolymers, HA-based scaffolds have the benefits of good biocompatibility, biodegradability, and versatile functionality. Since HA is a naturally occurring glycosaminoglycan, its excellent biocompatibility reduces its immunogenicity, which is an important consideration in clinical applications as the immune response can hinder tissue regeneration [42]. Moreover, HA also biodegrades into harmless metabolites, which allow the tissue incorporation and has a lower risk for complications than other traditional methods [41, 45]. The viscoelastic properties of HA enable the regeneration with better mechanical properties. It also promotes cell adhesion, proliferation, and migration required for tissue formation and growth [41]. In addition, HA can be adjusted chemically to improve mechanical stability. The unique combination of excellent biocompatibility along with multi-functional properties of HA further strengthens the promising scenario in next-generation scaffolding strategies to facilitate better patient outcomes in regenerative medicine [46].

12.1.3.3 Structure and Function of HA-Based Scaffolds

HA-based scaffolds provide a biomimetic environment and promote tissue regeneration. They have a porous, interconnected design that promotes nutrient and oxygen diffusion, fosters chondrocyte viability, and facilitates the integration of new tissue with native cartilage. HA-based scaffolds are adjustable with chemical alterations, such as cross-linking, to improve mechanical strength and stability [47].

Bioactive molecules have been used to promote cell adhesion, proliferation, and differentiation. HA-based scaffolds are bioactive platforms that regulate cellular performance for the purpose of tissue regeneration. They bind to cell surface receptors (for example, CD44, RHAMM) to modulate inflammatory responses, chondrocyte activation, and activity. These interactions facilitate the production of important cartilage matrix, most notably type II collagen and proteoglycans, that are necessary for biomechanical properties. The anti-inflammatory properties of HA can inhibit pro-inflammatory cytokines and oxidative stress, promoting a suitable microenvironment for repair [42].

HA-based scaffolds can be designed to deliver therapeutic agents as well, such as growth factors like TGF-β to facilitate localized release during repair. HA scaffolds can be utilized in combination with cellular and molecular therapies, providing a synergistic solution by fulfilling both structural and biological demands for cartilage repair. They are applicable to tendon and ligament repair, wound healing, and even soft tissue engineering due to their adaptability. Moreover, toward the next generation of regenerative therapies, scaffolds with smart materials and controlled-release systems are paving the way for future therapies.

12.1.3.4 Design Principles for HA-Based Scaffolds

HA-based scaffolds can be manufactured in a dry form and hydrated fluids pre- or intra-implantation. They must allow room for reparative cells to enter and proliferate, at the same time allowing for nutrition and differentiation. Scaffolds should be bioresorbable and degrade at an adequate rate for new tissue formation while demonstrating mechanical support for osteo/chondroconductive features [12].

Incorporation of bioactive molecules or stem cells within HA-based scaffolds is a strategic approach to promote structural and biological repair. Surface modifications of the scaffold can be made to adsorb bioactive agents to enhance regenerative potential. To integrate and function in a long-lasting manner, HA-based scaffolds must keep up immune tolerance and improved biocompatibility of anti-inflammatory properties. Scalability and reproducibility are important for clinical translation, and approaches such as bioprinting can create patient-specific scaffolds for mechanical support and delivery of bioactive factors. A pre-contoured scaffold complementing the defect would allow for the optimal placement. The in-situ retention time of the scaffold should be adequate to promote osteoconduction and osteoinduction and yield healing that would mimic a natural process [48].

12.1.3.5 Biocompatibility and Biodegradability of HA Materials

Biocompatibility and biodegradability of hyaluronic acid (HA) materials are influenced by their molecular structure and interactions with water, making them crucial for cartilage treatment and regenerative medicine [49]. HA changes conformation upon the varying of pH and ionic situations due to its carboxyl and hydroxyl groups. These groups contribute to HA's ability to interact with its environment [49]. Cross-linked HA, used in tissue engineering, faces instability from interchain bond breakage, which must reform during degradation to retain mechanical properties. This process encourages cell migration as mechanical load diminishes. Degradation byproducts may serve as bioactive signaling domains, aiding tissue regeneration [49].

Owing to its non-immunogenic properties, the risk of tissue rejection is minimal. Thus, HA yields a conducive microenvironment for cellular function, reassuring biocompatibility. Another advantage is controlled biodegradability. HA degrades by enzymatic processes or hydrolysis in times of implantation, releasing harmless degradation products, such as oligosaccharides. The degradation kinetics of these systems may be tuned by chemical modifications [49].

HA-based scaffolds are also the target of research that tries to maximize HA material changes and casting to get the best fitting properties, allowing for individualized patient solutions. Such advancements not only strengthen HA's involvement in cartilage repair but also expand its use in soft tissue regeneration.

12.1.4 Synergistic Effects of Hyaluronic-Acid Scaffolds with BMAC

BMAC integrated with HA-based scaffolds is an improved technique for cartilage diseases, combining their structural and biological advantages [50]. HA scaffolds and BMAC work in synergy, maximizing the benefits of both. The combination can significantly improve cell retention and tissue integration. Such retention is critical to the therapeutic efficacy of BMAC, providing a constant local reservoir of MSCs and a milieu of regenerative molecules promoting cartilage repair. The porous structure of HA-based scaffolds has been proven to promote the infiltration of the surrounding cells and the integration with the tissues by providing migration, proliferation, and differentiation of MSCs into chondrocytes as well as nutrient and oxygen exchange, which are the keys to cell survival in avascular cartilage. With HA scaffolds undergoing biodegradation, they can initially support the target structure and subsequently integrate into the surrounding tissue [51]. This localized retention reduces cell loss and sustains therapeutic effects over time, an important consideration when initiating and sustaining cartilage repair due to its inherent limited capacity for regeneration [52]. Furthermore, HA-based scaffolds provide a mechanical buffer for the cellular and molecular components of BMAC, protecting them from mechanical stress and degradation and thus enhancing their viability [53].

HA's anti-inflammatory properties work in tandem with BMAC's regenerative effects, modulating the local immune response. HA exhibits anti-inflammatory effects that complement the regenerative properties of BMAC, modulating the local immune response. HA promotes an anti-inflammatory stance by interacting with CD44 receptors, which reduces pro-inflammatory cytokines and promotes anti-inflammatory mediators, creating a homeostatic environment favorable for cartilage regeneration [54]. In addition, HA scaffolds enhance chondrogenic differentiation of MSCs and provide fundamental mechanical and biochemical cues for producing cartilage-specific components to repair damaged cartilage [52, 55]. The complementary effects of HA and BMAC also promote angiogenesis and vascular remodeling [33].

Controlled release of growth factors and bioactive molecules greatly amplifies the interactive effects of HA-based scaffolds with BMAC during regeneration of cartilaginous tissue [56]. The HA scaffolds proficiently bound bioactive components from BMAC (e.g., TGF-β, VEGF, and BMPs) and executed a sustained release. This continuous outpouring ensures that these molecules are present at the site of injury, creating a beneficial environment for not only mesenchymal stem cells (MSCs) but also other reparative cells [57]. HA scaffolds facilitate localized, sustained release of molecules [16]. Moreover, the ability of the scaffold to retain BMAC at the defect site acts as a source of bioactive molecules while preventing rapid degradation [56].

HA scaffolds have many variations currently being researched to refine mechanical properties, degradation rates, and biochemical functions to meet cartilage repair requirements. The pore size and interconnectivity of the scaffold can be tailored, which can facilitate cell infiltration and the diffusion of necessary nutrients. Novel fabrication approaches like 3D printing enable the design of scaffolds for specific defect geometries and clinical needs.

12.2 Current Applications in Medicine

12.2.1 Orthopedics (e.g., Cartilage Repair, Osteoarthritis)

Studies show that BMAC directly addressing joint cartilage defects (especially knee) is very effective [58]. In addition, BMAC appears to be effective in the treatment of osteoarthritis (OA), characterized by cartilage loss, inflammation, and pain. In contrast to traditional OA treatments that simply relieve symptoms, BMAC takes a more direct approach to underlying causes with its minimally invasive technique. The MSCs improve joint inflammation, thereby promoting regeneration and pain relief [33]. Growth factors, such as TGF-β and PDGF, promote both cell proliferation and matrix production. Clinical features are pain relief, mobility, and increased cartilage quality in OA patients treated with BMAC [59]. Other orthopedic applications of BMAC include tendon and ligament reconstruction, fracture healing, and spinal disc generation [28]. In tendon injuries, BMAC promotes collagen synthesis and accelerates healing by recruiting stem cells and providing a supportive environment [60]. In fractures, MSCs and growth factors promote regeneration and vascularization, especially for non-unions [61]. BMAC is revealed to be promising in returning disc structure in the treatment of spinal disc degeneration through stimulating repair of both the annulus fibrosus and the nucleus pulposus [62]. Challenges remain with regard to BMAC's application in terms of variability in outcomes based on age and health of the patient as well as quality of the harvest. Although it can be considered generally safe and minimally invasive, there is a need for standardization in preparation techniques to guarantee efficacy [63].

Continuous research and trials are necessary to maximize the utility of BMAC and to extend its applications. BMAC represents a major breakthrough in orthopedic medicine, providing a regenerative solution for diseases that are traditionally treated with only symptomatic relief or invasive surgeries. Its ability to generate cartilage, treat osteoarthritis, and support tendon, ligament, and bone healing underscores its game-changing potential for enhancing patient outcomes. BMAC is poised to drive further orthopedic innovation as research progresses.

12.2.2 Wound Healing and Soft Tissue Regeneration

BMAC is also an important component in wound healing and soft tissue regeneration. BMAC comes from the patient's own bone marrow and contains a high concentration of mesenchymal stem cells (MSCs), hematopoietic stem cells (HSCs), platelets, and growth factors VEGF, PDGF, and TGF-β [29].

One of the main advantages of BMAC is its anti-inflammatory properties. Chronic wounds like diabetic foot ulcers and pressure sores are most often affected by prolonged inflammation, which prevents healing. MSCs present in BMAC secrete immunoregulatory cytokines (e.g., IL-10), leading to a shift in infiltrating macrophage subtype ratios toward an anti-inflammatory M2 subtype, as opposed to an inflammatory M1 subtype [64]. Also, angiogenesis is promoted by such growth factors as VEGF, which improves blood circulation and ensures the oxygen and nutrient supply required for regeneration. BMAC offers an autologous and minimally invasive solution in the context of burn care and soft tissue repair [65]. BMAC has also demonstrated potential for soft tissue repair for muscles and ligaments, which have limited reconstructive ability. BMAC-derived MSCs can undergo myocyte and fibroblast differentiation and provide tissue repair, in addition to releasing bioactive molecules that can induce local cell proliferation and ECM remodeling [66].

BMAC is a significant improvement over the current management methods of chronic wounds, burns, and soft tissue injuries. It works by identifying and treating the factors that hinder healing and therefore incorporates stem cells, growth factors, and bioactive molecules for tissue healing. It may hold the key to future developments in wound management and soft tissue regeneration, which may offer patients alternative and better ways of treating complicated conditions.

12.3 The Healing Cycle and Its Optimization

12.3.1 Phases of the Healing Cycle

Three distinct physiologic phases constitute the healing cycle with cartilage repair: inflammation, proliferation, and remodeling [67–69]. The process starts with inflammation, which begins right after injury and is characterized by the diffusion of pro-inflammatory cytokines such as IL-1β and TNF-α in injured tissues from immune cells and damaged cells. Neutrophils and macrophages are recruited by these molecules and secrete growth factors (e.g., TGF-β, VEGF, PDGF). Although inflammation is critical for recovery, it can also impair healing if excessive. Thus, the healing process requires proper regulation of inflammatory responses [70].

The next phase after inflammation is the proliferation phase, and it includes the recruitment of mesenchymal stem cells (MSCs) and chondroprogenitor cells. Under the influence of TGF-β and BMPs, these cells rapidly proliferate and differentiate into chondrocytes that produce the major components of the extracellular matrix—type II collagen and proteoglycans. This step is essential for the healing of the cartilage tissue. HA-based scaffolds assist in ensuring retention of the cells and provide an ideal microenvironment for ECM formation [71].

Lastly, the remodeling phase includes the reorganization of the newly synthesized cartilage. Chondrocytes adjust the structure of ECM by extracting misaligned components. In osteochondral injuries, vascularization at the cartilage-bone interface promotes the delivery of nutrients. But due to the avascularity nature of cartilage tissue, it tends to heal as fibrocartilage rather than hyaline cartilage [72]. HA scaffolds and BMAC enhance this phase, offering mechanical support and supplying MSCs and growth factors for continued ECM synthesis and remodeling.

12.3.2 How BMAC and HA Interact with the Healing Cycle

12.3.2.1 Accelerating Inflammation Resolution

Bone marrow aspirate concentrate (BMAC) and hyaluronic acid (HA) work together in promoting inflammation resolution, which is critical for cartilage repair [73]. The inflammation phase is the initial phase, which eliminates the debris and brings in the repairing cells. However, inflammation can be aggravated to a level that hampers the healing of the tissue. BMAC and HA help in setting up an anti-inflammatory environment, which allows for the progression to the proliferation and regeneration phases. BMAC contains numerous stem cells, cytokines, and growth factors such as TGF-β, IL-10, and PDGF that also help in resolving inflammation [69].

The secreted factors polarize the macrophages from the pro-inflammatory M1 to the tissue restoring M2 phenotypes. It suppresses the pro-inflammatory cytokines IL-1β and TNF-α while increasing the anti-inflammatory cytokines IL-10 and TGF-β. This process reduces the local inflammation and thus protects the cartilage [69].

HA binds to cell surface receptors, including CD44 on the immune cells, which leads to reduction of pro-inflammatory cytokines and up-regulation of reparative factors [74]. Its viscoelastic nature provides a shield to the injured area, thus reducing the inflammatory cell infiltration. In managing the immune response, HA reduces oxidative stress and tissue degradation to allow for the progression to proliferation. Also, the combination of HA and BMAC also improves the cellular signaling. There is a possibility of settling BMAC by HA scaffolds, which results in continuous release of MSCs and their products to the injury site and therefore extends the period of anti-inflammatory effect and optimal levels of growth factors for cellular recruitment and regeneration. These interactions set the stage for the conditions that are necessary for cell proliferation as well as extracellular matrix synthesis in the repair of the cartilage [53].

Ultimately, BMAC and HA together offer a useful approach for managing the inflammatory healing phase. This approach enables the inflammation to resolve, thereby avoiding more damage to the tissues and, at the same time, creating a platform for the healing and regeneration of the tissues. Further development of the properties of the HA scaffold and the optimization of the BMAC may provide possibilities for enhancing these synergistic effects and, therefore, the outcomes of cartilage repair.

12.3.2.2 Promoting Angiogenesis and Tissue Regeneration

BMAC and HA work together in order to improve the healing process since they enhance angiogenesis and tissue regeneration, which is very important in the treatment of cartilage defects and joints [18]. Angiogenesis is the formation of new blood vessels, and this process is very important at the cartilage-subchondral bone interface, where nutrients and reparative cells are required. As we know, cartilage is avascular, and the subchondral bone plays a role in the nutrition and support of the healing tissue. BMAC and HA meet this challenge by promoting angiogenesis in the subchondral region and supporting the formation of avascular cartilage tissue [75].

VEGF, being released from MSCs present in BMAC, is a growth factor that stimulates endothelial cell growth and formation of vascular-like structures. PDGF acts to recruit pericytes and smooth muscle cells in order to stabilize the newly formed vessels, thus forming functional blood vessels. Angiopoietins released from MSCs help in the process of vascular development to supply nutrients and oxygen to the injured area. It is evident that the network provided by these vessels is necessary for the support of the metabolism of the regenerating cartilage and subchondral bone and thus accelerates the healing process [75].

HA also mediates angiogenesis through scaffolding that ensures that the bioactive molecules and cells are retained at the injury site. This hydrophilic polymer also controls the release of VEGF and PDGF in a sustained manner, which in turn enhances the bioavailability of these growth factors [76]. Also, HA has a porous structure that enables the movement of endothelial cells and MSCs in order to set up a platform for angiogenesis and tissue formation. HA binds to cell surface receptors, which results in the increased activity of MSC and endothelial cells and their proliferation as well as the production of proangiogenic factors [47]. Furthermore, HA regulates the inflammation process, thus avoiding the development of excessive immune responses that can interfere with the process of vascularization and tissue healing [77].

During angiogenesis, BMAC and HA facilitate the differentiation of MSCs into chondrocytes and osteoblasts of the BMAC. These cells are able to produce the extracellular matrix components required for the reconstruction of cartilage and subchondral bone. The HA scaffolds act as a temporary ECM by giving mechanical support and biochemical cues for the tissue to develop. Their degradation is sequential and matches the maturation of the newly formed tissues in order to ensure the connection with the native structures and to avoid the formation of fibrotic tissue [78].

The combination of BMAC and HA is useful in the treatment of focal cartilage defects since both are effective in the regeneration of the vascularized subchondral bone and the avascular cartilage. In focal cartilage defects, the mutual interaction of these components facilitates the repair of the osteochondral unit and, hence, the healing process. In conditions such as osteoarthritis, BMAC and HA therapy enhance the joint homeostasis by promoting angiogenesis, reducing inflammation, and enhancing the healing of cartilage. This dual effect enhances the healing process and the quality of the regenerated tissue, thus increasing its strength and functionality.

12.3.2.3 Supporting Long-Term Remodeling and Tissue Strength

The cooperation between BMAC and HA is very important in the remodeling stage. This phase involves integration of repaired cartilage into the surrounding structures and makes sure that these are able to withstand the physiological loads. BMAC and HA help in the formation of ECM, support the chondrocyte function, and may help in solving some of the problems that could have hindered healing. The MSCs present in BMAC release cytokines and become chondrocytes, which is useful in matrix formation. Growth factors regulate collagen formation and the repair of interfaces, enhancing the formation of stable repairs while controlling metalloproteinases to ensure that there is a balance between ECM synthesis and degradation. When HA breaks down, it is replaced by the native ECM, thus ensuring that the tissue is well integrated. HA binds with cellular receptors and initiates signaling pathways that include adhesion and matrix synthesis. It also helps in the processes of collagen organization and proteoglycan deposition, thus trying to attain the biomechanical characteristics of native cartilage.

A major challenge in the treatment of cartilage defects is the failure of the regeneration process, which results in the formation of fibrous cartilage instead of hyaline cartilage. BMAC and HA address this by providing the cues for hyaline cartilage restoration. The BMAC contains MSCs and growth factors that help in the differentiation of chondrocytes and production of type II collagen, whereas HA provides the necessary matrix. Some of the benefits of HA include reduction of inflammation, which helps in reducing the chronic inflammation that may lead to the formation of fibrous tissues. This combination ensures that there is the formation of durable and strong cartilage that can withstand loads.

From the clinical perspective, the combination of BMAC and HA is beneficial as it enhances the treatment of large cartilage defects and osteochondral injuries, which may result in poor healing when managed with conventional techniques. These improvements enhance the patient's outcome in the long term. Current research aims at enhancing the properties of HA scaffolds to enhance their role in remodeling. Furthermore, in the case of BMAC, it is also possible to enhance the results by increasing the number of cells in the sample or by adding specific growth factors. More clinical trials are required in order to determine the durability of the cartilage and its performance in the future.

12.3.3 Factors Influencing Success

12.3.3.1 Patient-Specific Variables (Age, Comorbidities, etc.)

The efficacy of bone marrow aspirate concentrate (BMAC) together with hyaluronic acid (HA)-based scaffolds in the treatment of cartilage injury depends on several factors, which include the patient's age, co-morbidities, general lifestyle, and the specific type of cartilage loss. Individualized treatment strategies are important in order to enhance the results at every stage of the healing process.

Age is a major factor that determines the success of BMAC-HA therapy since older people have fewer functional MSCs. Fewer and unfunctional MSCs may cause a delay in the cartilage healing process mainly during the proliferative and remodeling phases [79]. Such strategies as MSC enrichment or preconditioning may improve the results. Other diseases such as diabetes, obesity, and autoimmune diseases can have negative effects on healing. Diabetes can also affect the wound healing and angiogenesis processes, while obesity can cause inflammation and stress on the joints, which accelerate the degeneration [80]. These conditions can be treated to enhance the effectiveness of the treatment. The size and chronicity of the cartilage defects are also key factors that determine the success of the therapy. Chronic injuries often feature scar tissue that hinders repair, while acute injuries create a more favorable healing environment [81]. There are numerous lifestyle factors that can affect the healing process; these include smoking and activity levels. Smoking adversely affects angiogenesis and cellular activity, while an appropriate activity level can improve the results [82]. Specific rehabilitation is required for achieving the best results.

There are several advances in the field of personalized BMAC-HA therapies for elderly individuals or those with suboptimal MSCs such as the use of MSC enhancement and the addition of anti-inflammatory factors. The properties of HA scaffolds can be modified depending on the patient's defect. Some of the post-implantation factors include stability of the scaffold and management of the microenvironment. It has been suggested that the joint may require some immobilization followed by specific rehabilitation. Mechanical loading has to be maintained to an optimum level to enhance ECM synthesis without subjecting the tissue to high strain levels.

12.4 Challenges and Limitations

BMAC and HA-based scaffolds are also known to be potential candidates in the field of cartilage repair, but all of them have several limitations. The use of BMAC is influenced by several patient-specific factors, with the quality of MSCs harvested being a major factor of concern. These factors include the age of the patient and comorbid conditions, including diabetes and obesity, which affect the MSCs' function through reduction of proliferation and differentiation into chondrocytes. This can be compounded by chronic inflammation requiring specific management to improve results, which may include preconditioning of MSCs or boosting BMAC.

The quality of BMAC is also influenced by the harvesting site and processing techniques. Bone marrow is commonly extracted from the iliac crest, but if the techniques are not proper, then it may lead to a reduced number of MSCs and growth factors in the samples. There are certain standards that should be followed in processing protocols to ensure consistent therapeutic efficacy.

The design of the scaffold and the materials affect the cartilage repair. There are parameters that one has to consider, such as porosity, stiffness, and degradation rate of the scaffold. In load-bearing regions of the scaffold, there should be pores that can support the structure and at the same time allow for cell penetration. Degradation rates must also be controlled in a way that supports healing at the right time.

Technical challenges include the precise delivery of BMAC and scaffolds to defects. Ensuring local placement is critical for maximizing retention and bioactive molecule delivery. Large or irregularly shaped defects complicate uniform distribution, risking incomplete repair. Custom scaffolds, including 3D-printed options, can enhance integration but may complicate procedures.

There are advancements being made to enhance the BMAC and HA technologies. Better isolation techniques for MSCs, including density gradient centrifugation can enhance the quality of the isolated MSCs. Some treatments that have been found to enhance the function of MSCs include hypoxic pre-conditioning as well as the use of growth factors. In scaffold development, bioengineered materials are used. For instance, growth factor release systems as well as nanostructured surfaces that resemble natural cartilage may enhance the interactions between the tissue and the cells.

12.4.1 Potential Risks and Contraindications

There are certain risks and contraindications associated with the use of bone marrow aspirate concentrate (BMAC) and hyaluronic acid (HA)-based scaffolds in the treatment of cartilage injuries. Some of the risks include variability in the quality of BMAC, which depends on the harvesting techniques, site of harvesting, age, and general health of the patient. Contamination during preparation can lower the concentration of mesenchymal stem cells (MSCs) and bioactive molecules, reducing regenerative potential. HA scaffolds are biocompatible but may induce local inflammatory reactions in patients with sensitivity to HA products, leading to discomfort and edema. In addition, there are problems that may arise from the scaffold degradation rates, such as if the degradation is too fast, then there is a risk of loss of structural support, while if the degradation is slow, then there is a risk of non-integration of the tissue. The contraindications for BMAC-HA therapy are, therefore, active infections, which may worsen the outcome, and severe joint deformities or advanced osteoarthritis, which may not respond well. Some systemic diseases, including autoimmune diseases and cancer, can alter the immune responses and raise safety concerns of the treatment. Therefore, it is important to select the right patient, perform the procedures most appropriately, and develop scaffolds to suit the patient's needs to reduce risks. Current research in BMAC enhancement, scaffold development, and immunomodulation focuses on minimizing the adverse effects and increasing the versatility of BMAC-HA therapies.

12.5 Gaps in Clinical Evidence and Need for Further Research

There are still important gaps in the clinical evidence regarding the effectiveness of BMAC and HA-based scaffolds for cartilage repair, thus highlighting the need for more research. Many of the current studies also differ in the methods that they use in BMAC harvesting, processing, scaffold design, and delivery. There are no standardized outcome measures, thus making it difficult to compare results and make firm conclusions about the long-term effects of these treatments. Some important questions remain to be answered regarding the best number of mesenchymal stem cells (MSCs) to be used in BMAC, the most appropriate rates of degradation and mechanical properties of HA scaffolds, and how best to incorporate them into the healing process. Relevant clinical trials are necessary to assess the durability of cartilage regeneration and the resistance of the regenerated cartilage to the physiological loading. Further research is needed to assess the influence of other patient-specific factors, including age, comorbidities, and the duration of cartilage defects. There may be roles for advanced imaging and molecular diagnostics in the assessment of tissue incorporation and turnover to determine the mechanisms of action of BMAC-HA therapy. Investigating novel techniques such as bioengineered scaffolds, controlled release systems, and other personalized regenerative therapies may improve the effectiveness of BMAC-HA therapies.

12.6 Future Directions and Innovations in BMAC and Hyaluronic Acid-Based Scaffold Research

The future of bone marrow aspirate concentrate (BMAC) and hyaluronic acid (HA)-based scaffolds in cartilage repair is poised for groundbreaking advancements in biomaterials, stem cell biology, and regenerative medicine technologies. Addressing current limitations and optimizing these therapies will require innovative approaches that enhance their efficacy, safety, and adaptability.

Advancements in BMAC processing and cellular optimization focus on improving BMAC's quality and consistency, as current isolation methods for MSCs and bioactive substances from bone marrow lead to variable therapeutic results. Future efforts will aim for automated processing systems that enhance MSC yield and purity with reduced contamination. Techniques like density gradient centrifugation, magnetic cell sorting, and microfluidic separation are in development to enhance cell isolation. Additionally, preconditioning MSCs via hypoxic environments or growth factor exposure, as well as genetic modifications, is being investigated to boost their regenerative capacity. These innovations target the enhanced BMAC preparations to achieve better therapeutic outcomes.

In HA-based scaffold design, the need for optimized scaffolds that provide structural support and facilitate healing is recognized. Future designs could include bioactive nanomaterials to improve mechanical properties and bioactivity. Surface modifications, introducing integrin-binding peptides, will enhance scaffold-tissue interaction, promoting integration and regeneration. 3D bioprinting could produce patient-specific scaffolds with optimized characteristics from individual imaging data, enhancing repair success. Hybrid scaffolds using HA with other biomaterials like collagen will address complex repair challenges, including osteochondral lesions.

Combination therapies and adjunctive treatments are becoming essential in elevating regenerative outcomes with BMAC and HA scaffolds. For instance, incorporating platelet-rich plasma (PRP) into BMAC-HA systems adds growth factors and cytokines, boosting their regenerative effect. Alternatively, MSC-derived exosomes provide a cell-free treatment to retain stem cell benefits. Additionally, integrating anti-inflammatory agents or small molecules targeting pathways like NF-κB into HA scaffolds may optimize local repair conditions.

The integration of smart biomaterials and advanced monitoring presents new horizons in scaffold design. Such materials will dynamically respond to local tissue conditions, adjusting properties based on real-time feedback. Examples include pH-sensitive scaffolds releasing therapeutic agents in reaction to changes in inflammation. Advanced monitoring technologies with biosensors in scaffolds enable clinicians to observe integration and remodeling, allowing for therapy adjustments.

Clinical research and long-term validation will be crucial for translating BMAC-HA therapies into mainstream practice, requiring large-scale, multicenter trials with uniform protocols to evaluate efficacy and safety. Emphasis on long-term monitoring of regenerated cartilage's durability under physiological stress will be essential, alongside the development of imaging biomarkers and diagnostics to evaluate regeneration.

The future of BMAC and HA scaffolds lies in personalized medicine, utilizing patient-specific data to tailor therapies. Integrating genetic profiles, MSC quality, and cartilage defect characteristics can optimize treatment protocols and scaffold designs. This approach aims to improve BMAC-HA efficacy while minimizing complications.

12.7 Conclusion

With both BMAC and HA-based scaffold research findings, the future research is exciting as we see more and more advancements in the biomaterials and cellular engineering fields. By effectively addressing many of these challenges in a careful and strategic manner, it is anticipated that these novel and advanced therapies can fundamentally redefine cartilage repair in many transformative and impactful ways. This revolution means that patients get better and more tailored treatments. Also, further strengthening and sustaining the collaborative relationships between researchers, clinicians, and industry stakeholders and ensuring that there is adequate funding will be critical in realizing the potential of regenerative medicine. Thus, with every progress made in this regard, the possibility of successful treatment of cartilage diseases is ever increasing, a ray of light to the affected individuals.

References

1. Betz UAK, Arora L, Assal RA, Azevedo H, Baldwin J, Becker MS, et al. Game changers in science and technology—now and beyond. Technol Forecast Soc Chang. 2023;193:122588.
2. Mobarak MH, Islam MA, Hossain N, Al Mahmud MZ, Rayhan MT, Nishi NJ, et al. Recent advances of additive manufacturing in implant fabrication—a review. Appl Surf Sci Adv. 2023;18:100462.
3. De Francesco F, Zingaretti N, Parodi PC, Riccio M. The evolution of current concept of the reconstructive ladder in plastic surgery: the emerging role of translational medicine. Cells. 2023;12(21)
4. Beheshtizadeh N, Gharibshahian M, Pazhouhnia Z, Rostami M, Zangi AR, Maleki R, et al. Commercialization and regulation of regenerative medicine products: promises, advances and challenges. Biomed Pharmacother. 2022;153:113431.
5. Capponi S, Daniels KG. Harnessing the power of artificial intelligence to advance cell therapy. Immunol Rev. 2023;320(1):147–65.
6. Altyar AE, El-Sayed A, Abdeen A, Piscopo M, Mousa SA, Najda A, et al. Future regenerative medicine developments and their therapeutic applications. Biomed Pharmacother. 2023;158:114131.
7. Todros S, Todesco M, Bagno A. Biomaterials and their biomedical applications: from replacement to regeneration. Processes [Internet]. 2021;9(11)
8. Sun AR, Udduttula A, Li J, Liu Y, Ren P-G, Zhang P. Cartilage tissue engineering for obesity-induced osteoarthritis: physiology, challenges, and future prospects. J Orthop Transl. 2021;26:3–15.
9. Merimi M, El-Majzoub R, Lagneaux L, Moussa Agha D, Bouhtit F, Meuleman N, et al. The therapeutic potential of mesenchymal stromal cells for regenerative medicine: current knowledge and future understandings. Front Cell Dev Biol. 2021;9:661532.
10. Li R, Liu K, Huang X, Li D, Ding J, Liu B, et al. Bioactive materials promote wound healing through modulation of cell behaviors. Adv Sci (Weinh). 2022;9(10):e2105152.
11. Joyce K, Fabra GT, Bozkurt Y, Pandit A. Bioactive potential of natural biomaterials: identification, retention and assessment of biological properties. Signal Transduct Target Ther. 2021;6(1):122.
12. Kotla NG, Mohd Isa IL, Larrañaga A, Maddiboyina B, Swamy SK, Sivaraman G, et al. Hyaluronic acid-based bioconjugate systems, scaffolds, and their therapeutic potential. Adv Healthc Mater. 2023;12(20):e2203104.
13. Ding Y-W, Zhang X-W, Mi C-H, Qi X-Y, Zhou J, Wei D-X. Recent advances in hyaluronic acid-based hydrogels for 3D bioprinting in tissue engineering applications. Smart Mater Med. 2023;4:59–68.
14. Brittberg M. Treatment of knee cartilage lesions in 2024: from hyaluronic acid to regenerative medicine. J Exp Orthop. 2024;11(2):e12016.
15. Veronesi F, Zielli SO, Brogini S, Artioli E, Arceri A, Mazzotti A, et al. Scaffolds for osteochondral lesions of the talus: systematic review and meta-analysis of the last ten years literature. Bioengineering (Basel). 2024;11(10)
16. Liang J, Liu P, Yang X, Liu L, Zhang Y, Wang Q, et al. Biomaterial-based scaffolds in promotion of cartilage regeneration: recent advances and emerging applications. J Orthop Transl. 2023;41:54–62.
17. Wei Q, An Y, Zhao X, Li M, Zhang J. Three-dimensional bioprinting of tissue-engineered skin: biomaterials, fabrication techniques, challenging difficulties, and future directions: a review. Int J Biol Macromol. 2024;266(Pt 1):131281.
18. Kim GB, Seo MS, Park WT, Lee GW. Bone marrow aspirate concentrate: its uses in osteoarthritis. Int J Mol Sci. 2020;21(9)

19. Holton J, Imam MA, Snow M. Bone marrow aspirate in the treatment of chondral injuries. Front Surg. 2016;3:33.
20. Farag MM. Recent trends on biomaterials for tissue regeneration applications: review. J Mater Sci. 2023;58(2):527–58.
21. Lana J, da Fonseca LF, Macedo RDR, Mosaner T, Murrell W, Kumar A, et al. Platelet-rich plasma vs bone marrow aspirate concentrate: An overview of mechanisms of action and orthobiologic synergistic effects. World J Stem Cells. 2021;13(2):155–67.
22. Dabrowska S, Andrzejewska A, Janowski M, Lukomska B. Immunomodulatory and regenerative effects of mesenchymal stem cells and extracellular vesicles: therapeutic outlook for inflammatory and degenerative diseases. Front Immunol. 2020;11:591065.
23. Kwon M, Kim BS, Yoon S, Oh SO, Lee D. Hematopoietic stem cells and their niche in bone marrow. Int J Mol Sci. 2024;25(13)
24. Ribatti D, Tamma R, Annese T. The role of vascular niche and endothelial cells in organogenesis and regeneration. Exp Cell Res. 2021;398(1):112398.
25. Firmansyah Y, Sidharta VM, Wijaya L, Tan ST. Unraveling the significance of growth factors (TGF-β, PDGF, KGF, FGF, pro collagen, VEGF) in the dynamic of wound healing. Asian J Med Health. 2024;22(3):49–61.
26. Sharma P, Kumar A, Dey AD, Behl T, Chadha S. Stem cells and growth factors-based delivery approaches for chronic wound repair and regeneration: a promise to heal from within. Life Sci. 2021;268:118932.
27. Lana JF, Purita J, Jeyaraman M, de Souza BF, Rodrigues BL, Huber SC, et al. Innovative approaches in knee osteoarthritis treatment: a comprehensive review of bone marrow-derived products. Biomedicines [Internet]. 2024;12(12)
28. Husen M, Saris D. Regenerative medicine/cell therapy approaches (BMAC, PRP, and cellular based therapies). In: Sherman SL, Chahla J, LaPrade RF, Rodeo SA, editors. Knee arthroscopy and knee preservation surgery. Cham: Springer International Publishing; 2024. p. 915–31.
29. Mohammed RN, Aziz Sadat SA, Hassan SMA, Mohammed HF, Ramzi DO. Combinatorial influence of bone marrow aspirate concentrate (BMAC) and platelet-rich plasma (PRP) treatment on cutaneous wound healing in BALB/c mice. J Burn Care Res. 2024;45(1):59–69.
30. Gao M, Guo H, Dong X, Wang Z, Yang Z, Shang Q, et al. Regulation of inflammation during wound healing: the function of mesenchymal stem cells and strategies for therapeutic enhancement. Front Pharmacol. 2024;15:1345779.
31. Bouland C, Philippart P, Dequanter D, Corrillon F, Loeb I, Bron D, et al. Cross-talk between mesenchymal stromal cells (MSCs) and endothelial progenitor cells (EPCs) in bone regeneration. Front Cell Dev Biol. 2021;9:674084.
32. Stamnitz S, Klimczak A. Mesenchymal stem cells, bioactive factors, and scaffolds in bone repair: from research perspectives to clinical practice. Cells. 2021;10(8)
33. Balusani P Jr, Shrivastava S, Pundkar A, Kale P. Navigating the therapeutic landscape: a comprehensive review of platelet-rich plasma and bone marrow aspirate concentrate in knee osteoarthritis. Cureus. 2024;16(2):e54747.
34. Moreno-Garcia A, Rodriguez-Merchan EC. Orthobiologics: current role in orthopedic surgery and traumatology. Arch Bone Jt Surg. 2022;10(7):536–42.
35. Lee JS, Gillinov SM, Siddiq BS, Dowley KS, Martin SD. Surgical applications for bone marrow aspirate concentrate. Arthroscopy. 2024;40(9):2350–2.
36. Lucas D. Structural organization of the bone marrow and its role in hematopoiesis. Curr Opin Hematol. 2021;28(1):36–42.
37. Costela-Ruiz VJ, Melguizo-Rodríguez L, Bellotti C, Illescas-Montes R, Stanco D, Arciola CR, et al. Different sources of mesenchymal stem cells for tissue regeneration: a guide to identifying the most favorable one in orthopedics and dentistry applications. Int J Mol Sci. 2022;23(11)
38. Guillamat-Prats R. The role of MSC in wound healing, scarring and regeneration. Cells. 2021;10(7)
39. Karamanos NK, Theocharis AD, Piperigkou Z, Manou D, Passi A, Skandalis SS, et al. A guide to the composition and functions of the extracellular matrix. FEBS J. 2021;288(24):6850–912.
40. Yang KC, Yang YT, Wu CC, Hsiao JK, Huang CY, Chen IH, et al. Bioinspired collagen-gelatin-hyaluronic acid-chondroitin sulfate tetra-copolymer scaffold biomimicking native cartilage extracellular matrix facilitates chondrogenesis of human synovium-derived stem cells. Int J Biol Macromol. 2023;240:124400.
41. Marinho A, Nunes C, Reis S. Hyaluronic acid: a key ingredient in the therapy of inflammation. Biomolecules. 2021;11(10)
42. Menezes R, Vincent R, Osorno L, Hu P, Arinzeh TL. Biomaterials and tissue engineering approaches using glycosaminoglycans for tissue repair: lessons learned from the native extracellular matrix. Acta Biomater. 2023;163:210–27.
43. Vannini F, Berveglieri L, Boffa A, Filardo G, Viglione V, Buda R, et al. Hyaluronic scaffold transplantation with bone marrow concentrate for the treatment of osteochondral lesions of the talus: durable results up to a minimum of 10 years. Knee Surg Sports Traumatol Arthrosc. 2023;31(10):4551–8.
44. Jelodari S, Ebrahimi Sadrabadi A, Zarei F, Jahangir S, Azami M, Sheykhhasan M, et al. New insights into cartilage tissue engineering: improvement of tissue-scaffold integration to enhance cartilage regeneration. Biomed Res Int. 2022;2022:7638245.
45. Rosales P, Vitale D, Icardi A, Sevic I, Alaniz L. Role of hyaluronic acid and its chemical derivatives in

immunity during homeostasis, cancer and tissue regeneration. Semin Immunopathol. 2024;46(5):15.
46. He T, Li B, Colombani T, Joshi-Navare K, Mehta S, Kisiday J, et al. Hyaluronic acid-based shape-memory cryogel scaffolds for focal cartilage defect repair. Tissue Eng Part A. 2021;27(11–12):748–60.
47. Chen H, Xue H, Zeng H, Dai M, Tang C, Liu L. 3D printed scaffolds based on hyaluronic acid bioinks for tissue engineering: a review. Biomater Res. 2023;27(1):137.
48. Mahanani ES, Puspita S, Dewi AH. The proper design of scaffold porosity for bone regeneration (literature review). AIP Conf Proc. 2024;3127(1):020018.
49. Abatangelo G, Vindigni V, Avruscio G, Pandis L, Brun P. Hyaluronic acid: redefining its role. Cells. 2020;9:7.
50. Ow ZGW, Cheang HLX, Koh JH, Koh JZE, Lim KK-L, Wang D, et al. Does the choice of acellular scaffold and augmentation with bone marrow aspirate concentrate affect short-term outcomes in cartilage repair? A systematic review and meta-analysis. Am J Sports Med. 2022;51(6):1622–33.
51. Zhai P, Peng X, Li B, Liu Y, Sun H, Li X. The application of hyaluronic acid in bone regeneration. Int J Biol Macromol. 2020;151:1224–39.
52. Gao W, Chen K, He W, Zhao S, Cui D, Tao C, et al. Synergistic chondrogenesis promotion and arthroscopic articular cartilage restoration via injectable dual-drug-loaded sulfated hyaluronic acid hydrogel for stem cell therapy. Compos Part B. 2023;263:110857.
53. Whyte GP, Herman K, Gobbi A. One-step cell-based cartilage repair in the knee using hyaluronic acid-based scaffold embedded with mesenchymal stem cells sourced from bone marrow aspirate concentrate (HA-BMAC). In: Brittberg M, Slynarski K, editors. Lower extremity joint preservation: techniques for treating the hip, knee, and ankle. Cham: Springer International Publishing; 2021. p. 47–54.
54. Li M, Yin H, Yan Z, Li H, Wu J, Wang Y, et al. The immune microenvironment in cartilage injury and repair. Acta Biomater. 2022;140:23–42.
55. Zha K, Sun Z, Yang Y, Chen M, Gao C, Fu L, et al. Recent developed strategies for enhancing chondrogenic differentiation of MSC: impact on MSC-based therapy for cartilage regeneration. Stem Cells Int. 2021;2021:8830834.
56. Hernigou J, Vertongen P, Rasschaert J, Hernigou P. Role of scaffolds, subchondral, intra-articular injections of fresh autologous bone marrow concentrate regenerative cells in treating human knee cartilage lesions: different approaches and different results. Int J Mol Sci. 2021;22(8)
57. Djoudi A, Molina-Peña R, Ferreira N, Ottonelli I, Tosi G, Garcion E, et al. Hyaluronic acid scaffolds for loco-regional therapy in nervous system related disorders. Int J Mol Sci. 2022;23(20)
58. Pithadia P. BMAC and adipose-derived MSCs treatment for knee osteoarthritis: a systematic review. Int J Clin Case Rep Rev. 2021;
59. Langworthy M, Dasa V, Spitzer AI. Knee osteoarthritis: disease burden, available treatments, and emerging options. Ther Adv Musculoskelet Dis. 2024;16:1759720x241273009.
60. Blanton CM, Clougherty CO. The role of bone marrow aspirate in osseous and soft tissue pathology. Clin Podiatr Med Surg. 2021;38(1):1–16.
61. Ehlen QT, Costello JP 2nd, Mirsky NA, Slavin BV, Parra M, Ptashnik A, et al. Treatment of bone defects and nonunion via novel delivery mechanisms, growth factors, and stem cells: a review. ACS Biomater Sci Eng. 2024;10(12):7314–36.
62. Her YF, Kubrova E, Martinez Alvarez GA, D'Souza RS. The analgesic efficacy of Intradiscal injection of bone marrow aspirate concentrate and culture-expanded bone marrow mesenchymal stromal cells in discogenic pain: a systematic review. J Pain Res. 2022;15:3299–318.
63. Keeling LE, Belk JW, Kraeutler MJ, Kallner AC, Lindsay A, McCarty EC, et al. Bone marrow aspirate concentrate for the treatment of knee osteoarthritis: a systematic review. Am J Sports Med. 2021;50(8):2315–23.
64. Butler JJ, Dankert JF, Keller LE, Azam MT, Dahmen J, Kerkhoffs G, et al. Assessment of the monocyte subpopulations and M1/M2 macrophage ratio in concentrated bone marrow aspirate. Cartilage. 2024:19476035241304308.
65. Lee J-H, Parthiban P, Jin G-Z, Knowles JC, Kim H-W. Materials roles for promoting angiogenesis in tissue regeneration. Prog Mater Sci. 2021;117:100732.
66. Sundar DRA, Ak DP, Kumar DA, Nizar DAM, Subash DY. A study on bone marrow derived stem cells and its application on ACL graft regeneration in partial ACL tears. Int J Orthop Sci. 2023;
67. Gonzalez AC, Costa TF, Andrade ZA, Medrado AR. Wound healing—a literature review. An Bras Dermatol. 2016;91(5):614–20.
68. Hambly K, Silvers HJ, Steinwachs M. Rehabilitation after articular cartilage repair of the knee in the football (soccer) player. Cartilage. 2012;3(1 Suppl):50s–6s.
69. Landén NX, Li D, Ståhle M. Transition from inflammation to proliferation: a critical step during wound healing. Cell Mol Life Sci. 2016;73(20):3861–85.
70. Chen L, Deng H, Cui H, Fang J, Zuo Z, Deng J, et al. Inflammatory responses and inflammation-associated diseases in organs. Oncotarget. 2018;9(6):7204–18.
71. Chen H, Tan XN, Hu S, Liu RQ, Peng LH, Li YM, et al. Molecular mechanisms of chondrocyte proliferation and differentiation. Front Cell Dev Biol. 2021;9:664168.
72. Li Y, Xu L. Advances in understanding cartilage remodeling. F1000Res. 2015;4(F1000 Faculty Rev):642.
73. Gobbi A, Whyte GP. One-stage cartilage repair using a hyaluronic acid-based scaffold with activated bone marrow-derived mesenchymal stem cells compared with microfracture: five-year follow-up. Am J Sports Med. 2016;44(11):2846–54.

74. Weng X, Maxwell-Warburton S, Hasib A, Ma L, Kang L. The membrane receptor CD44: novel insights into metabolism. Trends Endocrinol Metab. 2022;33(5):318–32.
75. Madry H, Gao L, Eichler H, Orth P, Cucchiarini M. Bone marrow aspirate concentrate-enhanced marrow stimulation of chondral defects. Stem Cells Int. 2017;2017:1609685.
76. Alkabli J. Recent advances in the development of chitosan/hyaluronic acid-based hybrid materials for skin protection, regeneration, and healing: a review. Int J Biol Macromol. 2024;279:135357.
77. Yang P, Lu Y, Gou W, Qin Y, Tan J, Luo G, et al. Glycosaminoglycans' ability to promote wound healing: from native living macromolecules to artificial biomaterials. Adv Sci (Weinh). 2024;11(9):e2305918.
78. Radice M, Brun P, Cortivo R, Scapinelli R, Battaliard C, Abatangelo G. Hyaluronan-based biopolymers as delivery vehicles for bone-marrow-derived mesenchymal progenitors. J Biomed Mater Res. 2000;50(2):101–9.
79. Cavallo C, Boffa A, de Girolamo L, Merli G, Kon E, Cattini L, et al. Bone marrow aspirate concentrate quality is affected by age and harvest site. Knee Surg Sports Traumatol Arthrosc. 2023;31(6):2140–51.
80. Rohm TV, Meier DT, Olefsky JM, Donath MY. Inflammation in obesity, diabetes, and related disorders. Immunity. 2022;55(1):31–55.
81. Merkely G, Farr J, Saris D, Lattermann C. Cartilage surface treatment: factors affecting success and failure mechanisms. Oper Tech Sports Med. 2020;28(1):150711.
82. Chan AHP, Hu C, Chiang GCF, Ekweume C, Huang NF. Chronic nicotine impairs the angiogenic capacity of human induced pluripotent stem cell-derived endothelial cells in a murine model of peripheral arterial disease. JVS Vasc Sci. 2023;4:100115.

Cartilage Treatment with Adipose Mesenchymal Stem Cells

13

Simone Orazi, Angelo Boffa, Luca Andriolo, Alessandro Di Martino, and Stefano Zaffagnini

13.1 Introduction

Articular cartilage lesions and degenerative joint diseases remain a major challenge in orthopedic practice. The highly specialized architecture of hyaline cartilage, characterized by an abundant extracellular matrix, low cellular density, and an avascular, alymphatic, and aneural environment, accounts for its extremely limited intrinsic healing potential [1]. When structural integrity is disrupted by trauma, overload, or degenerative processes, restoration of native tissue architecture rarely occurs. Untreated focal defects may progress over time, contributing to persistent symptoms and potentially to the development or progression of osteoarthritis (OA) [2]. The understanding of OA has evolved from a purely mechanical and degenerative disorder to a complex disease involving the entire joint organ, including synovium and subchondral bone [3]. This conceptual shift has stimulated interest in orthobiologic strategies aimed not only at structural repair but also at modulation of the intra-articular environment. Among these, mesenchymal stromal cells (MSCs) have emerged as biologically appealing candidates due to their trophic and regulatory properties in addition to their multilineage differentiation potential [4].

MSCs can be isolated from several tissue sources, including bone marrow, synovium, periosteum, umbilical cord, and adipose tissue. Each source presents specific biological and practical characteristics [5]. In recent years, adipose tissue has attracted particular attention as a readily available and abundant reservoir of mesenchymal progenitor cells. Adipose-derived MSCs, contained within the stromal vascular fraction, can be harvested through minimally invasive procedures and provide a high cellular yield without mandatory culture expansion in selected settings [6, 7]. Beyond cellular abundance, adipose-derived products exhibit relevant immunomodulatory activity, which may be particularly valuable in OA, where low-grade synovial inflammation plays a central role in symptom generation and disease progression [8]. Clinically, these products have been applied both as intra-articular injections for symptomatic knee OA and as biological augmentation in focal cartilage repair procedures [9, 10].

The purpose of this chapter is to examine the biological rationale, technical aspects, clinical evidence, indications, and limitations of adipose-derived MSCs in cartilage treatment, with particular focus on OA and focal chondral lesions.

S. Orazi · A. Boffa (✉) · L. Andriolo · A. Di Martino · S. Zaffagnini
Clinica Ortopedica e Traumatologica 2, IRCCS Istituto Ortopedico Rizzoli, Bologna, Italy
e-mail: simone.orazi@studio.unibo.it; angelo.boffa@ior.it; luca.andriolo@ior.it; alessandro.dimartino@ior.it; stefano.zaffagnini@unibo.it

M. E. Erdil et al. (eds.), *Current Concept in Cartilage Treatment*,
https://doi.org/10.1007/978-3-032-27099-3_13

13.2 Biological Rationale of Adipose-Derived MSCs

MSCs are multipotent stromal cells defined by their capacity for trilineage differentiation and by a characteristic immunophenotypic profile. In joint disorders, however, their therapeutic relevance appears to depend less on direct differentiation and more on their regulatory activity within the local microenvironment [4]. MSCs can release a complex secretome composed of cytokines, growth factors, chemokines, and extracellular vesicles capable of modulating inflammation, apoptosis, angiogenesis, and matrix turnover [11]. Experimental evidence indicates that MSCs can influence macrophage polarization, promoting a shift toward anti-inflammatory phenotypes and attenuating catabolic signaling within the synovial environment. They may also provide trophic support to resident chondrocytes and endogenous progenitors [8]. Thanks to these properties, the therapeutic effect of MSCs appears predominantly regulatory, aimed at restoring intra-articular homeostasis rather than directly replacing damaged tissue. This paradigm forms the conceptual basis for their clinical application.

MSCs can be derived from multiple tissue sources, including adipose tissue, bone marrow, synovium, periosteum, infrapatellar fat pad, and perinatal tissues. Each source exhibits distinct biological characteristics in terms of cellular yield, proliferative capacity, differentiation potential, and secretory profile [5]. Among available MSC sources, bone marrow-derived MSCs represent the most extensively studied cell population in cartilage repair and OA and have historically constituted the reference standard in regenerative orthopedics [12].

In recent years, adipose tissue has gained particular interest due to its abundance, ease of access, and high progenitor yield. Adipose-derived mesenchymal MSCs are located within the stromal vascular fraction, a heterogeneous compartment enriched in perivascular progenitor cells. Compared with bone marrow aspirates, lipoaspirates provide a substantially higher number of nucleated and progenitor cells per unit volume of harvested tissue [6]. This difference becomes clinically relevant in older individuals, in whom bone marrow-derived progenitor populations demonstrate age-related decline in number and proliferative capacity [13]. In addition to quantitative aspects, adipose-derived stromal cells demonstrate relevant immunomodulatory properties, including the capacity to influence macrophage polarization within the osteoarthritic joint [8]. From a surgical standpoint, subcutaneous adipose harvesting through liposuction is minimally invasive and generally associated with limited donor-site morbidity. Combined with harvest feasibility and high cellular yield, these characteristics support adipose tissue as a clinically attractive MSC source. Moreover, some mechanical processing systems have been developed to preserve the native stromal niche and perivascular architecture while avoiding enzymatic digestion [14, 15]. Mesenchymal progenitor cells within adipose tissue are predominantly located in the perivascular niche. Preservation of this structural microenvironment during harvesting is biologically relevant, as excessive mechanical trauma may influence cellular viability and secretory behavior [14].

Comparative analyses suggest that no single tissue origin demonstrates unequivocal superiority across all clinical indications. Meta-analyses of intra-articular MSC therapies for knee OA reported consistent symptomatic improvement over available follow-up periods, while emphasizing variability in harvesting techniques, processing strategies, and outcome reporting [16–18]. This diversity complicates direct comparison between studies and interpretation of potential disease-modifying effects. Within this context, adipose-derived MSCs should be regarded as one component of a broader regenerative strategy rather than a universally superior alternative.

13.3 Harvesting and Processing Techniques

Adipose tissue is typically harvested through a minimally invasive liposuction procedure performed under local or regional anesthesia

(Fig. 13.1). The most commonly used donor site is the peri-umbilical abdominal subcutaneous fat, although other areas such as the flanks may be considered. After injection of a local anesthetic solution into the subcutaneous compartment to provide analgesia and vasoconstriction, adipose tissue is aspirated using blunt cannulas connected to low-pressure suction systems in order to minimize mechanical trauma to the stromal vascular compartment. Particular attention is paid to gentle handling of the lipoaspirate to preserve cellular viability and the integrity of the perivascular niche. Compared with bone marrow aspiration, adipose harvesting allows collection of larger tissue volumes and is generally associated with limited donor-site morbidity [6].

Following harvesting, adipose tissue requires processing before intra-articular injection or local application to cartilage defects. Enzymatic isolation of stromal vascular fraction, mechanical micro-fragmentation, and in vitro culture expansion represent the principal approaches currently used, each associated with distinct biological and regulatory implications.

- Collagenase-based enzymatic digestion allows isolation of the stromal vascular fraction, a heterogeneous suspension containing MSCs together with endothelial cells, pericytes, and other stromal components. Following enzymatic incubation and centrifugation, adipose tissue is dissociated into a cellular fraction that can be collected and prepared for intra-articular use or further in vitro expansion. This strategy enables enrichment of progenitor cells and facilitates cellular characterization prior to administration [7]. Enzymatic processing modifies the native structural organization of adipose tissue and is generally performed in a controlled laboratory setting. Within several regulatory frameworks, this type of manipulation is categorized as more-than-minimal, and its clinical use may therefore be subject to specific national regulations and authorization pathways [16].
- Culture expansion permits amplification and characterization of MSCs under controlled conditions. Nevertheless, ex vivo expansion introduces regulatory complexity and requires staged treatment. Prolonged culture may also influence replicative capacity, particularly in older donors [13].
- Mechanical processing systems generate injectable adipose clusters while preserving stromal and perivascular architecture [14, 15]. These systems typically rely on gentle mechanical forces, such as repeated passage through calibrated filters or grids and washing with saline solution, in order to reduce the size of adipose clusters and remove residual blood, oil, and cellular debris. The objective is to obtain a more homogeneous injectable product while maintaining the integrity of the stromal vascular niche. Unlike enzymatic digestion, mechanical pro-

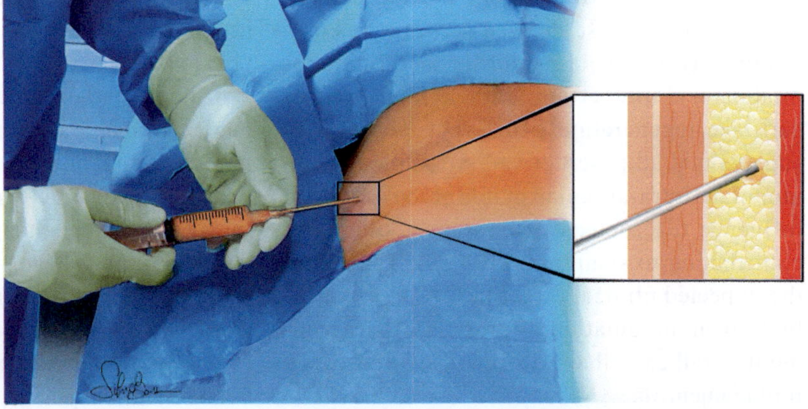

Fig. 13.1 Adipose tissue is harvested from the subcutaneous abdominal fat (usually the lower or lateral abdomen). The site is injected with adrenaline and lidocaine and then the adipose tissue is collected with a blunt cannula. Copyright of Silvia Bassini, 2026. All rights reserved

cessing does not involve chemical dissociation of the extracellular matrix. In several regulatory frameworks, this approach is therefore considered minimal manipulation, allowing intra-operative preparation and single-stage clinical use. Experimental data indicate that microfragmented adipose tissue retains secretory and immunomodulatory activity after processing, supporting its proposed biological rationale [15].

A relevant challenge in clinical interpretation relates to variability in harvesting techniques, processing devices, cellular quantification, and injection protocols. Methodological analyses have highlighted inconsistencies in product characterization and reporting transparency [16, 18]. At present, no universally accepted processing standard exists, and optimal cell composition, dosing, and delivery strategy remain to be defined.

13.4 Evidence in Osteoarthritis

13.4.1 Biological Rationale

OA is currently recognized as a whole-joint disease characterized by structural cartilage degeneration, synovial inflammation, subchondral bone remodeling, and alterations of the osteochondral unit [3]. Increasing evidence highlights the role of low-grade chronic inflammation and macrophage polarization in symptom generation and disease progression [19]. Within this framework, the therapeutic rationale for adipose-derived MSCs relies predominantly on their paracrine and immunomodulatory properties rather than direct cartilage regeneration [4]. Experimental data suggest that adipose-derived stromal cells can modulate intra-articular cytokine balance and influence macrophage phenotype, potentially contributing to symptom relief [8]. Therefore, the expected clinical effect in OA is primarily biological modulation of the joint environment rather than structural cartilage replacement.

Preclinical studies have reported potential disease-modifying effects of injectable adipose-derived cell-based therapies in OA models. A recent systematic review of 71 animal studies demonstrated that adipose-derived products exert structural and biological effects on joint tissues in both small and large animal OA models [20]. Treated joints showed macroscopic and histological improvement of cartilage surfaces, preservation of cartilage thickness, and reduced synovial membrane inflammation when compared with untreated OA controls. In addition to structural findings, reductions in serum and synovial fluid levels of inflammatory mediators and cartilage degradation markers were observed, suggesting modulation of the intra-articular inflammatory milieu. Functional improvements in clinical or behavioral measures were also reported in several models. Taken together, these data support a potential disease-modifying activity of adipose-derived products at the preclinical level. The extent to which these structural and biological effects translate into consistent and durable structural regeneration in humans remains to be fully clarified, as current clinical studies primarily report symptomatic improvement rather than robust imaging or biomarker-based disease modification.

13.4.2 Clinical Evidence

The clinical literature on intra-articular adipose-derived therapies for knee OA includes case series, randomized controlled trials, and systematic reviews, reporting overall short- to mid-term improvements in pain and functional outcomes [17, 18].

Clinical studies evaluating intra-articular enzymatic stromal vascular fraction administration have reported minimal adverse events together with reductions in pain and improvements in functional scores among patients with knee OA, despite most available evidence derives from case series lacking control groups [7]. In a recent randomized double-blind placebo-controlled trial including 39 individuals with knee OA, patients treated with enzymatic stromal vascular fraction exhibited significantly better clinical outcomes than controls during a follow-up period of up to 12 months, although magnetic resonance imaging failed to demonstrate measurable increases in cartilage thickness [21]. Furthermore, another randomized controlled trial involving 32 knee OA patients reported superior clinical and radiological outcomes at 12 months following intra-articular stromal vascular fraction injection compared with hyaluronic acid treatment [9]. Despite these encouraging results, the limited sample sizes of the currently available studies highlight the necessity for larger, high-quality trials to better define the actual therapeutic effectiveness of enzymatic stromal vascular fraction. Expanded adipose-derived MSCs have also shown symptomatic benefit in controlled settings, but heterogeneity across cell sources and study designs limits source-specific conclusions, and regulatory constraints restrict widespread application [22].

More robust clinical evidence derives from the use of adipose-derived products obtained through minimal manipulation approaches. Micro-fragmented adipose tissue injections showed promising results in the clinical practice in patients with knee OA, with a low number of adverse events and a significant improvement in pain, function, and quality of life. A recent systematic review of the literature documented 33 clinical studies focusing on the injective use of minimally manipulated adipose tissue approach for knee OA treatment, reporting safety and overall positive results up to 24 months of follow-up [23]. The authors also performed a meta-analysis exploring the comparison between micro-fragmented adipose tissue and platelet-rich plasma, with the inclusion of five randomized controlled trials. The analysis of the adverse events and clinical outcomes in terms of improvement in VAS score and KOOS subscales did not demonstrate a significant difference between the two orthobiologic approaches, except for the KOOS Symptoms and KOOS QOL subscales that demonstrated a significantly higher improvement in the adipose tissue group. This systematic review also highlighted a substantial methodological heterogeneity in processing techniques injected dose, OA severity, and follow-up duration, thus limiting conclusions regarding comparative superiority among orthobiologic strategies [23]. In this context, a high-level randomized controlled trial comparing micro-fragmented adipose tissue with platelet-rich plasma injections in 118 patients with knee OA showed that both treatments provided significant clinical improvement up to 24 months, with comparable changes in clinical scores, similar safety profiles, and no evidence of radiographic progression [24]. However, in patients with more advanced OA severity (Kellgren–Lawrence grade 3–4), micro-fragmented adipose tissue was associated with greater early IKDC improvement and a higher proportion achieving the minimal clinically important difference at 6 months, although these differences were not maintained at later follow-up and were not observed for KOOS pain. Beyond the direct comparison between these two orthobiologic approaches, their combined use has also been investigated in clinical practice with the aim of achieving potential synergistic effects in the treatment of OA. A recent systematic review specifically addressing the association of adipose-derived products with platelet-rich plasma analyzed both preclinical and clinical evidence of this combined approach, documenting encouraging experimental findings in terms of cartilage histology and biomarker modulation, which were not consistently reproduced in clinical practice [25]. Although case series suggested symptomatic benefits, controlled studies failed to demonstrate additional clinical or imaging advantages from platelet-rich plasma augmentation compared with adipose-derived products alone.

Across these studies, interpretation of results must also account for the substantial placebo effect associated with intra-articular injections in OA, which may persist over time and influence patient-reported outcomes [26]. Taken together, current evidence indicates that adipose-derived therapies are generally safe and capable of providing symptomatic improvement in selected patients with mild-to-moderate knee OA. However, consistent structural regeneration or definitive disease-modifying effects have not yet been conclusively demonstrated.

13.5 Evidence in Focal Cartilage Lesions

13.5.1 Biological Rationale

Focal chondral and osteochondral defects represent a clinical entity distinct from diffuse OA, typically affecting younger and active individuals and often arising from traumatic or sport-related injuries [2]. The limited intrinsic healing capacity of hyaline cartilage has historically led to the development of reparative and restorative strategies, including bone marrow stimulation, osteochondral transplantation techniques, and autologous chondrocyte implantation [27]. Among these, microfracture has been widely adopted as a first-line procedure for small to medium-sized lesions, relying on the recruitment of mesenchymal progenitor cells from the subchondral bone and the formation of a fibrin clot rich in marrow-derived elements. However, the repair tissue that develops is predominantly fibrocartilaginous, with biomechanical properties inferior to native hyaline cartilage and variable durability over time [28–30].

Within this framework, adipose-derived MSCs have been proposed as biological adjuncts aimed at enhancing the reparative environment rather than replacing established surgical techniques (Fig. 13.2). The rationale for combining adipose-derived MSCs with microfracture lies in supplementing the marrow-derived clot with additional progenitor and stromal elements capable of modulating the inflammatory and chondrogenic microenvironment. Experimental studies suggest that adipose-derived MSCs may support early chondrogenic differentiation and influence repair tissue organization through paracrine mechanisms [11]. Nevertheless, translation of these biological effects into consistent and durable hyaline-like cartilage regeneration in humans remains under investigation [12].

From a structural standpoint, histological and imaging analyses following bone marrow stimulation have consistently demonstrated fibrocartilaginous repair tissue with variable integration [29]. While the addition of adipose-derived cells has been hypothesized to improve tissue quality, robust histological confirmation of durable hyaline-like cartilage regeneration following adipose-derived therapies in humans remains limited [12, 31, 32]. Imaging evaluations have shown improved defect filling in some series, but standardized structural endpoints and long-term comparative data are lacking. Taken together, current evidence supports potential clinical improvement but does not conclusively demonstrate restoration of native hyaline cartilage [12].

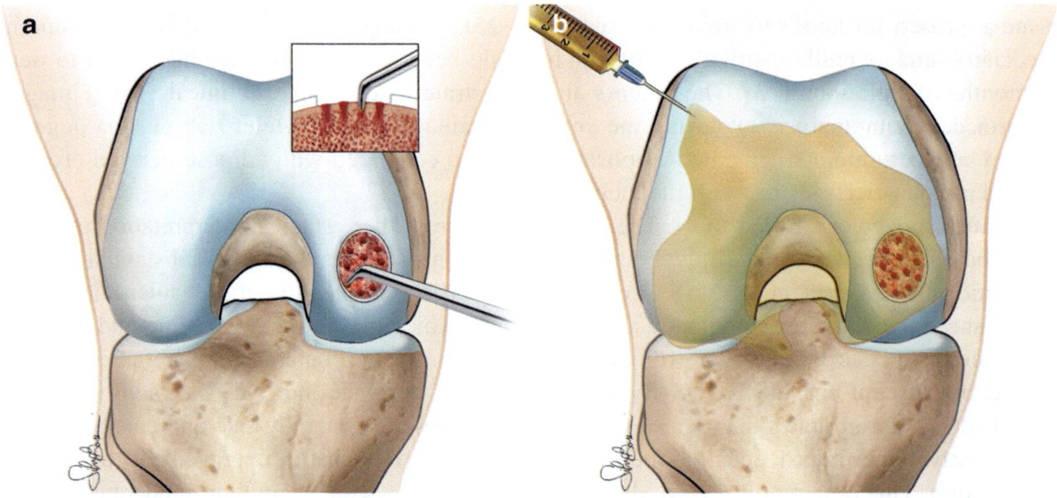

Fig. 13.2 Microfracture technique combined with adipose tissue product injection. Microfractures are performed (**a**), and then the injection of adipose tissue MSCs is performed (**b**). Copyright of Silvia Bassini, 2024. All rights reserved

13.6 Clinical Evidence

Clinical evidence evaluating adipose-derived MSC augmentation of marrow stimulation is still limited. A prospective randomized trial comparing microfracture alone with microfracture combined with intra-articular adipose-derived MSC injection in patients with knee chondral lesions reported greater improvement in pain and functional scores in the combined treatment group at mid-term follow-up, along with more complete defect filling on imaging assessment [30]. However, the study population was relatively small and the follow-up duration limited, restricting definitive conclusions regarding long-term durability and structural restoration. In this field, stronger clinical support has mainly emerged from studies investigating osteochondral lesions of the talus. Comparative clinical investigations evaluating the addition of adipose-derived MSCs to microfracture procedures have shown improved outcomes for the combined approach compared with bone marrow stimulation performed alone at short-term follow-up [31, 33]. In addition, Kim et al. [31] reported superior magnetic resonance imaging results in a cohort of 50 patients presenting unfavorable prognostic characteristics who underwent either microfracture treatment supplemented by a single intra-articular injection of adipose-derived stromal vascular fraction or microfracture alone.

Adipose-derived cells have also been incorporated into scaffold-based cartilage repair strategies within single-stage procedures, with the intent of delivering a progenitor-rich and trophically active environment within a structural matrix capable of supporting tissue organization [32]. Although clinical reports describe satisfactory mid-term outcomes in selected patients, most published studies consist of small case series without robust randomized comparison against established techniques [12].

Overall, currently available studies are characterized by limited sample size, heterogeneity in lesion characteristics and surgical techniques, and relatively short follow-up, and high-level randomized trials with standardized structural endpoints are still needed to clarify the magnitude and durability of clinical benefit [12, 31, 32]. In clinical practice, adipose-derived mesenchymal cell therapy in focal cartilage lesions should therefore be interpreted as a biological augmentation strategy rather than a substitute for established surgical techniques. Microfracture remains a cost-effective and technically accessible first-line option for small to medium-sized lesions [28], and the addition of adipose-derived products may enhance early clinical outcomes in selected patients. However, long-term superiority over marrow stimulation alone has not been conclusively established [12, 31]. Careful patient selection remains essential, with younger individuals presenting contained defects, stable joints, and corrected biomechanical alignment representing the most suitable candidates, whereas advanced degenerative changes or unaddressed instability represent unfavorable conditions for biological augmentation [34].

13.7 Conclusions

Adipose-derived mesenchymal stromal cell therapies represent a biologically sound and clinically feasible option within the evolving field of orthobiologics for cartilage disorders. Their proposed benefit relies predominantly on immunomodulatory and trophic mechanisms rather than direct structural regeneration. In knee OA, available evidence supports short- to mid-term symptomatic improvement in selected patients, with an overall favorable safety profile. However, consistent disease-modifying effects and durable structural cartilage restoration have yet to be clearly demonstrated. In focal cartilage lesions, adipose-derived products should be regarded as biological adjuncts rather than replacements for established surgical techniques. Although early clinical results are encouraging, definitive long-term superiority over conventional approaches has not been established. Careful patient selection, appropriate correction of biomechanical factors, and realistic expectation management remain central to clinical decision-making. Further well-designed randomized studies with standardized structural outcomes and adequate follow-up are needed to clarify the true long-term impact and optimal role of these therapies in cartilage pathology treatment.

References

1. Hunziker EB. Articular cartilage repair: basic science and clinical progress. Osteoarthr Cartil. 2002;10:432–63.
2. Flanigan DC, Harris JD, Trinh TQ, et al. Prevalence of chondral defects in athletes' knees: a systematic review. Med Sci Sports Exerc. 2010;42:1795–801.
3. Loeser RF, Goldring SR, Scanzello CR, Goldring MB. Osteoarthritis: a disease of the joint as an organ. Arthritis Rheum. 2012;64:1697–707.
4. Caplan AI. Mesenchymal stem cells: cell-based reconstructive therapy in orthopedics. Tissue Eng. 2005;11:1198–211.
5. Davies BM, Snelling SJB, Quek L, et al. Identifying the optimum source of mesenchymal stem cells for use in knee surgery. J Orthop Res. 2017;35:1868–75.
6. Aust L, Devlin B, Foster SJ, et al. Yield of human adipose-derived adult stem cells from liposuction aspirates. Cytotherapy. 2004;6:7–14.
7. Perdisa F, Gostynska N, Roffi A, et al. Adipose-derived mesenchymal stem cells for the treatment of articular cartilage: a systematic review. Stem Cells Int. 2015;2015:597652.
8. Manferdini C, Paolella F, Gabusi E, et al. Adipose stromal cells mediated switching of the pro-inflammatory profile of M1-like macrophages. Osteoarthr Cartil. 2017;25:1161–71.
9. Hong Z, Chen J, Zhang S, et al. Intra-articular injection of autologous adipose-derived stromal vascular fraction for knee osteoarthritis: a randomized trial. Int Orthop. 2019;43:1123–34.
10. Shanmugasundaram S, Vaish A, Chavada V, et al. Safety and efficacy of stromal vascular fraction for knee osteoarthritis: a systematic review. Int Orthop 2021.
11. Fortier LA, Barker JU, Strauss EJ, et al. The role of growth factors in cartilage repair. Clin Orthop Relat Res. 2011;469:2706–15.
12. Filardo G, Madry H, Jelic M, et al. Mesenchymal stem cells for the treatment of cartilage lesions. Knee Surg Sports Traumatol Arthrosc. 2013;21:1717–29.
13. Stolzing A, Jones E, McGonagle D, Scutt A. Age-related changes in human bone marrow-derived mesenchymal stem cells. Mech Ageing Dev. 2008;129:163–73.
14. Bianchi F, Maioli M, Leonardi E, et al. A new non-enzymatic method to obtain fat tissue derivative enriched in pericyte-like elements. Cell Transplant. 2013;22:2063–77.
15. Vezzani B, Shaw I, Lesme H, et al. Higher pericyte content and secretory activity of microfragmented adipose tissue. Stem Cells Transl Med. 2018;7:876–86.
16. Robinson PG, Murray IR, West CC, et al. Reporting of mesenchymal stem cell preparation protocols and composition. Am J Sports Med. 2019;47:991–1000.
17. Huang R, Li W, Zhao Y, et al. Clinical efficacy and safety of stem cell therapy for knee osteoarthritis: a meta-analysis. Medicine (Baltimore). 2020;99:e19434.
18. Filardo G, Previtali D, Napoli F, et al. PRP injections for knee osteoarthritis: a meta-analysis. Cartilage. 2021;13:364S–75S.
19. Zhang H, Lin C, Zeng C, et al. Synovial macrophage M1 polarisation exacerbates experimental osteoarthritis. Ann Rheum Dis. 2018;77:1524–34.
20. Perucca Orfei C, Boffa A, Sourugeon Y, et al. Cell-based therapies have disease-modifying effects on osteoarthritis in animal models. A systematic review by the ESSKA Orthobiologic initiative. Part 1: adipose tissue-derived cell-based injectable therapies. Knee Surg Sports Traumatol Arthrosc. 2023;31:641–55.
21. Garza JR, Campbell RE, Tjoumakaris FP, Freedman KB, Miller LS, Santa Maria D, et al. Clinical efficacy of intra-articular mesenchymal stromal cells for the treatment of knee osteoarthritis: a double-blinded prospective randomized controlled clinical trial. Am J Sports Med. 2020;48(3):588–98. Epub 2020/02/29.
22. Xia P, Wang X, Lin Q, Li X. Efficacy of mesenchymal stem cell injection for knee osteoarthritis: a meta-analysis. Int Orthop. 2015;39:2363–72.
23. Veronesi F, Andriolo L, Salerno M, Boffa A, Giavaresi G, Filardo G. Adipose tissue-derived minimally manipulated products versus platelet-rich plasma for the treatment of knee osteoarthritis: a systematic review of clinical evidence and meta-analysis. J Clin Med. 2024;13:67.
24. Zaffagnini S, Andriolo L, Boffa A, et al. Microfragmented adipose tissue versus platelet-rich plasma for the treatment of knee osteoarthritis: a prospective randomized controlled trial at 2-year follow-up. Am J Sports Med. 2022;50:2881–92.
25. Orazi S, Boffa A, Salerno M, et al. Adipose tissue-derived injectable products combined with platelet-rich plasma for the treatment of osteoarthritis: the promising preclinical results are not confirmed by the clinical evidence. EFORT Open Rev. 2024;9:1023–33.
26. Previtali D, Merli G, Di Laura FG, et al. Long-lasting effects of placebo injections in knee osteoarthritis. Cartilage. 2020;13:185S.
27. Steadman JR, Rodkey WG, Rodrigo JJ. Microfracture: surgical technique and rehabilitation to treat chondral defects. Clin Orthop Relat Res. 2001;391 Supp:S362–9.
28. Mithoefer K, McAdams T, Williams RJ, et al. Clinical efficacy of the microfracture technique for articular cartilage repair in the knee. Am J Sports Med. 2009;37:2053–63.
29. Knutsen G, Engebretsen L, Ludvigsen TC, et al. Autologous chondrocyte implantation compared with microfracture in the knee. J Bone Joint Surg Am. 2004;86:455–64.

30. Koh YG, Kwon OR, Kim YS, et al. Adipose-derived mesenchymal stem cells with microfracture versus microfracture alone for cartilage repair. Arthroscopy. 2016;32:97–109.
31. Kim YS, Lee HJ, Choi YJ, et al. Stromal vascular fraction and marrow stimulation in osteochondral lesions of the talus. Am J Sports Med. 2014;42:2424–34.
32. Giannini S, Buda R, Vannini F, et al. One-step bone marrow-derived cell transplantation in talar lesions. Clin Orthop Relat Res. 2009;467:3307–20.
33. D'Ambrosi R, Indino C, Maccario C, Manzi L, Usuelli FG. Autologous microfractured and purified adipose tissue for arthroscopic Management Of Osteochondral Lesions of the talus. J Vis Exp. 2018;23:56395. https://doi.org/10.3791/56395.
34. Gomoll AH, Madry H, Knutsen G, et al. The subchondral bone in articular cartilage repair. Knee Surg Sports Traumatol Arthrosc. 2010;18:434–47.

14 Articular Cartilage Preservation Surgeries

Matteo Innocenti and Mattia Chirico

14.1 Introduction

Osteotomies around the knee are corrective surgeries that aim to re-establish the biomechanical alignment of the joint, reducing the load on the damaged or deteriorating cartilage and slowing down the progression of osteoarthritis (OA), thereby preserving the cartilage [1]. These procedures are particularly useful in young, active patients with axial deformities of the knee, such as varus or valgus knees, where cartilage wear tends to be concentrated in one of the joint compartments [2].

The main objective of osteotomy is to restore a more balanced load on the articular surfaces, thus preserving the function of the knee and cartilage and avoiding or delaying the need for total arthroplasty [3]. For as easy as it is to say and imagine, such procedures are difficult. Osteotomies around the knee are technically demanding procedures that have traditionally relied on two-dimensional (2D) planning for what is essentially a complex three-dimensional (3D) surgery. When evaluating the potential benefits of an osteotomy around the knee for a patient, the two most crucial factors are appropriate patient selection and the precision of the mechanical axis correction achieved. The accuracy of this correction heavily depends on meticulous preoperative planning and precise surgical execution. Consequently, there has been a growing interest in incorporating computer technology and patient-specific instrumentation (PSI) during surgery to enhance surgical precision and optimize clinical outcomes.

Computer-assisted navigation (CAN) significantly improves the accuracy of the cuts made during an osteotomy, and its popularity has increased for both preoperative planning and intraoperative application [4, 5].

This technique was originally implemented in spinal surgeries and later successfully adopted in arthroplasty. Its success in guiding cuts for total knee arthroplasty led to the utilization of CAN for osteotomies to achieve more consistent deformity correction. CAN provides real-time enhancement of the accuracy and precision of correction angles in multiple planes while making osteotomy cuts (Fig. 14.1).

A key advantage of CAN is its ability to account for rotational components, which are typically difficult to assess with standard 2D radiographs, by providing a 3D evaluation.

Despite its effectiveness in preoperative planning, CAN offers limited control over tibial alignment or posterior tibial slope during osteot-

M. Innocenti (✉) ·
Department of Orthopedic Surgery, University Hospital of Florence, Florence, Italy
e-mail: matteo.innocenti@unifi.it

M. Chirico
Institute for Complex Arthroplasty and Revisions, Ifca - Villa Ulivella, Florence, Italy
e-mail: mattia.chirico@unifi.it

M. E. Erdil et al. (eds.), *Current Concept in Cartilage Treatment*,
https://doi.org/10.1007/978-3-032-27099-3_14

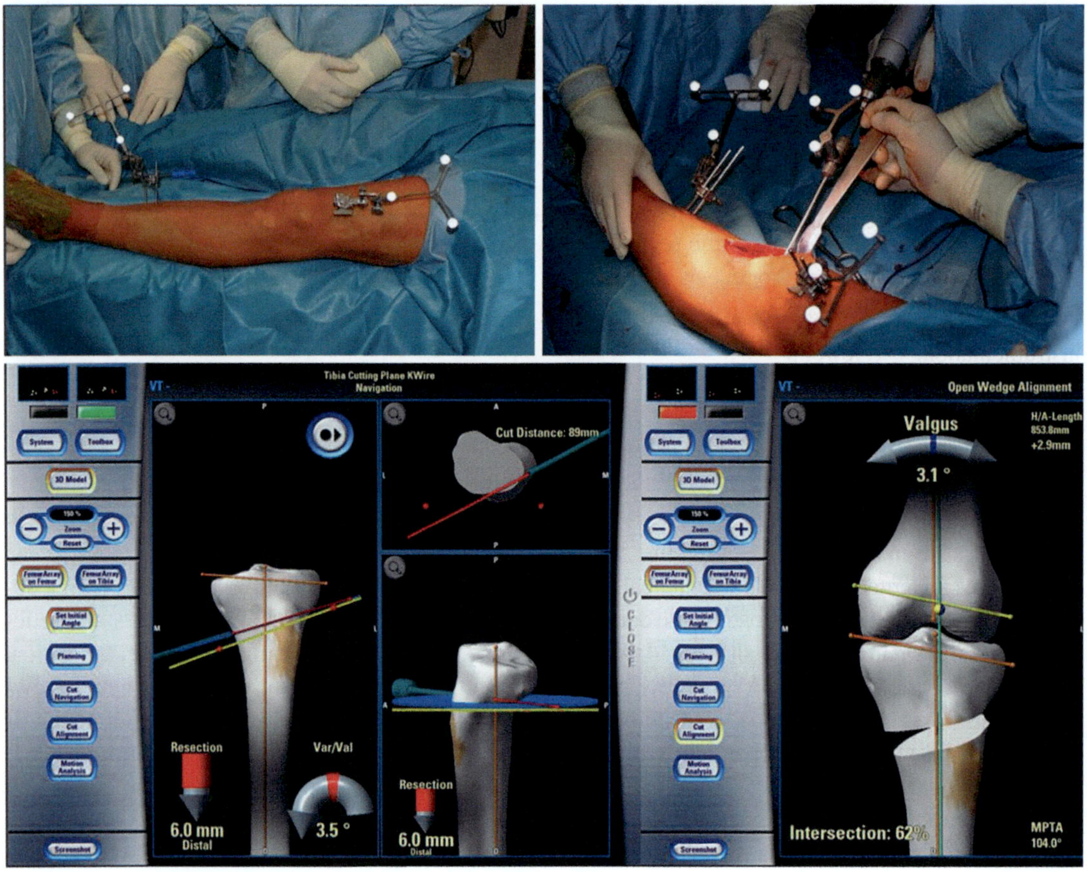

Fig. 14.1 The figure shows an osteotomy procedure assisted by computer navigation. In the upper part of the image, two scenes are visible: In the upper section, the leg is prepared for the procedure, with reference markers attached to the tibia and femur to enable position tracking through the navigation system. In the lower part of the image, the monitor of the navigation system is displayed, showing various real-time feedback screens

omy distraction and fixation. Unintended changes in the tibial slope can cause instability in the sagittal plane and increase stress on the cruciate ligaments, potentially impairing knee function.

This limitation has led to the adoption of PSI to better manage complex multiplanar deformities. PSI for osteotomies was initially developed for maxillofacial surgery, but in the past decade, its use has expanded in orthopedic surgery, showing promising preliminary outcomes in various operative contexts. Primary benefits of PSI include high accuracy without requiring external cameras and referencing systems, a rapid learning curve, and reduced overall exposure to fluoroscopy [6–8].

PSI involves customizing surgical tools and guides based on the individual's anatomy. This customization is achieved through preoperative imaging and advanced 3D modeling techniques. It consists of producing a patient-specific cutting guide to be used during surgery to achieve the planned cut and gap opening. Preoperative planning and customized tools streamline the procedure, reducing operating time.

Several authors have introduced this technique in their practice with excellent results [6, 9].

All patients listed for PSI mOW-HTO receive an additional preoperative CT scan to the conventional long-leg standing X-rays. CT scans are executed with the Activemotion CT protocol that involves a bilateral acquisition (right and left leg) of fields of view with the same spatial coordinates: 2 cm. long package (with 2 mm slices) located on the heads of the femurs, 15 cm long package (with 0.6 mm slices) from distal femur to proximal tibia;

5 cm long (with 0.6 mm slices) on the ankles with soft tissue viewing window. After bidimensional templating, the surgeon sends the company the description of the correction desired on coronal and sagittal planes. The company sends back a 3D reconstruction of the lower limb reproducing native alignment and new coronal and sagittal alignment after the planned HTO. The surgeon can then decide if further modifications are required or not.

After that the manufacturer produces the PSI instrumentation. (Newclip Technics, Haute Goulaine, France). It includes personalized cutting jigs, 3D bone model, patient-specific wedge to open the osteotomy cut. Cutting guides are made of biocompatible plastic material Nylon-PA2200. All the PSI are sterile and available for intraoperative use (Fig. 14.1). The company takes five weeks to produce the cutting guides from the moment the CT is performed. The cost of the procedure in our hospital is around €1500, including CT scan, PSI instruments, cutting guides, and fixation devices (plate and screws). As a matter of fact, developing and fabricating PSI tools can be more expensive than performing osteotomies with the traditional instrumentation. Moreover, not all surgical centers have access to the necessary imaging and 3D modeling technologies.

14.1.1 Future Directions in Knee Osteotomies

Future developments in knee osteotomies are likely to include the integration of artificial intelligence in surgical planning, advancements in imaging and modeling for even more precise surgical interventions, and the potential role of augmented reality (AR) in enhancing surgical visualization and accuracy.

14.2 Deformity Analysis

The evaluation of lower limb deformities begins by examining the patient's alignment in the coronal, sagittal, and axial planes. Coronal alignment is typically evaluated with full weight-bearing radiographs of the pelvis and limbs, including the hip and ankle joints. The mechanical axes of the femur (MAF) and tibia (MAT) are identified, and the angle between them is referred to as the mechanical tibiofemoral angle (mHKA). A varus angle between 0 and 3 degrees indicates neutral alignment. To pinpoint the deformity location in cases of coronal malalignment, measurements of the proximal tibial and distal femoral angles are taken. The medial proximal tibial mechanical angle (mMPTA) and the distal lateral femoral mechanical angle (mLDFA) are determined by the angles between their respective joint lines and mechanical axes, with typical values ranging from 85 to 90 degrees, averaging 88 for mLDFA and 87 for mMPTA (Fig. 14.2).

Accurate deformity analysis is crucial, as recent studies highlight that varus deformity is not solely tibial, nor is valgus deformity exclusively femoral, as was once thought. Performing an osteotomy at a site without deformity can result in a misalignment of the joint line obliquity (JLO) compared to the patient's natural alignment [10, 11]. JLO is the angle between a line drawn along the tibial plateau and the horizontal plane.

Another important consideration is the joint line convergence angle (JLCA), which reflects the condition of soft tissues and intra-articular structures. The JLCA is the angle formed by tangential lines to the distal femoral condyles and the tibial plateau, typically parallel in healthy knees (0–2 degrees). Assessing JLCA is critical because a high JLCA may result in overcorrection following an osteotomy. In addition to coronal alignment, the knee's sagittal alignment, represented by the posterior tibial slope (PTS), should also be assessed. This is best done using lateral radiographs of the proximal tibia or, ideally, a full-length tibial radiograph, with normal PTS values ranging from 6 to 11 degrees [12].

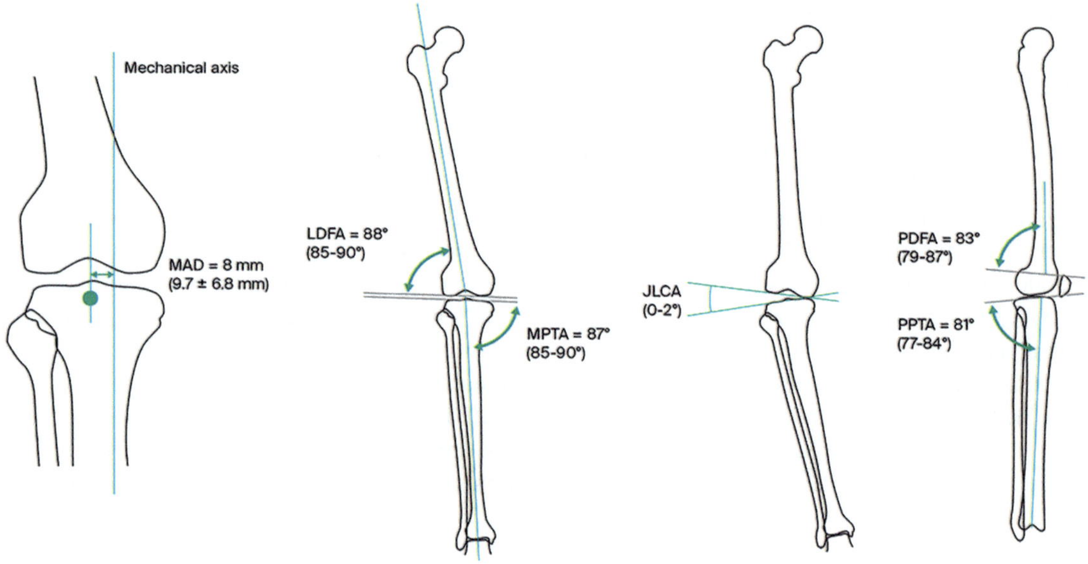

Fig. 14.2 This image illustrates the key mechanical angles used to assess lower limb deformities

14.3 Coronal Malalignment

14.3.1 Varus Deformity of Tibia

For patients presenting with varus alignment, a detailed deformity analysis is necessary to identify the specific location of the deformity. Since varus deformities are often linked to tibial abnormalities, a tibial-based osteotomy is typically the preferred treatment. This procedure is indicated for conditions such as medial compartment osteoarthritis, chronic ligament instability, meniscal insufficiency, and localized cartilage defects in the medial compartment; valgus-producing high tibial osteotomy (HTO) plays a role in managing multiple pathologies.

14.3.1.1 Surgical Indications

The primary objective of valgus-producing high tibial osteotomies (HTOs) is to offload the medial compartment in cases of significant metaphyseal deformity. By reducing the load on this compartment, the procedure helps alleviate pain, restore function for work or recreational activities, stabilize the joint, and slow the onset or progression of osteoarthritis. The most frequent indication for HTO is isolated medial compartment osteoarthritis in patients under 60 years old with full range of motion (ROM). Additional indications include varus alignment with medial compartment issues, chronic lateral ligament instability, failed anterior cruciate ligament reconstruction (ACL-R) in the context of excessive posterior tibial slope (PTS), varus or combined deformities, and instability of the posterior cruciate ligament (PCL) or posterolateral corner (PLC) [13–16].

Valgus-producing HTOs are also commonly performed alongside cartilage repair or meniscal procedures in the medial compartment. In joint preservation cases, correcting even minor varus malalignment is crucial to reduce stress on the reconstructed medial compartment. Relative contraindications for valgus-producing HTO include patients with patellofemoral or tricompartmental arthritis, severe medial compartment osteoarthritis (Kellgren-Lawrence grade IV), restricted knee ROM (such as flexion contracture greater than 10° or a total motion arc of less than 120°), and inflammatory arthritis [17].

14.3.1.2 Surgical Technique

When performing valgus-producing osteotomies, it is important to correct the existing varus deformity at its source, whether it originates in the tibia, femur, or intra-articular structures. Historically, tibial deformity has been considered the primary cause of knee varus alignment. Consequently, the two most commonly used techniques for addressing varus malalignment around the knee are the medial opening wedge (MOW) and lateral closing wedge (LCW) high tibial osteotomies. Although each method has its own unique benefits and limitations, both have been demonstrated to effectively reduce stress on the medial compartment by shifting the mechanical axis of the lower limb [18].

HTO Using the Medial Opening Wedge (MOW) Technique The MOW technique offers several benefits, including a faster, more precise procedure and the ability to preserve bone stock proximal to the tibial tubercle. However, it also has some drawbacks, such as the potential need for a bone graft when larger corrections are required. During HTO, it is crucial to evaluate the pre-operative and intended post-correction joint line obliquity (JLO), as certain cases may require a double-level osteotomy (DLO), where cuts are made both above and below the knee joint. Additionally, leg length discrepancy (LLD) should be carefully considered, since MOW-HTO tends to increase leg length compared to LCW-HTO, although this can vary based on the extent of the correction needed [19].

The position of the femoral joint also warrants attention, as MOW-HTO has been shown to lower patella height by approximately 7% and affect patellar inclination, especially when corrections exceed 15 degrees [20]. An alternative approach is an infra-tubercular biplanar osteotomy cut, which is less likely to disrupt the length-tension relationship of the extensor mechanism [21].

Lateral Closing Wedge (LCW) HTO One of the key benefits of LCW-HTO is the direct bone contact, which is believed to enhance healing and improve the stability of the construct. However, many surgeons find this technique less appealing due to the need to disrupt the proximal tibiofibular joint, perform dissection around the peroneal nerve, and execute multiple precise cuts. For larger corrections (greater than 10 mm), a proximal fibula osteotomy is required to fully close the osteotomy, and special care must be taken to protect the lateral collateral ligament during the procedure [22]. Despite these challenges, LCW-HTO remains a valuable option, particularly in cases involving significant leg length discrepancies or in patients with a higher risk of non-union, such as smokers.

14.3.1.3 Planning

Surgical planning for MOW-HTO is typically conducted using the Miniaci method. The process begins with drawing the Mikulicz line, which runs from the center of the femoral head to the center of the talus [23]. The next step is to determine the desired postoperative weight-bearing point and the hinge point (as shown in Fig. 14.2). The hinge point is located at the top of the fibular head within the lateral proximal tibial metaphysis. The correction angle is then calculated by drawing an angle between the line connecting the ankle's initial position to the hinge point and the line connecting the future ankle position to the hinge point—this forms the correction angle (Fig. 14.3).

For LCW-HTO, a similar approach can be used, but the hinge point is positioned at the medial proximal tibia, approximately 2 cm below the joint line and around 4–6 mm from the medial cortex [24].

Traditionally, valgus-producing HTOs were planned to correct alignment toward Fujisawa's point (62.5% across the tibial plateau). However, recent studies suggest that the degree of correction should be adjusted based on factors such as the severity of osteoarthritis, ligament instability, and the alignment of the contralateral limb [25]. Generally, the higher the osteoarthritis grade, ligamentous instability, or valgus in the opposite knee, the more substantial the correction should be (around 60–65%). Conversely, in procedures like meniscal transplant or cartilage restoration with minimal osteoarthritis and varus alignment in the contralateral knee, a lesser correction of around 50–55% may be sufficient.

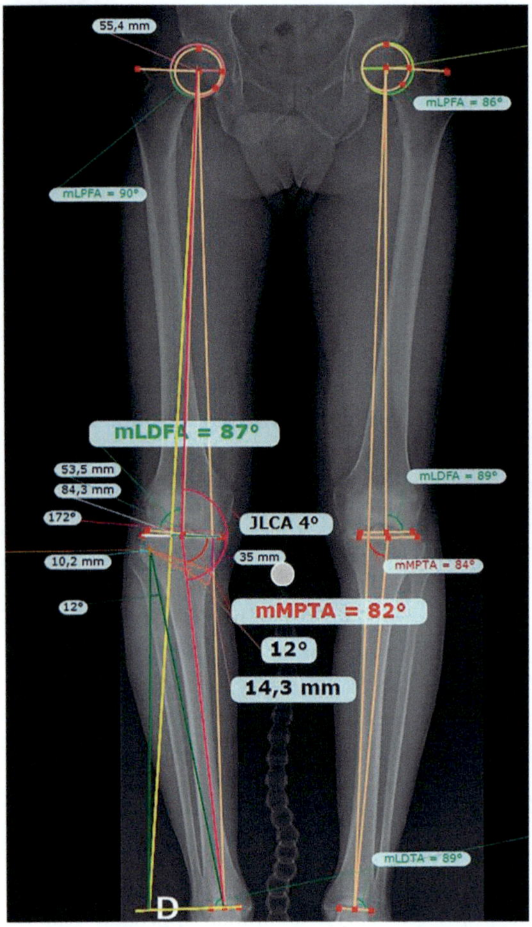

Fig. 14.3 This figure illustrates the planning and execution of a high tibial osteotomy (HTO) procedure using the Miniaci method

14.3.2 Valgus Deformity of Femur

A varus-producing distal femoral osteotomy (DFO) is commonly performed in cases of symptomatic isolated lateral compartment osteoarthritis, lateral meniscal deficiency, patellofemoral instability, or persistent medial collateral ligament insufficiency. For patients with lateral compartment osteoarthritis and valgus alignment, a deformity analysis is essential to identify the precise location of the deformity. Since valgus deformities are often linked to femoral abnormalities, a femur-based osteotomy is typically the preferred option. The distal femoral varus osteotomy can be executed using either a medial closing wedge (MCW-DFO) or a lateral opening wedge (LOW-DFO) approach, both of which will be discussed in this section.

14.3.2.1 Surgical Indications

The primary indication for a varus-producing distal femoral osteotomy (DFO) is isolated, symptomatic mild to moderate lateral compartment osteoarthritis with significant metaphyseal deformity. It is also commonly used in conjunction with other knee preservation surgeries, such as cartilage repair procedures and meniscal allograft transplants. In these combined cases, correcting even minor valgus malalignment can significantly reduce stress on the lateral compartment, easing the load on meniscal or cartilage transplants [26].

Additionally, while less common, a varus-producing DFO can be performed to address medial collateral ligament (MCL) insufficiency. Valgus deformity increases the abduction moment, putting more strain on the medial and posteromedial structures [27]. However, using a varus-producing DFO for MCL insufficiency is rare, and the literature on this procedure is limited.

Relative contraindications for varus-producing DFO include severe valgus deformity with tibial subluxation, significant knee instability, tricompartmental osteoarthritis, and flexion contractures greater than 15 degrees [28]. Other relative contraindications include severe patellofemoral osteoarthritis, rheumatoid arthritis, advanced age (over 65), considerable bone loss in the lateral compartment, and a history of septic arthritis in the knee.

In rare cases, valgus malalignment can also be corrected with a high tibial osteotomy (HTO) [29], utilizing either lateral opening or medial closing techniques.

14.3.2.2 Surgical Technique

MCW and LOW techniques can be performed for distal femoral osteotomies. The objective of a DFO-producing varus is typically to move the loading point within the 48–50% segment of the width of the tibial plateau, measured from the medial to the lateral side [30].

The MCW-DFO technique involves the correction of the mechanical axis by removing a wedge-shaped bone block from the medial distal femur and is typically fixed with a plate. Direct contact with the bone facilitates a faster healing process and the medial approach usually reduces soft tissue irritation [30]. Although MCW-DFOs are believed to have a lower rate of non-union or malunion than LOW-DFOs, there is currently no evidence of radiographic correction or healing when comparing MCW-DFOs and LOW-DFOs [31].

14.3.2.3 Planning

Surgical planning of DFO can be performed using methods similar to those described above for HTO (Fig. 14.4). The first step is to draw the Mikulicz line. Secondly, the desired postoperative weight-bearing point and the hinge point are defined. The hinge point for the MCW-DFO must be approximately 5 mm from the lateral cortical to ensure sufficient lateral hinge. The angle is then defined between a line connecting the center of the femoral head to the hinge point and a line connecting the future position of the center of the femoral head to the hinge point. This angle will be the desired correction angle (Fig. 14.3). A similar method can be used to determine the correction for a LOW-DFO; however, the hinge point will instead be close to the adductor tubercle on the medial femur, preserving a medial hinge of 1 cm [32].

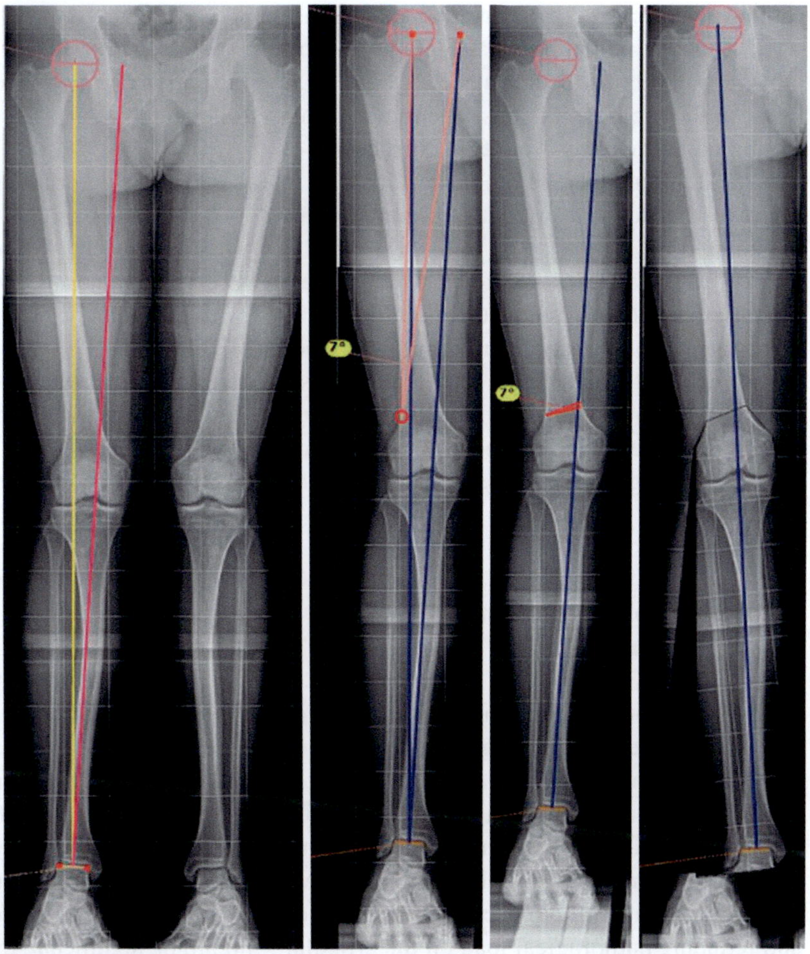

Fig. 14.4 This figure illustrates the planning and execution of a low femur osteotomy (LFO) procedure using the Miniaci method

14.4 Biplanar Osteotomy

Biplanar osteotomies can be used to correct coronal and sagittal malalignment in patients with more complex deformities in a single osteotomy procedure. Combined coronal and sagittal malalignment, in the form of increased PTS and varus knee alignment, is most commonly seen in patients with anterior cruciate ligament deficiency. Therefore, a biplanar MOW-HTO can be performed [33]. Although less commonly seen, combined varus-enhancing and posterior slope osteotomies can be performed for patients with valgus knee alignment and recurvatum. Similarly, in patients with varus knee osteoarthritis, PCL tears, and reduced PTS, biplanar osteotomies can be performed to correct varus and increase PTS. Another indication for a biplanar osteotomy is patients with chronic PCL and PLC tears; in these cases, it is possible to perform a combined osteotomy for the correction of varus and the increase of the posterior slope to improve the coronal and sagittal stability of the knee [34].

The advantages of biplanar osteotomies: increased rotational stability, mainly due to the presence of the anterior flange that does not allow a tilt greater than 5 degrees; possibility of opening independent of the plate shape; increase of the contact area; reduction of the existing gap; reduces the use of the graft [35].

14.5 Double Osteotomies Around the Knee

Double osteotomies represent an advanced surgical technique for treating significant knee deformities, particularly in cases of varus or valgus deformities involving both the distal femur and proximal tibia. This procedure aims to restore optimal lower limb alignment, reestablishing the natural biomechanics of the knee and reducing pathological load on the articular surfaces.

14.5.1 Preoperative Planning

The success of two-level osteotomies depends on meticulous preoperative planning, which includes detailed assessment of bony and joint deformities, definition of corrective goals, and selection of intervention sites.

It is crucial to identify the location and severity of the deformity, relying on comprehensive data, including mLDFA (medial Lateral Distal Femoral Angle), MPTA (Medial Proximal Tibial Angle), JLCA (Joint Line Convergence Angle), the Mikulicz line, and the new M-JL (Mechanical Joint Line).

14.5.2 Indications for Double Osteotomy

Indications for two-level osteotomies include the following:

- Complex deformities: Involvement of both the distal femur and proximal tibia.
- Altered M-JL: When the M-JL deviates from normal values (83–94°), a single-level correction might not provide optimal results (Fig. 14.5).
- Ligament instability: Deformities associated with medial or lateral ligamentous insufficiency.
- Significant correction: When correction exceeds 10 degrees, a single osteotomy may result in alterations to tibial slope or biomechanical complications.

14.5.3 Techniques for Double-Level Osteotomy

The choice of osteotomy type depends on the patient's condition and the surgeon's expertise. Current practice widely favors medial interventions on the tibia for both varus and valgus deformities. On the distal femur, literature does not highlight significant differences between techniques, making the approach largely surgeon-

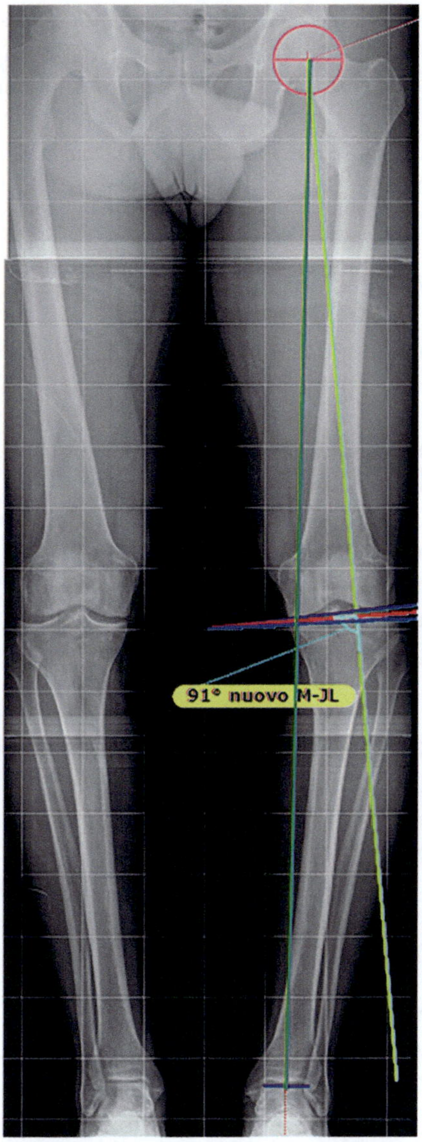

Fig. 14.5 The figure illustrates how to calculate the new M-JL. If M-JL < 83° or >94°, a double osteotomy is required

dependent. The following scenarios outline common approaches:

1. **Varus deformity:**
   - Tibial open-wedge osteotomy combined with lateral closing-wedge distal femoral osteotomy.
   - Tibial open-wedge osteotomy combined with medial opening-wedge distal femoral osteotomy.
2. **Valgus deformity**:
   - Tibial closing-wedge osteotomy combined with medial closing-wedge distal femoral osteotomy.
   - Tibial closing-wedge osteotomy combined with lateral opening-wedge distal femoral osteotomy.

In cases involving dual osteotomies, the biplanar technique is highly advantageous, offering superior sagittal and rotational stability, reducing the risk of malpositioning the tibial tuberosity, and minimizing intraoperative fractures. Additionally, the use of **customized cutting guides** based on patient-specific 3D models enhances precision in bony cuts and alignment correction. These techniques are essential to mitigate errors given the complexity of dual osteotomies.

14.5.4 Conclusion

Double-level osteotomies provide an effective solution for addressing complex knee deformities but require meticulous planning and advanced surgical skills. Personalized approaches supported by modern technologies, such as 3D modeling and custom cutting guides, optimize functional outcomes and minimize the risk of complications.

14.6 Complications

There are significant disparities in the literature regarding the reported complication rate after osteotomies. Complications can be differentiated into: intraoperative (hinge fractures, undercorrections, slope alterations, patella baja, neurovascular); early (infections, thrombosis, and pulmonary embolism); late (delayed union, late overcorrections) [30] (Fig. 14.6).

A systematic review reported rates of 8% and 23% for hardware removal after MCW- and LOW-DFO, respectively [31]. The higher rate of hardware removal in patients undergoing LOW-DFO may be due to irritation of the iliotibial band.

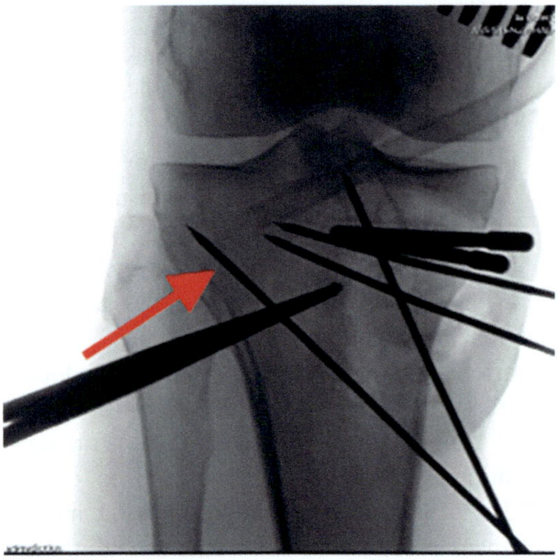

Fig. 14.6 This figure shows an intraoperative radiograph where it is possible to note the positioning of the lateral Kirshner wire to protect the hinge (arrow)

Hinge fractures are a known complication in valgus-producing HTOs, but measures can be taken to mitigate their occurrence and/or severity. Hinge fractures are divided according to the Takeuchi classification [36]. In the case of MOW-HTO, ensuring that the osteotomy cut stops 5–10 mm from the lateral margin at the level of the upper third of the tibiofibular joint margin helps reduce the rate and severity of hinge fractures [37]. More recently, the addition of a Kirschner wire just medial and parallel to the lateral tibial cortex has been shown to increase the maximum failure load by up to 880% (Fig. 14.4). Hinge fractures are more likely to occur with larger corrections, particularly when gaps reach and exceed 11 mm [38]. The osteotomy space should be opened slowly intraoperatively with stacked osteotomes or an opening device to minimize the risk of a hinge fracture.

14.7 Let's Step Into the Operating Room Together

Knee osteotomy is an advanced surgical procedure used to correct lower limb deformities, redistribute joint loads, and improve knee function. This chapter provides a step-by-step guide, from patient positioning to the completion of the procedure, including key points, precautions, and essential techniques, presenting an HTO case as an example.

14.7.1 Patient Positioning

Proper positioning is critical to ensure precision during the procedure:

- Operating table: Use a radiolucent table and position it as distally as possible.
- Knee support: Apply an ipsilateral leg press to maintain knee flexion.
- Surgeon visibility: Ensure the lead surgeon has a direct frontal view of the surgical field (Fig. 14.7).

14.7.2 Identifying Anatomical Landmarks

Before making the incision, the following anatomical landmarks must be identified:

1. Patella.
2. Tibial tuberosity.
3. Patellar tendon.
4. Medial femoral condyle.
5. Posterior edge of the tibia (Fig. 14.8).

These landmarks serve as guides for precise incisions and optimal access to bony and ligamentous structures.

14.7.3 Surgeon and Fluoroscope Positioning

- The fluoroscope should be positioned ipsilateral to the operated limb.
- The monitor should be placed contralaterally for clear and accessible visualization throughout the procedure.

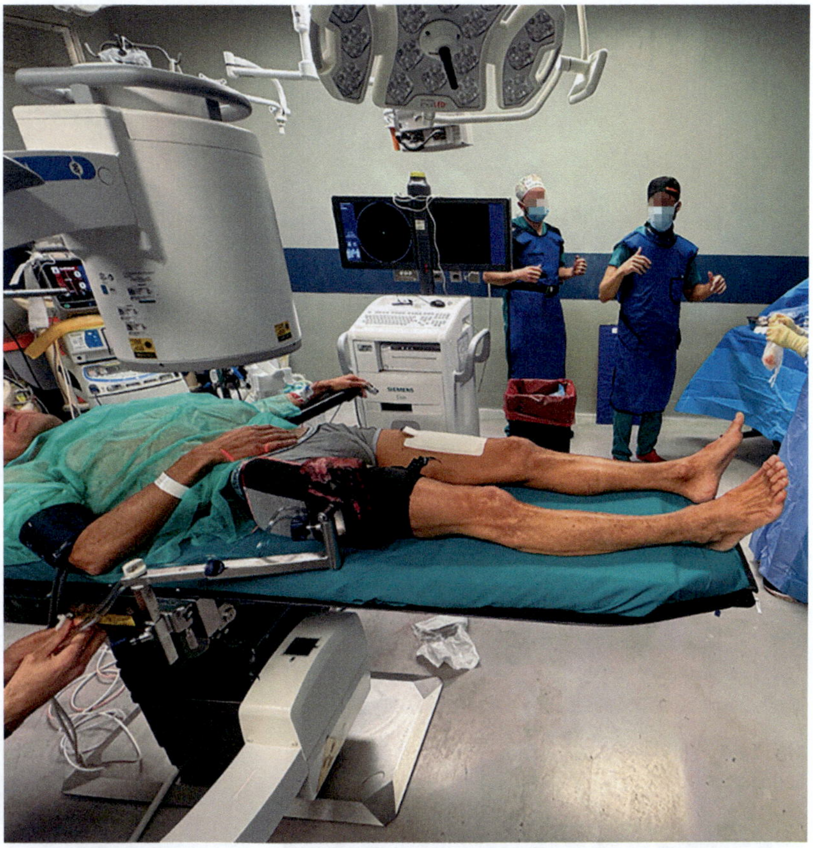

Fig. 14.7 This figure shows correct position of patient and knee supports

14.7.4 Leg Positioning During Incision

- Position a triangular support under the knee to stabilize the limb and create space for manipulation.
- Place a bolster under the ankle to elevate the limb, free the popliteal fossa, and protect posterior vascular structures (Fig. 14.9).

14.7.5 Incision and Tissue Exposure

- Make sequential incisions through the layers to expose the osteotomy site while respecting the following:
  1. Medial collateral ligament.
  2. Hamstring tendons.
- Take care to preserve surrounding vascular and neural structures (Fig. 14.10).

14.7.6 Pre-Cutting and Hinge Protection

Before performing the bone cut:

- Position custom-made cutting guides to ensure precise and controlled cuts.
- Insert Kirschner wires (K-wires) above and below the anticipated cutting site to protect the hinge.
- Use a posterior Hohmann retractor to safeguard vascular structures and minimize intraoperative risk (Fig. 14.11).

14.7.7 Performing the Bone Cut

- Execute the bone cut using appropriate instruments, guided by the templates.
- Ensure hinge stability by leaving at least 5 mm of intact lateral cortical bone.
- Confirm the accuracy of the cut with fluoroscopic imaging (Fig. 14.12).

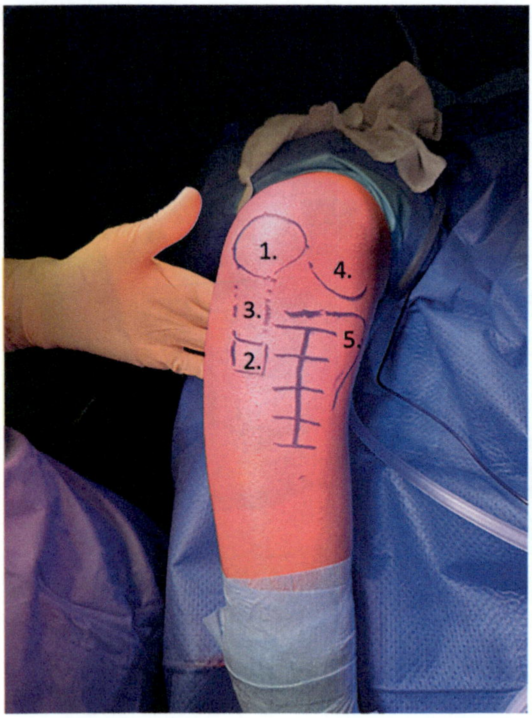

Fig. 14.8 This figure shows correct position of patient and knee supports

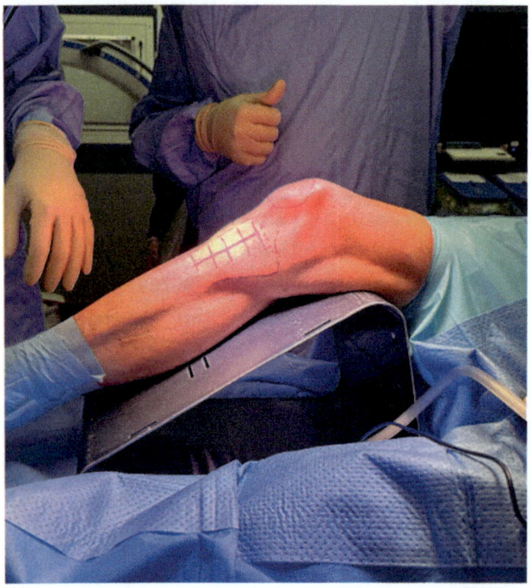

Fig. 14.9 This figure shows the correct position of knee

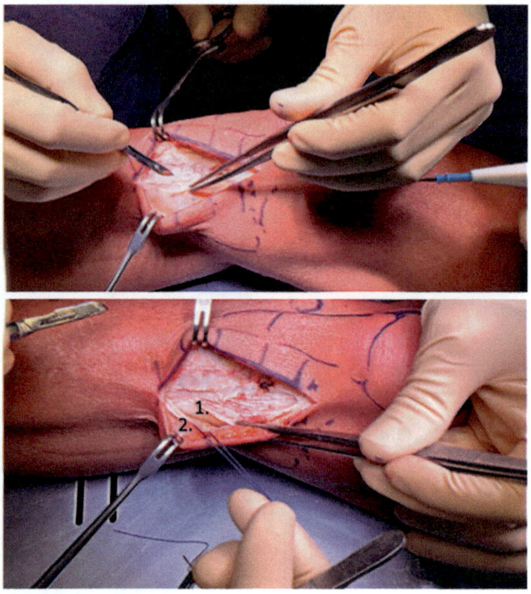

Fig. 14.10 Surgical incision view showing the presence of the medial collateral ligament and the hamstrings

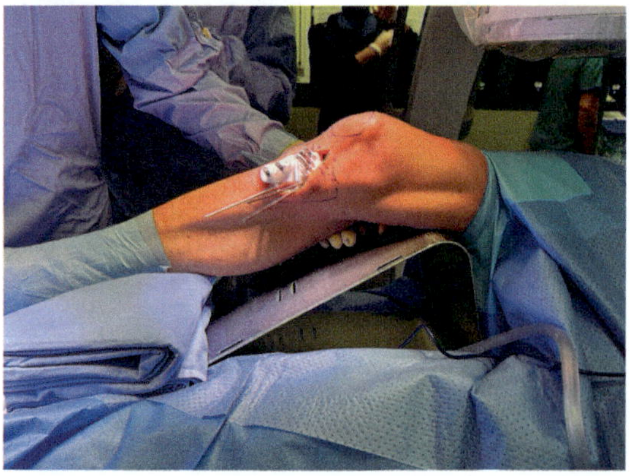

Fig. 14.11 Pre-cutting and hinge protection

14.7.8 Closure and Fixation

- Following the bone cut, open or close the osteotomy as indicated (open-wedge or close-wedge technique).
- Fix the osteotomy using angular stability plates or other suitable fixation devices.
- Verify the final correction with fluoroscopy, ensuring alignment matches the preoperative plan.

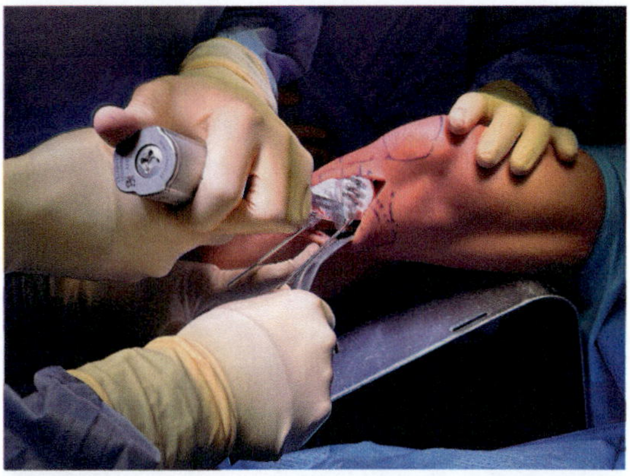

Fig. 14.12 Guided bone cut execution using a custom-made cutting and oscillating saw

14.7.9 Postoperative Monitoring

- Obtain immediate postoperative radiographs to confirm correct positioning and fixation stability.
- Monitor the patient for any immediate complications, such as vascular injury or mechanical instability.

14.7.10 Final Considerations

Knee osteotomy is a complex procedure requiring a systematic approach and meticulous preparation. Protecting critical structures, employing personalized tools, and performing precise cuts are essential for procedural success and minimizing complications.

14.8 Case Report: Lengthening Osteotomy and Closing Wedge Varus Osteotomy Using a Custom-Made Mask

14.8.1 Introduction

Lengthening osteotomies are surgical procedures used to correct bone deformities and improve limb functionality. This case report describes a procedure performed with a custom-made mask to optimize alignment following bone deformity caused by a road traffic accident and a previous lengthening osteotomy.

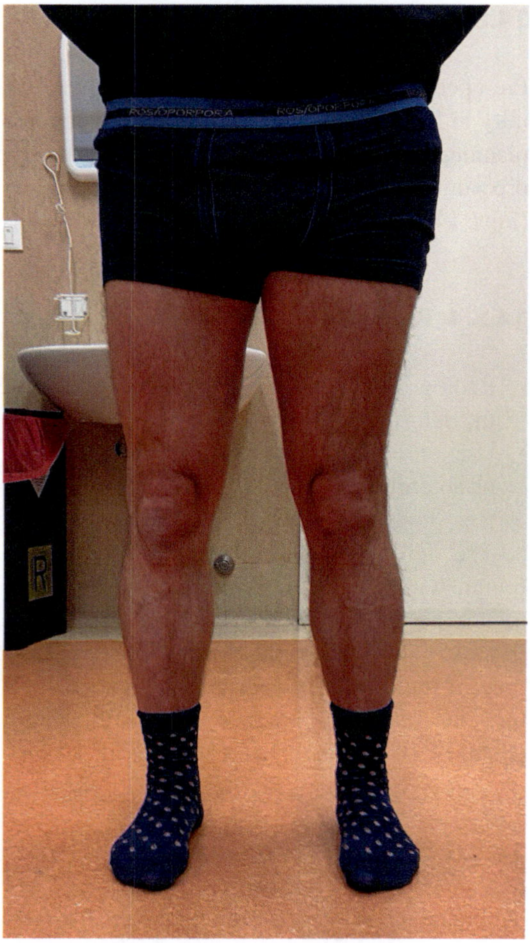

Fig. 14.13 Lower limbs under load

14.8.2 Case Presentation

- Patient: Male, 55 years old (Fig. 14.13).
- Condition: Distal left femur fracture in 1987, initially treated with a DCS plate, which was removed after 5 months due to breakage. Residual sequelae included a distal left femur fracture with a 3 cm limb length discrepancy and valgus deformity, treated with an extendable nail.
- Indication: Surgical correction of the limb length discrepancy through a lengthening osteotomy and axis correction via a varus osteotomy of the femur.

14.8.3 Pre-Operative Examinations

Pre-operative X-rays revealed a significant deformity in the affected bone, necessitating detailed planning to ensure proper alignment during the procedure following the lengthening osteotomy (Figs. 14.14 and 14.15).

14.8.4 Preoperative Planning

- Radiographic study to determine the extent of the deformity.
- Use of custom-made tools to facilitate the osteotomy execution and plate positioning.

The deformity was entirely located in the femur, with an LDFA of 97. Given the hypermetria of the left lower limb and significant femoral valgus, a medial closing wedge osteotomy of the distal femur was performed to correct the axis and reduce the limb length (Figs. 14.16 and 14.17).

14.8.5 Surgical Procedure

1. Technique Used: Distal femur varus osteotomy performed with a custom-made cutting guide to ensure precise osteotomy execution (Figs. 14.18 and 14.19].

14.8.6 Postoperative Examinations

The postoperative X-rays show the achievement of good limb alignment and the restoration of proper limb length (eumetry) (Fig. 14.20).

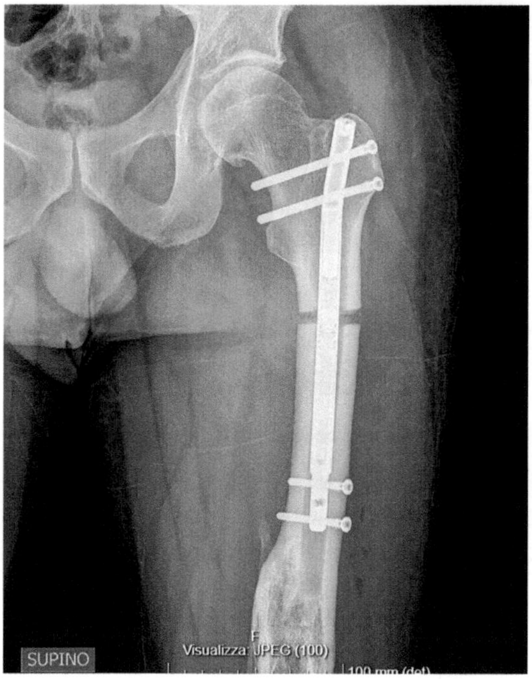

Fig. 14.14 Intermediate radiographic evaluation of the lengthening osteotomy using an extendable nail

14.8.7 Follow-Up

One-month check-up: Good implant stability and progress in osteotomy healing (Fig. 14.21).

14.8.8 Conclusions

The use of custom-made guides in osteotomy procedures is an effective option to enhance surgical precision and postoperative outcomes. This case highlights the importance of thorough preoperative planning and technological innovation in orthopedic surgery.

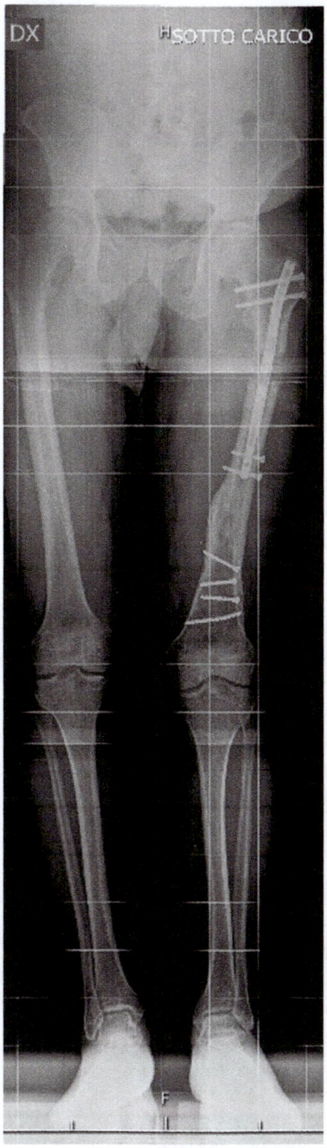

Fig. 14.15 Pre-operative X-rays of the distal femur varus osteotomy

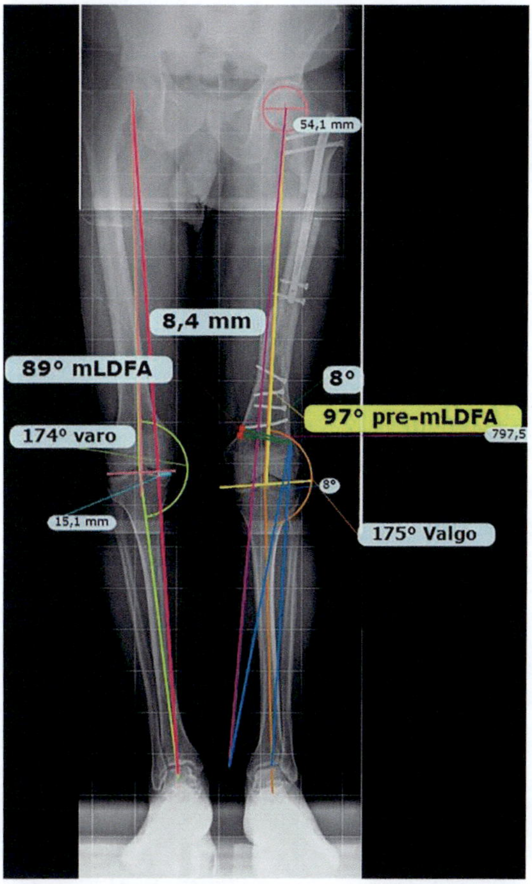

Fig. 14.16 Preoperative planning on X-rays

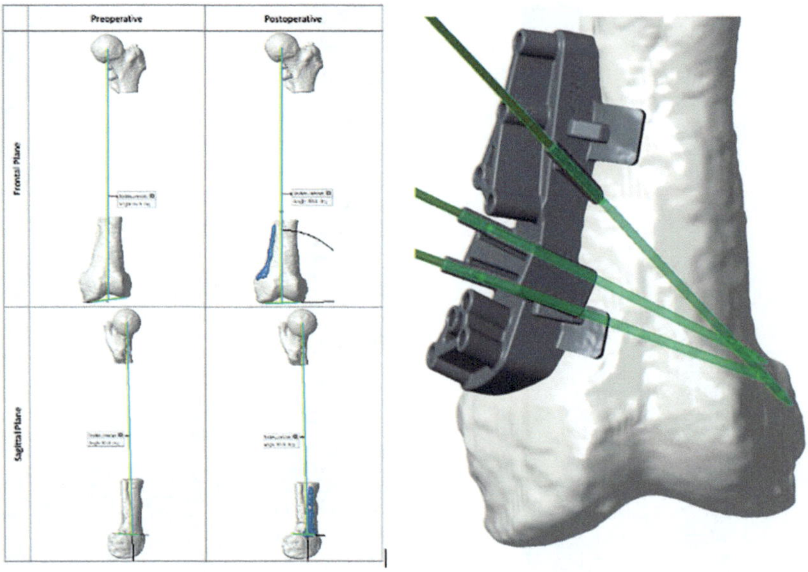

Fig. 14.17 Preoperative and postoperative images are presented, illustrating the alignment of the lower limb obtained through 3D graphic reconstructions

Left section:

– Frontal view: Shows the alignment of the mechanical axis of the limb before and after the procedure. The mechanical axis (green line) is traced through the center of the hip, knee, and ankle, highlighting any corrections made during the surgery

– Lateral view: Shows the lateral projection of the axis, emphasizing the improvement in anatomical and functional orientation. Correction of any sagittal deformities is visible

Right section:

A 3D model of the distal part of the tibia is shown, with a surgical guide specifically designed for screw positioning mounted on it

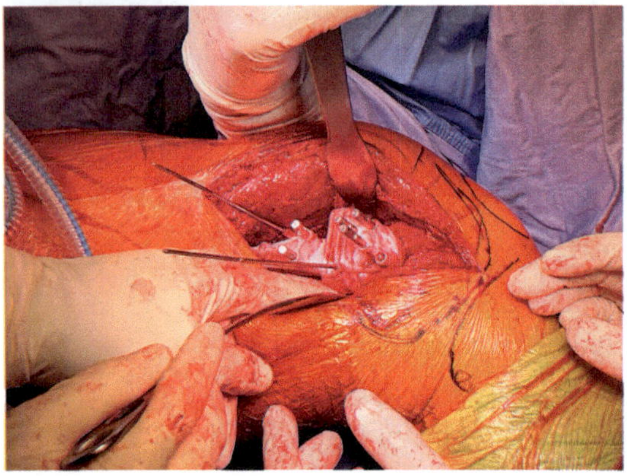

Fig. 14.18 Proper placement of the custom-made cutting guide for accurate osteotomy execution

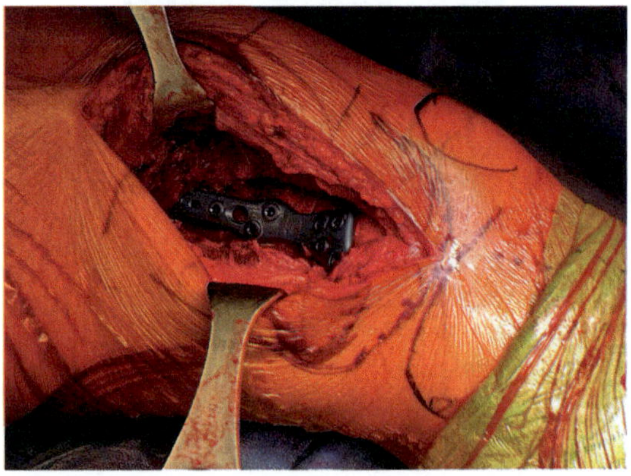

Fig. 14.19 Placement of the final plate

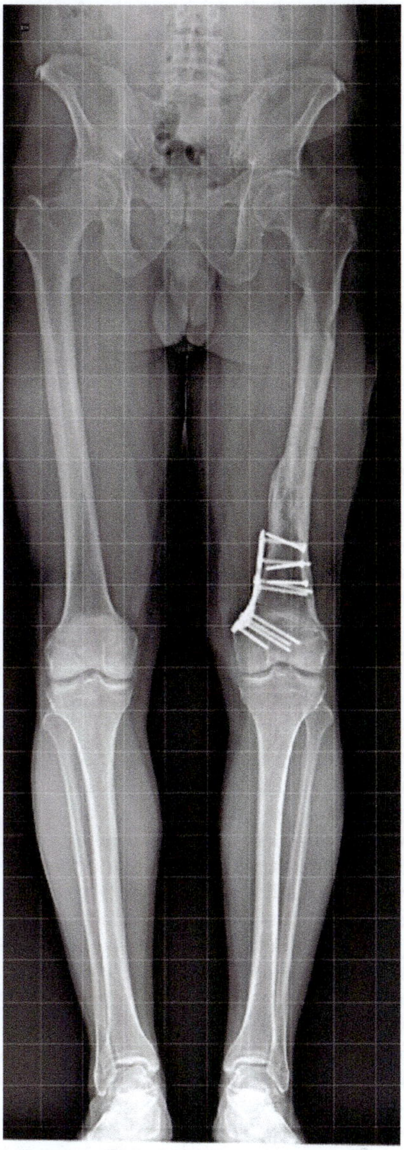

Fig. 14.20 Postoperative X-rays demonstrated proper bone alignment and satisfactory plate positioning

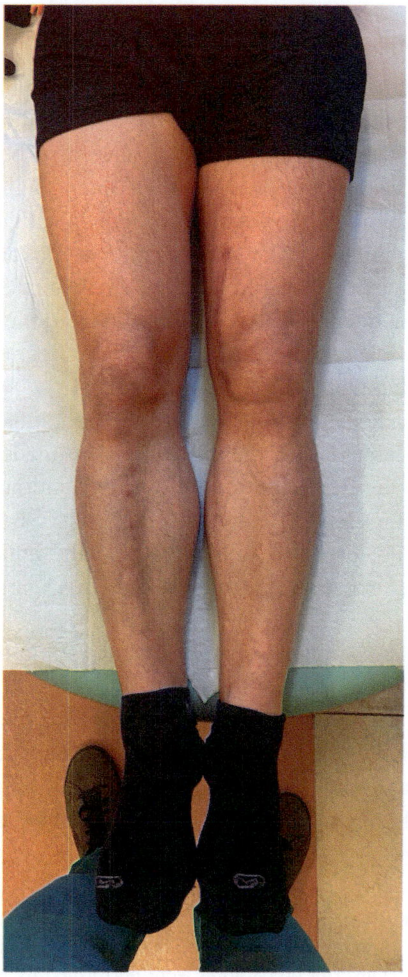

Fig. 14.21 Aligned limbs and restoration of leg length equality

14.9 Conclusions

As studies increasingly emphasize the multifaceted nature of lower extremity alignment, osteotomy planning and technique have also become more individualized. This chapter highlights techniques for correcting coronal misalignment through tibial and/or femoral osteotomies and the outcomes of these procedures. For patients with misalignment, DLO or biplanar osteotomies may be necessary to correct the degree of misalignment.

Surgical techniques are now becoming more personalized with the use of custom-made templates and templates based on information gathered through preoperative CT scans; PSIs allow for more precise osteotomies and the ability to correct existing deformities with less margin of error.

Knee surgeons should have a solid understanding of sagittal, coronal, biplanar, double-level, and derotation osteotomies. Preoperative digital 3D planning, PSI and navigation tools, as well as future robotics and artificial intelligence will likely help improve clinical outcomes for patients.

Author Contributions All listed authors have contributed substantially to this work: literature search and primary manuscript preparation were performed by MI and MC. MC and MI assisted with editing and finalizing the manuscript. All authors have read and approved the final manuscript to be submitted and published.

References

1. Smith JO, Wilson AJ, Thomas NP. Osteotomy around the knee: evolution, principles and results. Knee Surg Sports Traumatol Arthrosc. 2013;21(1):3–22.
2. Primeau CA, Birmingham TB, Leitch KM, Willits KR, Litchfield RB, Fowler PJ, et al. Total knee replacement after high tibial osteotomy: time-to-event analysis and predictors. Can Med Assoc J. 2021;193(5):E158–66.
3. Ackermann J, Merkely G, Arango D, Mestriner AB, Gomoll AH. The effect of mechanical leg alignment on cartilage restoration with and without concomitant high Tibial osteotomy. Arthroscopy : The Journal of Arthroscopic & Related Surgery. 2020;36(8):2204–14.
4. Xu K, Wang W, Wang Q, Sun J, Fang C, Sun Y, et al. Comparison of computer-assisted navigated technology and conventional technology in high tibial osteotomy (HTO): a meta-analysis. Comput Assist Surg. 2022;27(1):63–73.
5. Neri T, Myat D, Parker D. The use of navigation in osteotomies around the knee. Clin Sports Med. 2019;38(3):451–69.
6. Stimolo D, Leggieri F, Matassi F, Barra A, Civinini R, Innocenti M. Learning curves for high tibial osteotomy using patient-specific instrumentation: a case control study. Innov Surg Sci. 2024;9(3):123–31.
7. Chaouche S, Jacquet C, Fabre-Aubrespy M, Sharma A, Argenson JN, Parratte S, et al. Patient-specific cutting guides for open-wedge high tibial osteotomy: safety and accuracy analysis of a hundred patients continuous cohort. Int Orthop. 2019;43(12):2757–65.
8. Jacquet C, Sharma A, Fabre M, Ehlinger M, Argenson JN, Parratte S, et al. Patient-specific high-tibial osteotomy's "cutting-guides" decrease operating time and the number of fluoroscopic images taken after a brief learning curve. Knee Surg Sports Traumatol Arthrosc. 2020;28(9):2854–62.
9. Van Genechten W, Van Tilborg W, Van den Bempt M, Van Haver A, Verdonk P. Feasibility and 3D planning of a novel patient-specific instrumentation technique in medial opening-wedge high tibial osteotomy. J Knee Surg. 2021;34(14):1560–9.
10. Feucht MJ, Winkler PW, Mehl J, Bode G, Forkel P, Imhoff AB, et al. Isolated high tibial osteotomy is appropriate in less than two-thirds of varus knees if excessive overcorrection of the medial proximal tibial angle should be avoided. Knee Surg Sports Traumatol Arthrosc. 2021;29(10):3299–309.
11. Micicoi G, Grasso F, Kley K, Favreau H, Khakha R, Ehlinger M, et al. Osteotomy around the knee is planned toward an anatomical bone correction in less than half of patients. Orthop Traumatol Surg Res. 2021;107(4):102897.
12. Alaia MJ, Kaplan DJ, Mannino BJ, Strauss EJ. Tibial sagittal slope in anterior cruciate ligament injury and treatment. J Am Acad Orthop Surg. 2021;
13. Minzlaff P, Saier T, Brucker PU, Haller B, Imhoff AB, Hinterwimmer S. Valgus bracing in symptomatic varus malalignment for testing the expectable "unloading effect" following valgus high tibial osteotomy. Knee Surg Sports Traumatol Arthrosc. 2015;23(7):1964–70.
14. Noyes FR, Barber-Westin SD, Hewett TE. High tibial osteotomy and ligament reconstruction for varus angulated anterior cruciate ligament-deficient knees. Am J Sports Med. 2000;28(3):282–96.
15. Tischer T, Paul J, Pape D, Hirschmann MT, Imhoff AB, Hinterwimmer S, et al. The impact of osseous malalignment and realignment procedures in knee ligament surgery: a systematic review of the clinical evidence. Orthop J Sports Med. 2017;5(3):232596711769728.
16. Klek M, Dhawan A. The role of high Tibial osteotomy in ACL reconstruction in knees with coronal and sag-

ittal plane deformity. Curr Rev Musculoskelet Med. 2019;12(4):466–71.
17. Cantivalli A, Rosso F, Bonasia DE, Rossi R. High Tibial osteotomy and anterior cruciate ligament reconstruction/revision. Clin Sports Med. 2019;38(3):417–33.
18. Lu J, Tang S, Wang Y, Li Y, Liu C, Niu Y, et al. Clinical outcomes of closing- and opening-wedge high tibial osteotomy for treatment of anteromedial unicompartmental knee osteoarthritis. J Knee Surg. 2019;32(08):758–63.
19. Kim JH, Kim HJ, Lee DH. Leg length change after opening wedge and closing wedge high tibial osteotomy: a meta-analysis. PLoS One. 2017;12(7):e0181328.
20. Bito H, Takeuchi R, Kumagai K, Aratake M, Saito I, Hayashi R, et al. Opening wedge high tibial osteotomy affects both the lateral patellar tilt and patellar height. Knee Surg Sports Traumatol Arthrosc. 2010;18(7):955–60.
21. Krause M, Drenck TC, Korthaus A, Preiss A, Frosch KH, Akoto R. Patella height is not altered by descending medial open-wedge high tibial osteotomy (HTO) compared to ascending HTO. Knee Surg Sports Traumatol Arthrosc. 2018;26(6):1859–66.
22. Park JY, Kim JK, Han HS, Lee MC. Proximal tibiofibular division in lateral closing wedge high tibial osteotomy does not increase varus instability of the knee. Knee. 2019;26(6):1299–305.
23. Micicoi G, Martz P, Jacquet C, Fernandes LR, Khakha R, Ollivier M. High Tibial osteotomy with Miniaci planning using manual and Semiautomated digital measures. Video J Sport Med. 2021;1(6):263502542110329.
24. Lott A, James MG, Kaarre J, Höger S, Kayaalp ME, Ollivier M, et al. Around-the-knee osteotomies part II: surgical indications, techniques and outcomes—state of the art. J ISAKOS. 2024;9(4):658–71.
25. Kanakamedala AC, Hurley ET, Manjunath AK, Jazrawi LM, Alaia MJ, Strauss EJ. High tibial osteotomies for the treatment of osteoarthritis of the knee. JBJS Rev. 2022;10(1)
26. Sherman SL, Thompson SF, Clohisy JCF. Distal femoral varus osteotomy for the management of valgus deformity of the knee. J Am Acad Orthop Surg. 2018;26(9):313–24.
27. Feucht MJ, Tischer T. Kniegelenknahe Osteotomien bei Bandinsuffizienzen. Orthopade. 2017;46(7):601–9.
28. Wang JW, Hsu CC. Distal femoral varus osteotomy for osteoarthritis of the knee. J Bone Joint Surg. 2005;87(1):127–33.
29. Duerr RA, Harangody S, Magnussen RA, Kaeding CC, Flanigan DC. Technique for medial closing-wedge proximal tibia osteotomy in the valgus knee. Arthrosc Tech. 2020;9(7):e925–33.
30. Peng H, Ou A, Huang X, Wang C, Wang L, Yu T, et al. Osteotomy around the knee: the surgical treatment of osteoarthritis. Orthop Surg. 2021;13(5):1465–73.
31. Wylie JD, Jones DL, Hartley MK, Kapron AL, Krych AJ, Aoki SK, et al. Distal femoral osteotomy for the valgus knee: medial closing wedge versus lateral opening wedge: a systematic review. Arthroscopy : The Journal of Arthroscopic & Related Surgery. 2016;32(10):2141–7.
32. Duerr RA, Harangody S, Magnussen RA, Kaeding CC, Flanigan DC. Technique for medial closing-wedge proximal tibia osteotomy in the valgus knee. Arthrosc Tech. 2020;9(7):e925–e33.
33. Müller S, Frosch KH, Frings J, Berninger M, Krause M. Biplanar high tibial osteotomy for the combined correction of varus and posterior tibial slope malalignment. Orthop Traumatol Surg Res. 2023;109(4):103339.
34. Savarese E, Bisicchia S, Romeo R, Amendola A. Role of high tibial osteotomy in chronic injuries of posterior cruciate ligament and posterolateral corner. J Orthop Traumatol. 2011;12(1):1–17.
35. Pape D, Lorbach O, Schmitz C, Busch LC, Van Giffen N, Seil R, et al. Effect of a biplanar osteotomy on primary stability following high tibial osteotomy: a biomechanical cadaver study. Knee Surg Sports Traumatol Arthrosc. 2010;18(2):204–11.
36. Takeuchi R, Ishikawa H, Kumagai K, Yamaguchi Y, Chiba N, Akamatsu Y, et al. Fractures around the lateral cortical hinge after a medial opening-wedge high tibial osteotomy: a new classification of lateral hinge fracture. Arthroscopy: The Journal of Arthroscopic & Related Surgery. 2012;28(1):85–94.
37. Nakamura R, Komatsu N, Fujita K, Kuroda K, Takahashi M, Omi R, et al. Appropriate hinge position for prevention of unstable lateral hinge fracture in open wedge high tibial osteotomy. Bone Joint J. 2017;99-B(10):1313–8.
38. Lee SS, Celik H, Lee DH. Predictive factors for and detection of lateral hinge fractures following open wedge high tibial osteotomy: plain radiography versus computed tomography. Arthroscopy: The Journal of Arthroscopic & Related Surgery. 2018;34(11):3073–9.

15 Osteochondral Allograft Transplantation for Cartilage Repair and the Healing Cycle

Gokhan Meric and Behic Celik

15.1 Introduction

Cartilage damage and degeneration can be a debilitating and painful condition, often limiting the mobility and quality of life for those affected. Knee chondral injuries are a regular occurrence. About 60% of patients had high-grade cartilaginous abnormalities with lesion depths involving 50% or more of the cartilage surface, according to research analyzing over 30,000 arthroscopic surgeries [1]. However, recent advancements in medical science have opened up new avenues for treatment, one of which is osteochondral allograft transplantation. This innovative procedure holds promise in restoring damaged cartilage, offering hope to individuals suffering from conditions like osteoarthritis and traumatic injuries. In this chapter, we will touch upon the concept of cartilage repair with osteochondral allografts, the procedure's mechanics, benefits, and potential implications for patients seeking a path to recovery and improved joint function.

Surgical treatment of those chondral injuries includes arthroscopic chondral debridement, microfracture application, mosaicplasty, autologous chondrocyte implantation, and fresh osteochondral allograft transplantation. Transferring size-matched allograft cartilage and subchondral bone into chondral or osteochondral lesions of the knee is known as a fresh osteochondral allograft (OCA) transplant. OCAs can be used to transplant viable chondrocytes within mature hyaline cartilage in addition to replenishing bone stock that has been damaged or is not available. OCA has been utilized to treat difficult lesions in various joints, such as the shoulder and ankle, during primary and salvage surgeries [2].

OCA is a safe and effective treatment option for a number of difficult knee and ankle pathologies, including extensive chondral or osteochondral lesions, focal osteonecrosis, and specific types of post-traumatic arthritis, according to basic science and clinical investigations [3, 4].

Surgical treatment of articular cartilage lesions has gained popularity as a result of the development of techniques like autologous chondrocyte implantation and advancements in osteochondral autograft and allograft transplantations.

The use of osteochondral allografts has increased due to their adaptability. Osteochondral allografts can be utilized to treat lesions of diverse sizes, locations, and shapes even though they are typically only suggested for lesions larger than 2 cm^2. Osteochondral allografts are conducted in a single stage and can be used to treat osteochondral or simply articular surface abnormalities, in contrast to other restorative methods such as autologous cartilage implantation [5].

Autologous chondrocyte implantation (ACI), subchondral marrow stimulation (SMS), osteochondral autograft (OAT), and osteochondral

G. Meric · B. Celik (✉)
Yeditepe University School of Medicine, Orthopedics and Traumatology, Istanbul, Turkey

M. E. Erdil et al. (eds.), *Current Concept in Cartilage Treatment*,
https://doi.org/10.1007/978-3-032-27099-3_15

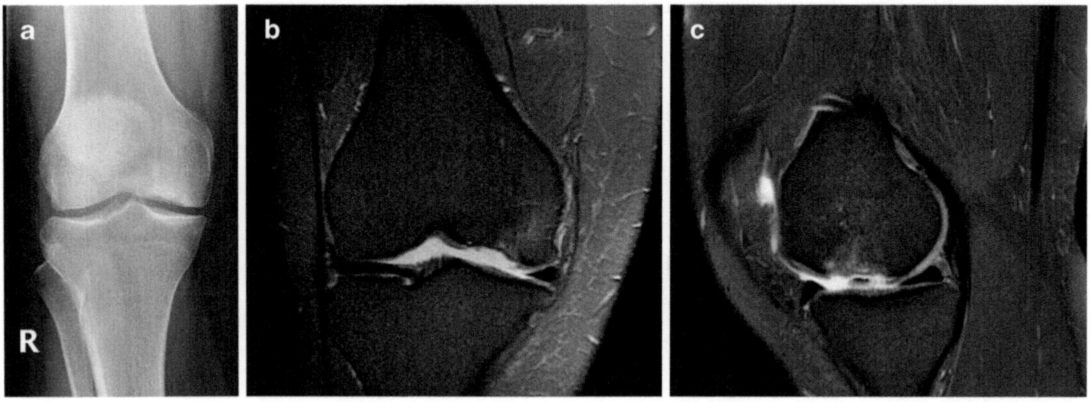

Fig. 15.1 X-ray and MRI are used as preoperative evaluation tools for the patients. (**a**) Preoperative AP X-ray of the right knee of a—year old patient. (**b**) Preoperative MRI views of the coronal and (**c**) sagittal planes, showing a cartilage defect zone which is >4cm^2

allograft (OCA) transplantation are a few of the cartilage procedures that have been discussed.

If the attempts on a cartilage repair case is unsuccessful, further cartilage repairs are carried out in accordance with a number of documented therapy algorithms.

It is significant to remember that the subchondral bone may be harmed by naive attempts at cartilage regeneration and as the number of the attempts rise, so does the lesion size [6]. Other conditions like osteochondritis dissecans (OCD), avascular necrosis (AVN), and trauma can also result in large cartilage lesions. These cartilage defects with regions larger than 2–4 cm^2 are linked to broken subchondral bone and are thought to be a sign that an OCA transplant is necessary [7].

Preoperative evaluation with X-ray and MRI is essential to determine lesion size, depth, location, and subchondral bone involvement before OCA transplantation (Fig. 15.1). In these circumstances, the OCA method can restore the cartilage's structural integrity by transferring a size-matched fresh osteochondral allograft containing viable hyaline cartilage and supporting subchondral bone.

15.2 Preoperative Planning

The candidate patient profile for the OCA treatment is as follows: age <50 years and if the chondral damage is located in either the femur or the patella. There may be accompanying alignment problems which may include the femorotibial axis and/or the patellofemoral joint. These need to be fixed firsthand. If there is any posttraumatic meniscal or ligamentous injury, these pathologies may be dealt with simultaneously or taken into consideration first, leaving the chondral transfer for later sessions.

15.3 Storage of the Graft

The standardization of graft storage can be directly linked to the increase in the usage of osteochondral allografts. The American Association of Tissue Banks and the US Food and Drug Administration worked together in 1998 to develop guidelines for refrigeration, storage mediums, and the maximum period of time tissues could be held before chondrocyte death occurred. These regulations gave tissue banks the push to start offering fresh osteochondral allografts for sale, which sped up the usage of these tissues in more applications [8]. The upper limit of the storage time is about 28 days, when samples are kept in +4 °C. The samples are studied and stored in Good Manufacturing Practice (GMP) laboratories, in which pharmaceutical products are consistently produced and controlled according to quality standards. These labs are approved by the Ministry of Health and are regulated by law. Serological and bacteriological tests are run twice for samples within 14 days' interval.

15.4 Surgical Method

A medial or lateral parapatellar arthrotomy was used for all procedures. The lesion's size was noted, and the nonviable tissue was removed via reamerization to a depth of 8–10 mm or so that allowed for a uniform bleeding surface of the subchondral bone. Then the lesion was prepared in a geometric format to a suitable depth. The immunogenic components of the marrow from the osseous surface were removed with a pulsatile lavage to reduce the immunogenicity of the graft. The graft was custom-made to fit the lesion, and trial fits were carried out until the graft was successfully placed. Press-fit fixation was used to secure the grafts. Press-fit fixation was used to secure the grafts. In some cases, fixation was augmented with a bioabsorbable pin (Figs. 15.2 and 15.3). Postoperative MRI was used to evaluate graft incorporation and cartilage viability during follow-up (Fig. 15.4).

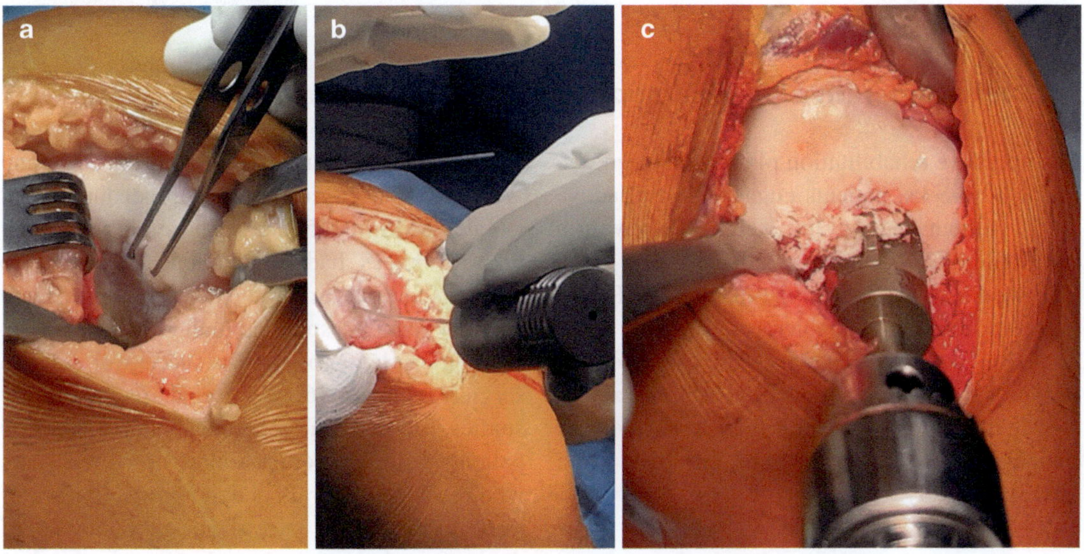

Fig. 15.2 Intraoperative photograph of the damaged cartilage zone in the medial femoral condyle. (**a**) A medial arthrotomy is performed, and the defected area is identified. (**b**) The K-wire is centrally inserted on the defective area through the sizer. (**c**) The defected area is reamerized to a depth of 8–10 mm, reaching the bleeding subchondral bone (Fig. 15.2)

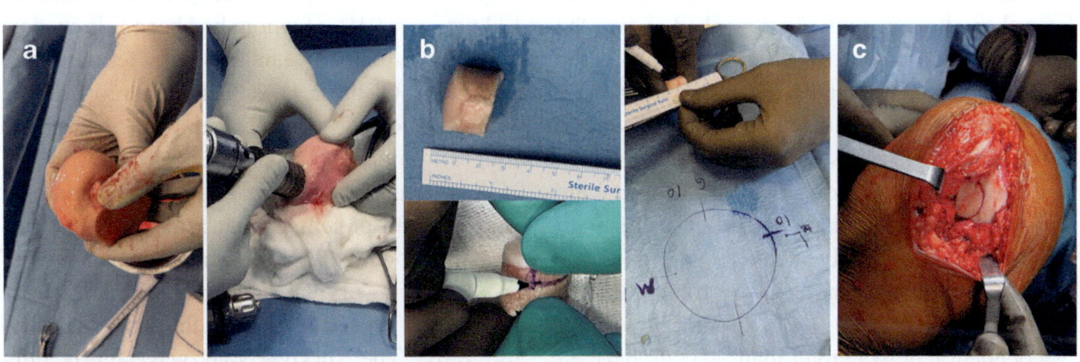

Fig. 15.3 Intraoperative photograph of the preparation of the osteochondral graft from the donor tissue. (**a**) The matching anatomical area of the defected area is located and reamerized to a depth of 10 to 12 mm of depth. (**b**) The four poles of the defected area and the graft are matched and the depth measurements are noted and marked on the graft. After this, the graft is cut and prepared for implantation according to the corresponding measurements (Fig. 15.3). (**c**) Implantation of the graft via 'press-fit' technique, the flash surface of the joint and bone-to-bone cooperation is seen

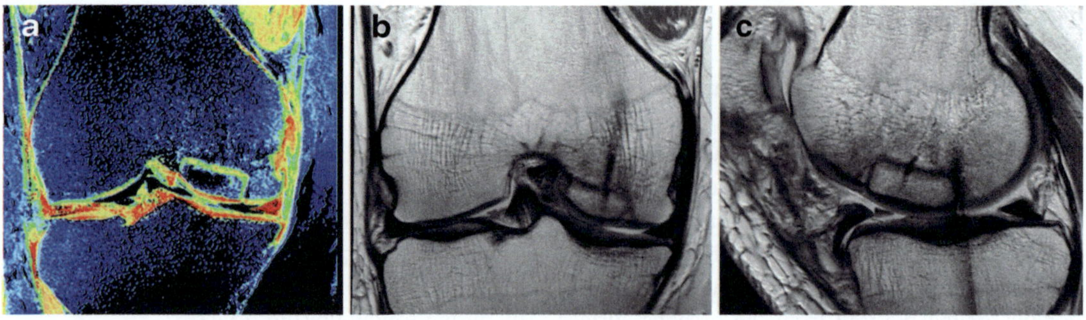

Fig. 15.4 Postoperative MRI views of the knee on (**a**) T2 mapping coronal plane, showing viable cartilage tissue; (**b**) coronal and (**c**) sagittal planes

15.5 Postoperative Rehabilitation

Postoperative rehabilitation plan was carried out. For 8–12 weeks, patients engaged in full active ROM without bearing any weight. Following a patellofemoral transplant, patients were given 3–4 weeks of passive range-of-motion (ROM) and weightbearing as tolerated with the knee locked in extension. Patients were often permitted to engage in recreational and athletic activities after 6 months. Up until the graft healed, all patients were followed up clinically and radiographically.

15.6 Discussion

Cartilage lesion treatment becomes increasingly unreliable and continues to be a problematic issue for orthopedic surgeons. As described above, the osteochondral allograft technique removes the damaged cartilage and adjacent subchondral bone to a depth sufficient to reach healthy subchondral bone. The excised osteochondral unit is then replaced with donor bone and cartilage, making this technique particularly useful in cases with subchondral bone involvement.

Osteochondritis dissecans, traumatic or degenerative cartilage lesions, and any other osteochondral defect larger than 2–4 cm^2 have all been treated with OCA transplantation as a salvage procedure, especially if there has been bone loss greater than 6 mm in depth.

In a study that assessed the outcome of osteochondral allograft (OCA) transplantation as a salvage procedure after various cartilage repair surgeries, out of 163 patients, 164 knees underwent OCA transplantation after SMS, OAT, and ACI. The majority of previous procedures were isolated SMS in 145 knees. The study found that 68% of knees had reoperations, 18.9% were allograft failures, and the median time to failure was 2.6 years. Despite the high reoperation rate, OCA transplantation was a successful salvage surgical treatment [6]. Gross et al., in one of their studies, followed and reported about a total of 60 patients with an average follow-up of ten years who received femoral condylar grafts. Twelve of those grafts failed, later requiring removing of the graft in three patients and conversion to total knee replacement in nine patients. The percentage of OCA transplant recipients who survived after 10 years ranged from 76% to 91% with long-term follow-up [4]. Levy et al. examined 122 patients, 91% of whom had been followed up on for more than 10 years following femoral condyle OCA. Of these, 47% had had a reoperation, with 24% of those cases being attributable to allograft failure [9].

A systematic review of 19 studies, including a total of 1036 patients found a mean 5-year survival rate of 86.7%, a 10-year survival rate of 78.7%, and a survival rate of 72.8% at 15 years and 67.5% at 20 years of the osteochondral allografts. The survival rate was significantly improved from preoperatively to postoperatively. However, revision cases, patellar lesions, and bipolar lesions were associated with worse survival rates. The study concludes that improved patient-reported outcomes can be expected after

OCA transplantation, with a survival rate of 78.7% at 10 years [10].

In conclusion, osteochondral allograft transplantation of the knee represents a promising and effective surgical option for individuals suffering from articular cartilage defects and joint degeneration. This innovative procedure offers the potential for pain relief, improved joint function, and a significant enhancement in the quality of life for patients who may otherwise face limited treatment options. While challenges such as graft availability, potential immune reactions, and long-term durability exist, ongoing advancements in tissue preservation and surgical techniques continue to improve the outcomes of osteochondral allograft procedures. As research and clinical experience in this field evolve, the future holds great promise for addressing the complex and debilitating issue of knee joint cartilage damage through osteochondral allograft transplantation.

References

1. Moyad TF. Cartilage injuries in the adult knee: evaluation and management. Cartilage. 2011;2(3):226–36. https://doi.org/10.1177/1947603510383973. PMID: 26069581; PMCID: PMC4300813
2. Sherman SL, Garrity J, Bauer K, Cook J, Stannard J, Bugbee W. Fresh osteochondral allograft transplantation for the knee: current concepts. J Am Acad Orthop Surg. 2014;22(2):121–33. https://doi.org/10.5435/jaaos-22-02-121.
3. Görtz S, De Young AJ, Bugbee WD. Fresh osteochondral allografting for steroid-associated osteonecrosis of the femoral condyles. Clin Orthop Relat Res. 2010;468(5):1269–78.
4. Gross AE, Shasha N, Aubin P. Long-term followup of the use of fresh osteochondral allografts for post-traumatic knee defects. Clin Orthop Relat Res. 2005;435:79–87.
5. Torrie AM, Kesler WW, Elkin J, et al. Osteochondral allograft. Curr Rev Musculoskelet Med. 2015;8:413–22.
6. Gracitelli GC, Meric G, Pulido PA, McCauley JC, Bugbee WD. Osteochondral allograft transplantation for knee lesions after failure of cartilage repair surgery. Cartilage. 2015;6(2):98–105. https://doi.org/10.1177/1947603514566298. PMID: 26069712; PMCID: PMC4462254
7. Gomoll AH, Farr J, Gillogly SD, Kercher JS, Minas T. Surgical management of articular cartilage defects of the knee. Instr Course Lect. 2011;60:461–83.
8. Garrity JT, Stoker AM, Sims HJ, Cook JL. Improved osteochondral allograft preservation using serum-free media at body temperature. Am J Sports Med. 2012;40(11):2542–8.
9. Levy YD, Görtz S, Pulido PA, McCauley JC, Bugbee WD. Do fresh osteochondral allografts successfully treat femoral condyle lesions? Clin Orthop Relat Res. 2013;471(1):231–7.
10. Familiari F, Cinque ME, Chahla J, Godin JA, Olesen ML, Moatshe G, LaPrade RF. Clinical outcomes and failure rates of osteochondral allograft transplantation in the knee: a systematic review. Am J Sports Med. 2018;46(14):3541–9. https://doi.org/10.1177/0363546517732531. Epub 2017 Oct 17

16 Use of 3D Bioprinters in Cartilage Repair and Engineering

Feza Korkusuz and Batuhan Erhan Aktaş

16.1 The Structure and Function of Articular Cartilage

Articular cartilage is a highly specialized connective tissue with distinct viscoelastic properties and lubrication. Its smooth and gliding surface maintains a low friction articulation and it facilitates the transfer of loads to the subchondral bone that is separated by a tidemark. One of the remarkable qualities of articular cartilage is its capacity to endure intense repetitive frictional forces without showing any significant signs of damage or degenerative alteration for decades and even throughout life under normal conditions [1]. The hyaline articular cartilage is located at the ends of long bones. It additionally works as a shock-absorbing structure that disperses forces generated during motion. The thickness of its layers in adult humans is typically around 1.0–2.0 mm, although it may differ across various regions of the joint (Fig. 16.1) [2]. The highest thickness is usually observed at the knee joint that is about 8.0 mm. It is a unique tissue as it lacks blood circulation, peripheral nerve endings, and lymphatic drainage. It is mainly made up of a dense extracellular matrix (ECM) containing specialized cells called chondrocytes. The ECM primarily contains synovial fluid, collagen, and proteoglycans, with a smaller quantity of non-collagenous proteins and glycoproteins and is constantly undergoing turnover [3]. About 70% of its wet weight is synovial fluid. Nourishment and waste disposal of cells is all through the synovial fluid that is synthesized by the synovium (Table 16.1). Dry-weight components of articular cartilage include inorganic ashes (principally hydroxyapatite), collagens, non-collagenous matrix proteins, lipids, saccharides, and chondronectin (Fig. 16.2) [4–6].

16.1.1 Chondrocytes

Chondrocytes, which make up around 2% of the total volume of articular cartilage, are the specialized and metabolically active cells that reside within this tissue. They originate from mesenchymal stem cells and have a distinct role in the development, maintenance, and restoration of the ECM. The primary method of nutrient delivery to the articular cartilage is the diffusion of synovial fluid into the tissue as blood vessels in articular cartilage are missing. Joint movement help to facilitate this diffusion process. The ratio of cells to ECM is extremely low in articular cartilage. Due to this situation, homeostasis and regeneration capacity of articular cartilage is limited. The shape, quantity, and size of chondrocytes in articular cartilage differ based on their zones. In the superficial zone, the

F. Korkusuz (✉) · B. E. Aktaş
Department of Sports Medicine, Hacettepe University, Ankara, Turkey

M. E. Erdil et al. (eds.), *Current Concept in Cartilage Treatment*,
https://doi.org/10.1007/978-3-032-27099-3_16

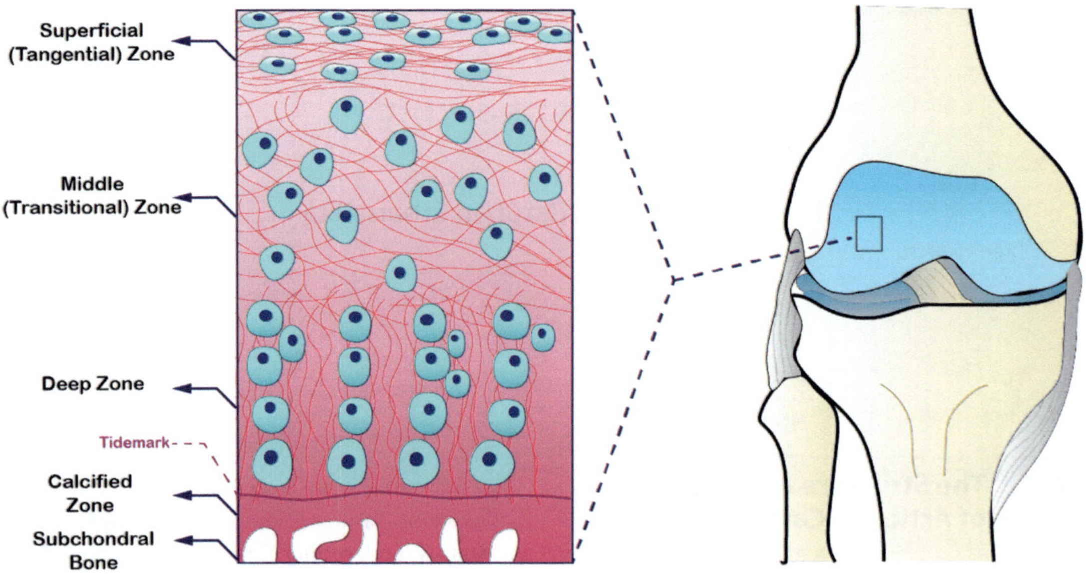

Fig. 16.1 Zonal organization of articular cartilage. The structural and functional properties of normal articular cartilage in a joint are derived from its composition of three distinct zones (superficial, middle, and deep) and the presence of a tidemark supported by the underlying calcified and subchondral bone zones

Table 16.1 The structure and function of articular cartilage

• Highly specialized connective tissue. Type II hyaline cartilage
• Hyaluronan is the link protein
• Distinct zonal layers
• Thickness (in the knee joint) about 8.0 mm
• No blood circulation
• No peripheral nerve endings
• No lymphatic drainage
• Cells: Chondrocytes
• Nourishment through synovial fluid
• 70% of its wet weight is synovial fluid
• Chondrocyte/extracellular matrix (ECM) ratio is about 1/100
• Distinct viscoelastic properties. Mainly lubrication
• Endures intense repetitive frictional forces
• Limited or no regenerative capacity

chondrocytes are aligned to the surface, longitudinal, fibrinoid, and flatter with a higher density compared to those in the deeper regions. Each chondrocyte creates a distinct microenvironment and is accountable for maintaining the extracellular matrix in its close surroundings. This microenvironment acts as a barrier that confines the chondrocyte within its own matrix, preventing migration to the neighboring regions of articular cartilage [7].

Chondrocytes generally do not establish direct cell-to-cell connections for signal transduction and communication with other cells. They can, however, react to various stimuli such as growth factors, mechanical loads, piezoelectric forces, and hydrostatic pressures. Chondrocytes engage in intercellular communication through diverse signaling pathways, orchestrating their actions and shaping the maturing cartilage during the process of cartilage development and endochondral ossification. Bone morphogenetic proteins (BMPs), vascular endothelial growth factor A (VEGF), and receptor activators of nuclear factor kappa-B ligand (RANKL) notably play a role in the hypertrophic growth plate zone. The role of VEGF, however, is not well-defined. Chondrocytes produce these signaling molecules, which act on adjacent cells, influencing their behavior. Bone morphogenic proteins for instance, facilitate chondrocyte differentiation and maturation. RANKL conversely participates in bone resorption that is a necessary process for replacing cartilage with bone during endochondral ossification [8]. The gene and protein expressions that define chondrocytes are closely tied to the specific matrix

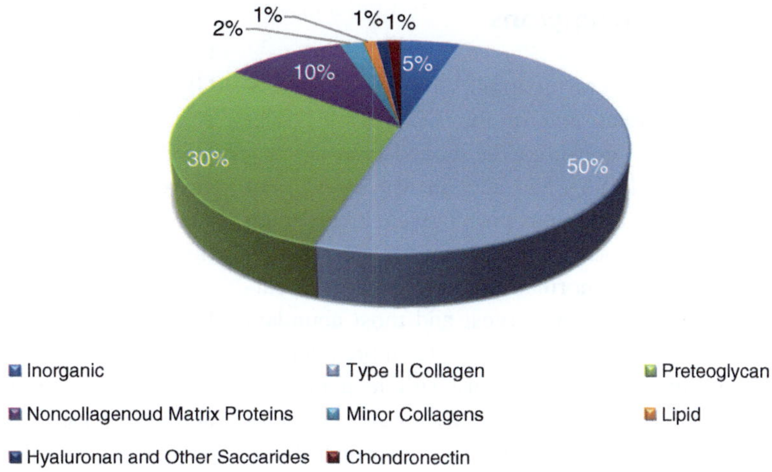

Fig. 16.2 Biochemical composition of articular cartilage

constituents present in articular cartilage and recent cellular therapies aim to evoke a response of regeneration by stimulating such factors, including VEGF and platelet-derived growth factor (PDGF). These factors are known to decrease inflammation and stimulate regeneration. The ability of chondrocytes to replicate is unfortunately limited, which can hinder the intrinsic healing capacity of cartilage after injury. Chondrocytes require an ideal chemical and mechanical environment to endure [9].

Table 16.2 Collagens present in articular cartilage [11]

Collagen type	Classification	Percentage
Type I	Fibril-forming collagen	0%
Type II	Fibril-forming collagen	90–95%
Type III	Fibril-forming collagen	n/a
Type IV	Network-forming collagen	n/a
Type V	Fibril-forming collagen	n/a
Type VI	Beaded filament collagen	1–2%
Type IX	FACIT	1–5%
Type X	Network-forming collagen	1%
Type XI	Fibril-forming collagen	1–5%

FACIT Fibril-associated collagens with interrupted triple helices, *n/a* no studies have been found to support it

16.1.2 Collagens

The extracellular matrix of articular cartilage is predominantly composed of collagen, which accounts for approximately 60% of the dry weight of cartilage. Type II collagen is the most abundant one, representing 90% to 95% of the collagen in the matrix, and is intertwined with proteoglycan aggregates to form fibrils and fibers. Other collagen types, such as I (either existing in minimal quantities or completely lacking in hyaline cartilage), IV, V, VI, IX, and XI, are also present but in smaller amounts and help to form and stabilize the type II collagen fibril network. There are over 15 distinct collagen types that make up at least the 29 polypeptide chains, each containing a triple helix structure of three α-chains. The amino acid composition of the polypeptide chains is primarily glycine and proline, with hydroxyproline providing additional stability through hydrogen bonding along the length of the molecule. These features contribute to the shear and tensile properties of articular cartilage, which are important for maintaining matrix stability (Table 16.2) [10].

The orientation of collagen fibers in articular cartilage varies depending on the depth, with the superficial zone containing tangentially arranged fibers, the deep zone containing radially oriented fibers, and the middle zone having a combination of arcade-like structure and randomly oriented fibers, serving as a transitional zone between the other zones. Articular cartilage acquires its distinctive biomechanical properties from the interaction between collagens, proteoglycans, and a charged fluid environment [12].

16.1.3 Proteoglycans

Proteoglycans are monomers of heavily glycosylated proteins and in the ECM of articular cartilage, they constitute the second-largest group of macromolecules and account for 10–15% of the wet weight. Various proteoglycans, including aggrecan, decorin, biglycan, and fibromodulin, are essential for normal function in articular cartilage. Aggrecan, the largest and most abundant proteoglycan by weight, possesses more than 100 chondroitin sulfate and keratin sulfate chains and contains a hyaluronan core with numerous glycosaminoglycan side chains. The proper functioning of cartilage tissue depends on the conglomeration of numerous proteoglycans into large macromolecules [13].

16.1.4 Synovial Fluid

The primary fluid component in articular cartilage and synovial fluid within the joint capsule is serum. In addition, synovial fluid contains significant amounts of inorganic salts such as sodium, potassium, calcium, and chloride. While most water in cartilage tissue is held within the extracellular matrix's molecular pore space, it also permeates throughout the tissue. Chondrocytes receive nutrients via diffusion from the joint space, with interstitial fluid serving as the primary carrier responsible for transporting both nutrients and waste within the tissue (Table 16.3) [14].

Many non-collagenous proteins and glycoproteins are found in the articular cartilage. Glycoproteins are essential for maintaining the structure and function of articular cartilage. They have significant involvement in various processes, including organizing the cartilage matrix, stabilizing collagen, and responding to conditions like osteoarthritis [16].

One noteworthy glycoprotein in articular cartilage is Matrilin-1, which was initially identified in association with aggrecan. Matrilin-1 levels change during cartilage maturation and increased amounts have been observed in osteoarthritis, suggesting its role in the disease [17]. Another important glycoprotein in articular cartilage is cartilage oligomeric protein (COMP), belonging to the thrombospondin family. COMP contributes to organizing and stabilizing collagen fibers in the extracellular matrix. It has been utilized as a diagnostic marker in serum to assess the degradation of the matrix in osteoarthritis [18]. The presence of these glycoproteins emphasizes their significance in maintaining the integrity and function of articular cartilage. Glycoproteins ensure the mechanical properties necessary for cartilage to withstand joint movement forces by contributing to collagen fiber organization and stabilization. Their involvement in pathological conditions such as osteoarthritis moreover suggests their potential as targets for therapeutic interventions aimed at preserving or restoring cartilage health. Glycoproteins found in articular cartilage therefore play a crucial role in its structure, function, and response to pathological conditions.

Table 16.3 Composition of the synovial fluid [15]

Characteristic	Mean or representative value	Characteristic	Mean or representative value
Volume	0.13–3.5 mL (adult knee)	**γ globulin**	0.38 g/dL
pH	7.3–7.4	**Immunoglobulin G**	13% of serum value
Relative viscosity	235	**Immunoglobulin M**	5% of serum value
Cl, HCO_3^-	Slightly higher than serum	**Immunoglobulin E**	22% of serum value
Na, K, Ca, Mg	Slightly lower than serum	**α_2-Macroglobulin**	3% of serum value
Glucose	Serum value ±10%	**Transferrin**	24% of serum value
Total protein	1.7–2.1 g/dL	**Ceruloplasmin**	16% of serum value
Albumin	1.2 g/dL	**CH50**	30–50% of plasma value
α_1 globulin	0.17 g/dL	**Hyaluronic acid**	300 mg/dL
α_2 globulin	0.15 g/dL	**Cholesterol**	7.1 mg/dL
β globulin	0.23 g/dL	**Phospholipid**	13.8 mg/dL

16.1.5 Zones

The thin outer layer of articular cartilage, known as the superficial or tangential zone, accounts for about 10–20% of the total thickness and is vital in shielding the underlying layers from shear stresses. The collagen fibers, predominantly type II and IX collagens, are densely packed and oriented parallel to the joint surface. The flattened chondrocytes are more abundant in this zone and its structural integrity is crucial for maintaining the health of the deeper layers. This layer is in direct contact with the synovial fluid and plays a significant role in the cartilage's tensile properties that enable it to withstand the compressive, tensile, and shear forces associated during joint movement, including walking, jumping, and running. The specialized proteins secreted by cells in the superficial zone are believed to resist and overcome the tissue's wear and tear properties [19].

The central transitional zone, which is beneath the superficial zone, plays an important role in connecting the superficial and deep zones anatomically and functionally. This zone accounts for a significant portion (40% to 60%) of the total cartilage volume and contains thicker collagen fibrils and proteoglycans. Collagen fibers in the middle zone have an arcade-like structure, with randomly oriented fibers interspersed throughout. Chondrocytes in this layer are at low density and have a spherical shape [20].

The primary role of the deep zone is to resist compressive forces, which it accomplishes through the perpendicular arrangement of collagen fibrils. This zone has the highest proteoglycan content, the lowest water concentration, and the largest diameter collagen fibrils in a radial pattern. The chondrocytes in the deep zone are arranged in columns parallel to the collagen fibers and perpendicular to the joint line and are present in low density. This zone constitutes approximately 30% of the total cartilage volume and represents the last purely hyaline tissue before reaching the bone. The tide mark separates the deep zone from the calcified cartilage, which plays a critical role in anchoring the collagen fibrils of the deep zone to the subchondral bone. The chondrocytes in this zone are hypertrophic and the cell population is scarce [3]. The subchondral bone, that is almost always involved in diseases and injuries, is very important to maintain the integrity and function of the articular cartilage. Recent surgical procedures aim to restore the subchondral bone to cope with the regeneration process.

16.1.6 Regions

The extracellular matrix of articular cartilage can be further divided into different regions based on its composition, proximity to chondrocytes, and organization of collagen fibers. These regions include the pericellular region, which is immediately surrounding the chondrocytes and contains a high concentration of proteoglycans and type VI collagen; the territorial region, which surrounds the pericellular region and has a lower concentration of proteoglycans but a higher concentration of type II collagen; and the interterritorial region, which makes up the majority of the ECM and contains a mix of collagen types, primarily types II, IX, and XI. These different regions contribute to the overall mechanical properties and function of articular cartilage. The matrix region that lies adjacent to the cell membrane is called the pericellular matrix and it envelops the chondrocyte completely. It primarily consists of proteoglycans and also includes glycoproteins and other non-collagenous proteins. This area of the matrix is thought to have a functional role in initiating signal transduction within the cartilage in response to load bearing [21]. The territorial matrix is situated around the pericellular matrix and consists mainly of fine collagen fibrils, which are arranged in a basket-like network around the chondrocytes [22]. It is thicker than the pericellular matrix and is thought to serve as a protective layer for the cartilage cells against mechanical stresses. It is additionally believed to play a crucial role in the resilience of the articular cartilage structure [23]. The largest one, the interterritorial region, plays the most significant role in determining the biomechanical properties of articular cartilage [24]. It is

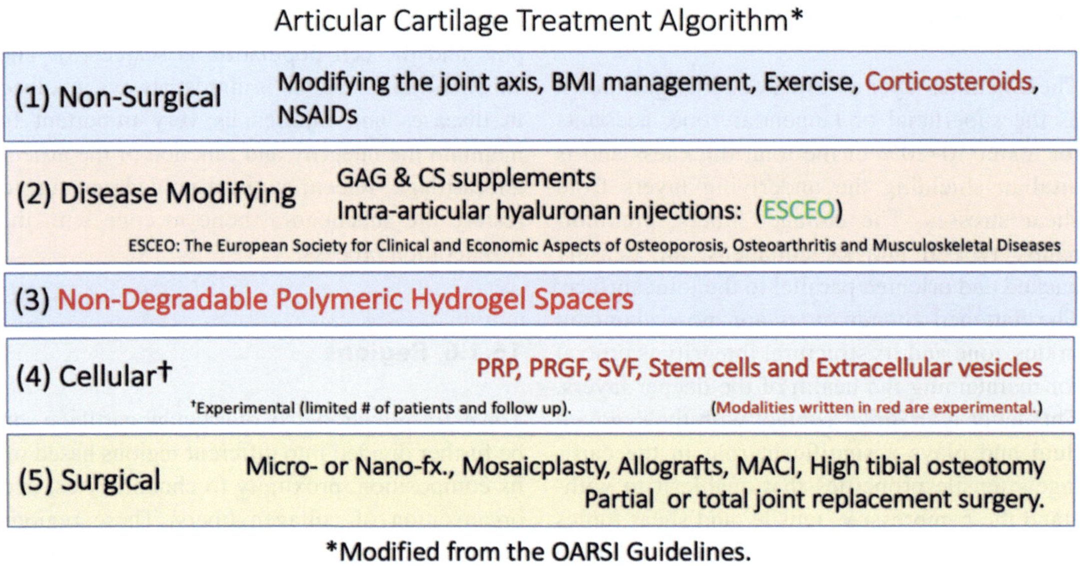

Fig. 16.3 Treatment algorithm of osteoarthritis and articular cartilage injuries

distinguished by a large number of randomly arranged bundles of collagen fibrils, which vary in orientation depending on the depth of the zone: parallel to the articular surface in the superficial zone, obliquely in the middle zone, and perpendicular in the deep zone. The presence of a significant amount of proteoglycans is also a characteristic feature of the interterritorial zone, which contributes heavily to the biomechanical properties of the articular cartilage [25].

Understanding the complexity of the articular cartilage structure is essential for developing effective strategies to prevent or treat joint disorders that involve cartilage damage or degradation. Articular cartilage repair and regeneration, however, is a challenging process with limited success. Chondrocytes do not generate an effective healing response and even with temporary functional restoration, the mechanically weaker repair tissue may eventually degenerate, leading to pain and disability. True and lasting functional restoration is rare while some degree of healing can occur. As a result, the absence of a complete healing response suggests that cartilage repair remains an ongoing challenge in the field of musculoskeletal science. Tissue engineering perspective that combines biomaterials, cells, and signaling molecules therefore is expanding its basic and clinical research in articular cartilage regeneration (Fig. 16.3).

16.2 Sport-Related Articular Cartilage Injuries, Osteochondritis Dissecans (OCD): Current Treatments and New 3D Printing-Related Approaches

16.2.1 Osteochondritis Dissecans: Definition, Incidence, and Variation Across Populations

Osteochondritis Dissecans (OCD) is described as a localized and yet unexplained change in the subchondral bone, which can pose a risk of destabilizing and damaging nearby articular cartilage, ultimately leading to the early onset of osteoarthritis [26]. Most OCD patients describe a major or minor direct or indirect sport-related injury to their joints. The treatment for OCD mainly depends on the maturity of the skeletal system and the stability of the lesion, which is determined by the presence or absence of fracture in the articular cartilage and the separation of the subchondral bone. The primary objectives of treatment are to provide relief from symptoms and preserve joint health [27].

Osteochondritis dissecans can be classified into juvenile and adult forms, which are distinguished based on the maturity of the skeletal system at the time of diagnosis. Although most adult cases are believed to be unresolved juvenile lesions, instances of de novo adult OCD have also been reported. Adult OCD mainly affects the ankles, followed by the knees and has an incidence rate of 3.42 cases per 100,000 person-years. Juvenile OCD is more prevalent, with a frequency of 9.5–29 cases per 100,000 knees, 2.2 cases per 100,000 elbows, and 2–4.6 cases per 100,000 ankles [28–31]. Osteochondritis dissecans commonly affects physically active children and young adults, particularly those who participate in high-level athletics. The knee is the most commonly affected joint in these athletes, with a prevalence of 55–60%, followed by the elbow (84%) and talus (67.4%) [32, 33]. Elbow OCD is commonly observed in athletes involved in throwing sports and gymnastics. Knee and talar OCD patients in contrast are frequently linked to sports such as soccer, football, and basketball [34, 35]. The observed trend of OCD presenting at a younger age may be associated with earlier involvement or specialization in sports, as well as the rising prevalence of childhood obesity [36, 37]. According to a recent systematic review, it is probable that the etiopathogenesis of OCD involves a combination of biological and mechanical factors [38]. The development of OCD due to acute trauma, specifically lateral talar osteochondral lesions resulting from ankle sprains, is considered as a separate condition. Treatment for both types of OCD nevertheless is similar. The prevalent theory for the etiology of OCD in these cases suggests that repetitive loading causes vascular compromise, which is often associated with athletic activities, accounting for a prevalence rate of 55–60% [39, 40]. In throwing athletes and gymnasts, capitellar OCD mainly affects the dominant arm and is usually associated with valgus or axial stress. Knee OCD in baseball catchers conversely occurs at a younger age and is situated more posteriorly in the knee compared to non-catchers, likely due to loading in hyperflexion [41]. The most frequent occurrence of juvenile OCD in the femoral trochlea is observed in basketball, football, and soccer players who experience forces across the patellofemoral joint. Some researchers have also proposed a relationship with anatomical variations, such as narrower intercondylar width, a larger tibial spine, greater posterior-medial tibial slope, dysmorphic femoral condyles and a more distal femoral attachment of the posterior cruciate ligament [42–46]. Research has linked meniscal injury with the occurrence of OCD less frequently in the lateral aspect of the femoral condyle. There is additionally a correlation between knee OCD and alignment, with genu varum being associated with medial condylar lesions and genu valgum being linked with lateral condylar lesions. A significant association between unstable knee lesions and mechanical axis deviation furthermore has been identified.

16.2.2 Operative Treatment

Patients who have unstable lesions, unsuccessful non-surgical treatment, or unfavorable nomogram predictions are primarily recommended for surgery. The surgical approach used depends on the characteristics of the lesion. Surgical correction additionally may be necessary to address any accompanying pathology, such as limb malalignment and joint instability. There are multiple approaches available for managing chondral lesions and OCD, aiming to alleviate symptoms and improve functions. These methods comprise non-surgical strategies like physical immobilization and nonsteroidal anti-inflammatory medications, as well as surgical techniques, including osteotomy, abrasion arthroplasty, autograft implantation, mosaicplasty, microfracture, autologous chondrocyte implantation (ACI), and matrix-assisted autologous chondrocyte implantation (MACI) (Fig. 16.4). Arthroscopic debridement and microfracture are often utilized as initial treatments for symptomatic focal chondral lesions or OCD, while ACI and osteochondral grafting are considered second-line options.

Recent studies, however, suggest that ACI as a second-line measure, after failed microfracture, may result in a poorer outcome compared to using ACI as the primary intervention [47]. While the previously mentioned treatment methods are effective in reducing pain and improving the quality of life in patients, their long-term effectiveness is limited. ACI, MACI, and microfracture procedures often result in the formation of fibrocartilage tissue rather than true articular cartilage, which can negatively impact joint function. Cell- and tissue-based allografts have been proposed as a material-free repair strategy as an alternative. There is, however, a risk of disease transmission associated with the use of allografts, which is a concern for treatment [48].

Newer and more advanced treatment options, such as tissue-engineered strategies, have emerged as promising alternatives for the repair and regeneration of osteochondral lesions. This is due to the limited regeneration ability of articular cartilage and the need for more effective and favorable solutions. These strategies aim to mimic the structure and function of the damaged tissues and are considered a promising option for the thorough healing of both subchondral bone damage and cartilage lesions [49]. Various regenerative medicine and tissue engineering approaches have been proposed and implemented for the repair and regeneration of OCD. These strategies include scaffold-free methods that involve tissue-specific cells, genetically modified cells (e.g., Induced Pluripotent Stem Cell) and progenitor cells (e.g., Bone marrow-derived mesenchymal stem cells, Adipose-derived stem cells, Tendon-derived stem cells). Scaffold-based approaches, including monophasic, biphasic and multiple-phasic scaffolds, as well as gradient-designed scaffolds, are also utilized. Incorporating and releasing different bioactive factors and drugs through various delivery systems is furthermore another method used in OCD treatment. Marrow stimulation techniques, such as microfracture or nano-fracture, can be used for small chondral lesions or OCD less than two centimeters. This involves drilling the subchondral parts to stimulate an influx of MSCs from the bone marrow into the OCD [50]. Several grafts derived from periosteum and perichondrium, which contain progenitor cells, have also been applied. Their outcomes, however, have not been very promising so far [51]. Another technique, called mosaicplasty or osteoarticular transfer system (OATS), involves the transplantation of autologous osteochondral plugs. These plugs contain both the upper hyaline cartilage and the lower subchondral bone from non-weight-bearing areas of the patient's joints [52]. Causing an injury in the healthy articular cartilage is a drawback of this approach. Allografts can be preferred in mosaicplasty; however, their limitations should be considered.

Tissue engineering techniques have been increasingly utilized in recent years for the treatment of chondral lesions. Autologous chondrocyte implantation involves expanding chondrocytes from non-weight-bearing regions in a monolayer culture and then transplanting them with a periosteal flap [53]. This method has been improved by creating matrix-assisted autologous chondrocyte implantation, in which chondrocytes are seeded into various scaffolds. It should be noted that some treatments used for chondral defects, such as microfracture, however, may cause injury to the underlying bone, resulting in a new bone defect and potentially another OCD. Despite these treatments showing partial or temporary success, they are not completely effective [54]. There is currently no effective method to regenerate a durable and long-lasting osteochondral tissue. Some existing approaches even have negative side effects. Debridement and subchondral drilling in example, can cause fibrocartilage formation, while perichondral or periosteal grafting does not consistently attain hyaline cartilage. Autologous chondrocyte transplantation involves multiple operations and may cause problems due to different types of scaffolds and biomaterials. Although autologous osteochondral transplantation is the only clinically used surgical treatment that targets both hyaline cartilage and subchondral bone, it is sometimes associated with donor site morbidity, graft apoptosis, and contour mismatch, regardless of the availability of the grafts. Mosaicplasty and ACI additionally have variable clinical outcomes according to prospective randomized clinical trials [55].

Regenerative medicine, particularly in the field of articular cartilage repair, shows promise with the emergence of Induced Pluripotent Stem Cell (iPSC) therapies. iPSCs are a type of stem cell that can be generated from adult cells through a process called reprogramming. This method involves introducing specific transcription factors that revert the cells to a pluripotent state, enabling them to differentiate into various cell types, including chondrocytes. iPSCs possess the ability to differentiate into chondrocytes and promote the regeneration of damaged cartilage. Researchers have devised differentiation protocols that guide iPSCs toward chondrogenic lineages, leading to the production of iPSC-derived chondrocytes that closely resemble those naturally found in healthy cartilage [56]. iPSCs also allows for personalized treatment strategies and enhanced comprehension of cartilage-related disorders. Several challenges need to be addressed although iPSC therapies hold considerable potential. One such concern is the risk of tumorigenicity, where iPSCs may give rise to tumors.

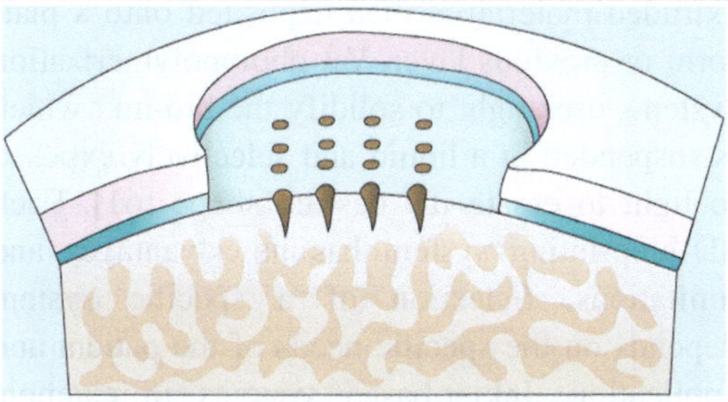

- **Microfracture**
  - Formation of fibrocartilage
  - Repaired tissue is susceptible to damage and usually declines in quality within approximately 18–24 months after the surgical procedure
  - Perforations trigger the activation of a secondary center of ossification, leading to the formation of intralesional osteophytes
  - Threefold-to-sevenfold increase in the failure rate of ACI when performed after prior microfracture

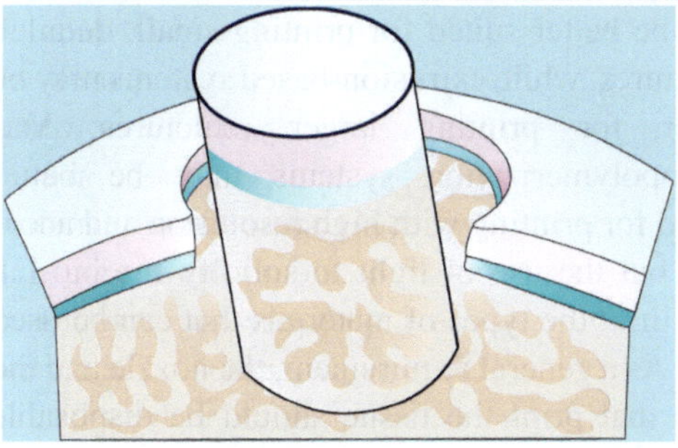

- **Osteochondral Autograft Transplantation**
  - In larger defects, mosaicplasty requires the transfer of multiple small cylinders (osteochondral plugs) to the defect
  - Restricted graft disposal and donor site-related morbidity

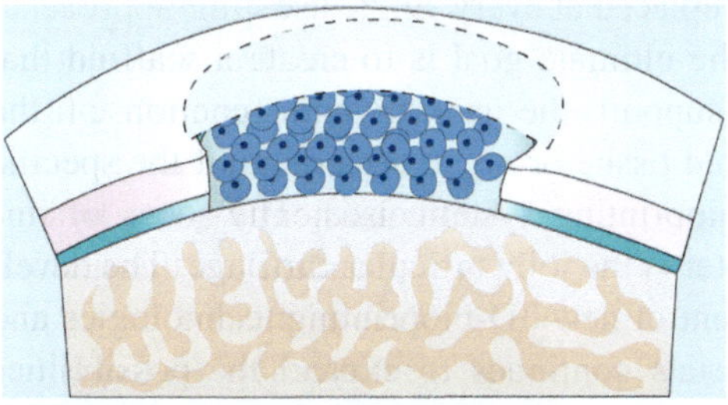

- **Autologous Chondrocyte Implantation (ACI)**
  - Two surgical procedures are needed
  - A long recovery time (6–12 months)
  - Hypertrophy of the periosteal flap

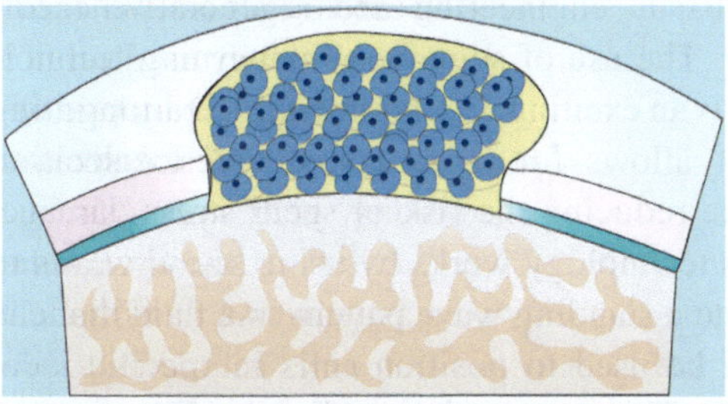

- **Matrix-induced Autologous Chondrocyte Implantation (MACI)**
  - Similar to ACI, MACI requires two surgical procedures but has a lower rate of hypertrophy of the graft
  - Expensive

16.2.3 3D-Bioprinting for OCD Repair

3D-bioprinting is a type of additive manufacturing method that can incorporate cells, growth factors, and biomolecules into biocompatible materials like "bio-ink" to create complex biological structures layer by layer. These structures are designed to closely mimic the intricate hierarchical architectures and compositions of their natural counterparts. The development of 3D-bioprinting technologies therefore has greatly expanded and been extensively investigated in the field of tissue engineering and regenerative biomaterials over the past few decades. This advancement has facilitated the rapid advancement of creating osteochondral scaffolds that replicate the multi-material composition and native architecture of natural tissue more accurately than traditional manufacturing techniques [57].

A typical bioprinting process, as discussed in the next section, involves a standard series of steps, although there are various types available. Firstly, 3D medical imaging (such as CT or MRI) is used to provide exact dimensions of the tissue. Secondly, a software is used to generate a 3D solid model which is arranged into thin cross-sections in stereolithography (STL) file format for printing. Thirdly, bio-ink is used which usually combines tissue-specific living cells or progenitor stem cells with a cytocompatible base that is usually of gelatin, collagen, silk, hyaluronan, nanocellulose alginate, or their composites to provide nutrients and scaffolding for cell growth. Fourthly, the printing machine deposits the bio-inks in a layer-by-layer manner with a thickness of around 0.5 mm per layer, with the bio-ink as a highly viscous fluid coming out of the nozzle. Finally, the layer solidifies to maintain its structure and shape until more layers are deposited continuously [58, 59]. The tuning of the nozzle structure and speed is therefore very important. Very liquid or solid injections should be avoided by optimization of the nozzle. The process of blending and solidification, also known as cross-linking, can be facilitated through UV light, heat, or specific chemicals. While using heat or chemicals, attention to prevent tissue damage should be prioritized. Advanced 3D-bioprinting technologies, with a precise and rigid printing program, allow the fabrication of osteochondral scaffolds with complex multi-material architectures. This approach is superior to conventional fabrication methods, which are often process-dependent and lack the required accuracy to create biomimetic osteochondral scaffolds with complex architecture and composition [60]. Inkjet-based 3D-bioprinting systems deposit droplets of bio-ink through a nozzle, similar to an inkjet printer, to build up the 3D structure layer by layer. Extrusion-based systems push the bio-ink through a nozzle or syringe and the extruded material is then deposited onto a platform or previous layer. Vat-photopolymerization systems uses light to solidify the bio-ink, which is suspended in a liquid and selectively exposed to light to create the desired shape [61]. Each 3D-bioprinting system has its advantages and limitations. Selection of a specific system depends on the specific needs of the patient and application. Inkjet-based systems in example may be better suited for printing small, detailed structures, while extrusion-based systems may be better for printing larger structures. Vat-photopolymerization systems may be better suited for printing with high resolution and accuracy but the use of light to solidify the bio-ink may limit the types of materials that can be used [62]. As a general requirement, the nozzle and the parts that print the tissue should be disposable and replaced at every single use.

The ultimate goal is to create a scaffold that can support the growth and function of the desired tissue or organ regardless of the specific 3D-bioprinting system used. The focus of this chapter is the joint articular cartilage. The development of new 3D-bioprinting technologies and materials continues to expand the possibilities for tissue engineering and regenerative medicine. The use of soundwave patterning technology is an exciting development in 3D-bioprinting as it allows for more gentle cell localization while reducing the risk of shear stress damage. This technology works by using sound waves to create a standing wave pattern in a fluid that can then be used to position cells in specific locations. This approach is effective for creating complex structures with multiple cell types and it has the potential to improve the accuracy and reliability of 3D-bioprinting for tissue engineering applications [63]. A recent study [64] described the manufacturing process and mechanical characteristics of a dual gradient scaffold for OCD repair and regeneration. These scaffolds are prepared of a blend of polycaprolactone (PCL) and hydroxyapatite and are designed to mimic the natural structure of the osteochondral interface. The use of a multi-material extrusion-based 3D-bioprinting system allowed for precise control over the composition and architecture of the scaffolds, which is important for creating biomimetic structures that can effectively support tissue growth and regeneration. The mechanical properties of the scaffolds were also carefully characterized to ensure that they could withstand the stresses and strains of the osteochondral environment. This approach represents an important step forward in the development of 3D-bio-printed scaffolds for tissue engineering applications.

Extrusion-based 3D-bioprinting technique is used to create a tri-layered osteochondral construct composed of GelMA/nHA hydrogels in some studies [65–67]. The construct displayed a suitable degradation rate, swelling ratio, mechanical properties, and a good biocompatibility. In vivo results showed improved integration with host tissues, a smoother joint surface and an increased expression of cartilage-specific extracellular matrix proteins and collagen type II. A recent study introduced a novel bio-fabrication method that involves guiding the growth of cellular spheroids within arrays of inkjet-based 3D-bio printed polymeric microchambers, enabling the engineering of structurally organized tissues [68]. Using a multi-tool bio-fabrication approach, they were able to create anatomically precise, human-sized osteochondral templates by incorporating a microchamber system onto a hypertrophic cartilage region designed to support endochondral bone formation. The entire construct was then cultured in a bioreactor for long-term culture, offering a scalable and versatile method for engineering structured articular cartilage tissues for joint resurfacing applications. It is important to note that despite significant scientific progress in 3D-bioprinting, no regulatory bodies have yet approved the clinical use of 3D-bioprinted products. This research field is still relatively new and we believe that 3D-bioprinting technologies will eventually have a significant role in the clinical repair and regeneration of OCD [69].

16.3 3D Articular Cartilage Printing Technologies (Fig. 16.4)

Three-dimensional bioprinting typically comprises three components: cells, growth factors, and printed scaffolds in cartilage tissue engineering. These scaffolds, composed of diverse bio-inks, play a crucial role in this technology. Creating scaffolds that accurately mimic articular cartilage necessitates advanced design and manufacturing techniques to develop anisotropic in vitro structures. These scaffolds should be capable of replicating the hierarchical biochemical, biophysical, and geometric properties observed in the native cartilaginous tissue, which vary in the depth-dependent arrangement [70, 71]. The hydrogel-based bio-inks employed in 3D bioprinting create a temporary microenvironment resembling the extracellular matrix, enabling enclosed cells' survival, proliferation, and differentiation rates. Several studies [72–75] have demonstrated the ability to customize hydrogel properties through various manufacturing methods. Hydrogels can be tailored to achieve specific goals in articular cartilage regeneration by adjusting factors such as cross-linking, polymerization, and printing. An ideal bio-ink should possess certain characteristics to ensure successful 3D printing and scaffold functionality. It should exhibit shear thinning properties, allowing for a decrease in viscosity during printing while enabling extrusion. Simultaneously, it should have the ability to cross-link immediately after printing to maintain its shape and provide mechanical stability to the printed construct [76]. The 3D printed scaffold furthermore should have sufficient porosity to facilitate cell attachment,

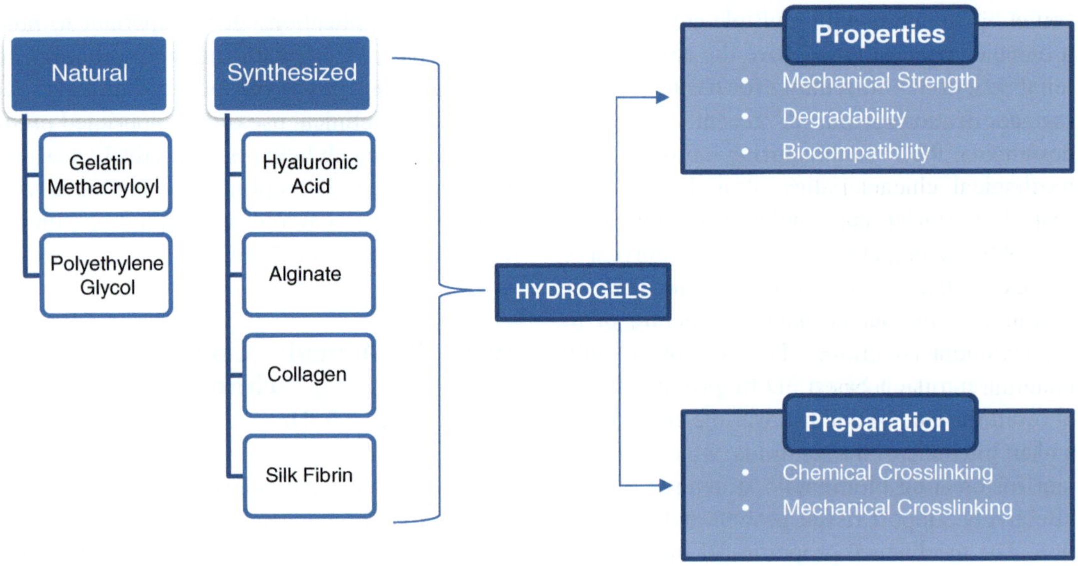

Fig. 16.4 Sources of Bio-inks

proliferation, and differentiation. It should allow for solute and nutrient diffusion as well as the deposition of extracellular matrix. The polymer concentration or cross-link density of the bio-ink can influence scaffold porosity [77, 78]. The bio-ink and the resulting scaffold moreover should be biodegradable at a rate that matches the regenerating tissue to allow for the gradual replacement of the scaffold with native cell-deposited ECM. Both the bio-ink and its degradation products must be non-toxic and non-immunogenic to ensure biocompatibility [79]. The construct furthermore should also be resistant to frictional forces. Hydrogels exhibit outstanding biocompatibility, thereby serving as a favorable transient environment for the sustained growth and specialized development of the encapsulated cells. Various materials are employed for 3D bioprinting for cartilage repair. These include natural substances like hyaluronic acid (HA), alginate, collagen (COL), and silk fibroin (SF), as well as synthetic polymers like gelatin methacryloyl (GelMA) and polyethylene glycol (PEG) [80–86]. Creating scaffolds that accurately mimic articular cartilage necessitates advanced design and manufacturing techniques to develop anisotropic in vitro structures. These scaffolds should be capable of replicating the hierarchical biochemical, biophysical, and geometric properties observed in the native cartilaginous tissue, which vary in a depth-dependent arrangement.

Three crucial criteria must be considered when selecting a suitable bio-ink. Firstly, the bio-ink should exhibit a mechanical strength comparable to that of native cartilage. Secondly, it must possess excellent biocompatibility to avoid cytotoxicity. Lastly, the bio-ink should degrade at a rate aligned with the speed of cartilage regeneration, as the scaffolds serve as temporary extracellular matrix. Natural resource-based inks generally offer good biocompatibility but often lack mechanical strength, whereas bio-inks comprising synthetic polymers tend to have the opposite characteristics. The printed structures should provide adequate mechanical and structural support by employing the appropriate bio-inks, as well as a sufficient nutrition supply. A combination of native progenitor cells, stem cells, and cartilage scaffolds are widely utilized to enhance cartilage repair and address defects to generate functional and high-quality neocartilage. Preserving the viability of living cells, maintaining the sensitivity of growth factors, and preserving the activity of bioactive substances pose significant challenges to in situ 3D bioprinting technology [87–89]. Lubricin, also known as

PRG4, is a lubricating glycoprotein naturally present in synovial fluid and cartilage. Its primary function is to reduce friction between the surfaces of cartilage during joint movement. The presence of PRG4 in the outer layers of the scaffold is a significant indication of the scaffold's ability to imitate the lubrication properties of natural cartilage in the context of 3D bioprinting. The expression of PRG4 varies in a gradient pattern across the four layers of the scaffold. This suggests that the bio-printed construct has the potential to offer lubrication across a wide range of joint movements and loading conditions [90].

The concept of lateral integration holds immense significance in the realm of osteochondral engineering. It refers to the ability of newly formed cartilage tissue to seamlessly bond and merge with neighboring native cartilage. This integration plays a pivotal role in ensuring the success of osteochondral regeneration, as it provides stability, load distribution, and the necessary mechano-transduction for optimal function [91]. Achieving lateral integration, however, poses numerous challenges that demand attention. Articular cartilage, with its low metabolic activity and dense extracellular matrix, exhibits anti-adhesive properties that blocks the adhesion of cells. Proteins encoded by the proteoglycan 4 gene, responsible for reducing friction in cartilage, along with glycosaminoglycans may directly inhibit cell adhesion. The surgical preparation of defects further complicates integration, as it leads to cell death at the defect margins, creating barriers to effective bonding. Biomechanical properties of the implanted scaffolds moreover often differ from those of native articular cartilage, resulting in stress concentration and impaired integration. This mismatch between the scaffold and the surrounding tissue can cause damage and inhibit or delay the integration process [92, 93]. A demarcation line between the normal and implanted and/or printed tissue can be seen in most of the scaffold applications. Researchers have explored various strategies to enhance lateral integration in light of these challenges. These include the use of anti-apoptotic agents to prevent cell death at the defect edge, matrix-degrading enzymes to counteract the anti-adhesive properties of the ECM, and functionalization of scaffolds to enable direct bonding to adjacent cartilage. These approaches, however, have primarily been studied in controlled laboratory settings or small animal models, lacking validation in larger animals or the context of tissue-engineering approaches [94, 95]. There is a pressing need to develop rehabilitation protocols and effective strategies that promote and enhance lateral integration consequently. Overcoming the obstacles to lateral integration is vital for achieving stable biologic fixation, ensuring proper load distribution and enabling the necessary mechano-transduction for successful osteochondral regeneration. In a study [96], researchers proposed a solution to address the problem of lateral integration in osteochondral repair. They developed a bilayer scaffold combined with a TGF-β3-loaded methacrylated silk fibroin sealant (Sil-MA) hydrogel. Researchers used rabbits as animal models to evaluate the repair capacity of their approaches. They created an osteochondral defect in the knee joint, ensuring that the defect extended to the subchondral bone. When the bilayer scaffold was implanted initially, blood oozed from the defect, indicating that the scaffold did not fit tightly into the defect. This lack of tight fit posed a challenge to achieving effective integration. They injected the Sil-MA hydrogel into the gap between the scaffold and the surrounding tissue and then applied UV irradiation to facilitate photocuring to overcome this issue. Bleeding from the defect ceased as a result, indicating the successful sealing of the cartilage layer of the scaffold and the surrounding tissue by the Sil-MA hydrogel. Adhesive properties of the Sil-MA hydrogel were attributed to a combination of factors. First, mechanical interlocking occurred as the Sil-MA solution penetrated the irregular surface of the tissue and the surface of the tissue surface of the scaffold. The covalent bonding of radicals generated during the photopolymerization process additionally contributed to the adhesive strength. Hydrophobic/hydrophilic and electrostatic interactions between the tissue surface and the Sil-MA solution were furthermore believed to enhance adhesion. The precise mechanism of adhesion of Sil-MA, however, has not been fully elucidated and requires further investigation. In the future, innovative techniques such as the approach demonstrated by these researchers, hold the potential to overcome the challenges associated with lateral integration in osteochondral repair (Table 16.4).

Careful consideration must be given to the cell density when formulating a cell-loaded bio-ink injectable as multiple studies have demonstrated its notable impact on both the bio-ink itself and the resulting printout. The density of primary chondrocytes in example has been observed to affect the gelation rate and storage modulus of collagen bio-inks during extrusion printing, with higher cell densities resulting in decreased rates and elastic modulus. The cells in example, mesenchymal stem cells, including adipose-derived stem cells, and bone marrow-derived mesenchymal stem cells (BMSCs), are multipotent stem cells capable of rapid proliferation and promising for cartilage regeneration. They are mixed with hydrogel materials to create a bio-ink that can be loaded into a 3D bioprinter and printed into a desired structure. The cells can then grow and

Table 16.4 Sources of Hydrogels [97–122]

- **Hyaluronic Acid:**
  - Is a polymeric glycosaminoglycan (GAG) that comprises duplicated ß-1,4-d-glucuronic acid-ß-1,3-N-acetyl-D-glucosamine residues.
  - Significantly facilitates chondrogenesis
  - Gelation methods include chemical agents, photocross-linking, electropolymerization
  - Has moderate biocompatibility
  - Has bioactive properties but poor mechanical strength which can be improved by cross-linking
  - Implants made of fragmented or low-molecular-weight HA do not interact effectively with cells and surrounding tissue, leading to inflammation and scaffold degradation. To overcome this, chemical-modified HA derivatives have been developed.
- **Alginate:**
  - Derives from the cell wall of brown seaweed
  - Gelation method includes cation adding
  - Has high biocompatibility
  - Has rapid degradation rates
  - Has shear-thinning capability and flexibility but poor stability
  - The oxidation of alginate has been found to enhance the in vivo biodegradability of alginate-based inks by generating additional reactive sites
- **Collagen:**
  - Gelation methods include chemical agents and physical methods(heating, drying, etc.)
  - Has high biocompatibility
  - Good biocompatibility, inferior viscosity and mechanical properties, cross-linking with chemicals may involve toxic agents, such as glutaraldehyde and 1-ethyl-3-(3-(dimethylamino)propyl) carbodiimide.
  - By incorporating other materials or modifying its fibrillogenesis, such as through enzymatic processes, the properties of collagen (COL) can be adjusted or fine-tuned
- **Silk fibroin:**
  - Produced by Bombyx mori silkworms, is composed of 43% glycine, 30% alanine, and 12% serine
  - Gelation methods include chemical agents and cryogelation
  - Has moderate biocompatibility
  - Lower immune response, modifiable degradation and elasticity, cross-linking with chemicals may involve toxic agents
  - B. Mori silk without sericin has low immune reactivity, compatible degradation rates, and high elasticity
  - Can be blended with gelatin and other biopolymers to create bioinks for scaffolds with customizable mechanical properties and controlled pore sizes
- **GelMA:**
  - A derivative of gelatin, primarily consists of methacrylamide groups with a smaller portion of methacrylate groups
  - Gelation method include photocross-linking
  - Has high biocompatibility
  - Fast gelation, low cytotoxicity but poor mechanical strength
  - Additionally, it demonstrates a notable swelling rate, leading to increased wound pressure and insufficient stability necessary for maintaining the required space for cartilage regeneration

differentiate within the printed structure to form functional tissue [91, 123, 124].

Bio-inks commonly incorporate additives that serve various purposes:

1. Additives that improve biocompatibility and repair efficacy.
2. Additives that enhance hydrogel cross-linking and mechanical properties.
3. Additives that refine printing resolutions.

Growth factors are also important additives of bio-inks, as they are essential for inducing cellular response, stimulating cell differentiation and tissue regeneration, enhancing chondrogenesis, and inhibiting chondrocyte hypertrophy [80, 87, 89].

The most widely applied growth factors for 3D bioprinting include [125–131]:

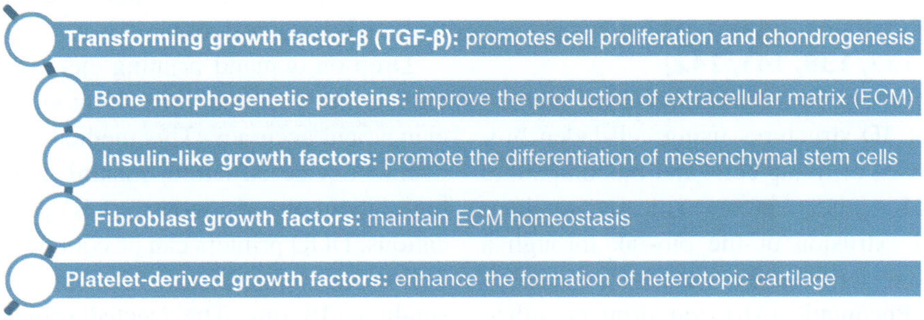

These growth factors are important additives in bio-inks for 3D bioprinting, as they can induce a cellular response, stimulate cell differentiation and tissue regeneration, and enhance chondrogenesis. Incorporation of nanomaterials such as graphene, nano clay, and ceramic nanoparticles furthermore is commonly used to enhance the strength and durability of hydrogel-based bio-inks. Additives are utilized additionally to improve the printing resolution of the resulting structures. Introduction of click reactions between thiols and alkene groups in the bio-ink polymers enables immediate solidification during 3D printing, facilitating the creation of intricate and high-quality constructs. Photo absorbers like tartrazine are moreover widely used as additives to enhance cross-linking and improve the resolution of photo-cross-linkable hydrogels [132–136].

Different 3D printing techniques are associated with different bio-inks. One of the commonly used methods is the extrusion-based bio-printing (EBP), which involves loading the bio-ink into plastic or stainless-steel cartridges and extruding it through a printing nozzle onto a platform. Extrusion-based bio-printing is suitable for 3D printing with cell-loaded bio-inks and produces printouts with moderate resolution. Mechanical extrusion printing allows for both bio-ink deposition and withdrawal, facilitating clean cuts, and the correction of printing errors, resulting in improved shape fidelity of the printouts. Bio-inks, however, used in EBP must have a sufficiently high viscosity to prevent shape collapse. Shear thinning characteristics are necessary to protect the cells from shear stress when exiting the nozzle for cell-encapsulated bio-inks. Gelation methods such as temperature/pH change and photo-cross-linking can be applied during deposition depending on the materials [137, 138]. Another widely employed technique is light-based 3D printing using digital light processing (DLP) technology. DLP generates the printout from a reservoir filled with liquid bio-ink, which attaches to the platform above in contrast to EBP. As the platform moves up, the height of the 3D structure increases. DLP offers superior vertical structure fidelity and high printing resolution compared to other 3D printing methods. This, however, typically requires bio-inks to be photo-cross-linkable and the viscosity of the bio-inks must be maintained within a specific range to ensure proper adhesion to the build plate or the layer above without detaching from the bottom of the build vat [139, 140]. In addition to the aforementioned techniques, drop-on-demand 3D printing has also found applications in cartilage tissue engineering.

16.3.1 Ex Vivo Bioprinting (Fig. 16.5)

Several 3D printing techniques can be used for bioprinting, including:

16.3.1.1 Extrusion-Based 3D Printing [137, 138, 141, 142]

Extrusion printing is a commonly used method for creating 3D structures using cell-laden bio-inks composed of living cells and biocompatible materials. This process involves the pneumatic or mechanical extrusion of the bio-ink through a nozzle onto a sterile surface or within a suspension bath. Pneumatic extrusion printers utilize pressurized air (5–800 kPa) to extrude bio-inks with relatively low viscosity (30–6 × 10^7 mPa s). On the other hand, mechanical-based printers are suitable for bio-inks with higher viscosity (>6 × 10^7 mPa s) and directly dispense the bio-ink from a material cartridge.

The extruded filaments, typically cylindrical with an average diameter of 150–350 μm, can be further cross-linked using light, heat, enzymes, or chemicals to form mechanically robust 3D structures. Despite the widespread use of extrusion-based printers in implant applications, they still face certain challenges. High pressure or mechanical force exerted by the nozzle can induce shear stress, leading to reduced cell viability. Bio-inks with special rheological properties, such as shear thinning behavior, have been incorporated into the 3D printing process to prevent cell damage to address this issue. Additionally, compared to other 3D printing methods, extrusion printing has lower resolution capabilities, typically ranging from 200 to 1000 μm.

16.3.1.2 Inkjet-Based 3D Printing [99, 143–146]

Inkjet printing has gained significant attention as a precise 3D fabrication method, offering efficient and high-resolution deposition of polymers, biomolecules, electronic components, and living cells. Two main types of inkjet printing methods can be distinguished based on the formation of ink droplets: continuous inkjet (CIJ) printing and drop-on-demand (DOD) inkjet printing. Continuous inkjet printing involves the continuous flow of liquid ink from the nozzle, forming individual droplets due to the Rayleigh-Plateau instability of the liquid. CIJ printing, however, has limitations due to device complexity, bio-ink waste, and potential material contamination, making it less preferred.

Drop-on-demand printing ejects ink droplets only when necessary, resulting in higher efficiency and accuracy. This method simplifies the overall device structure, making it suitable for both laboratory and industrial 3D printing applications. DOD printers can be equipped with multiple nozzle and the nozzle diameter can be as small as 18 μm. The ejected droplets have a diameter of less than 30 μm, enabling high-resolution printing for precise tissue construction. Currently, commercially available DOD printers utilize various actuation mechanisms, including thermal, piezoelectric, and electrostatic actuation, to deposit ink droplets through nozzles.

16.3.1.3 Laser-Based 3D Printing [124, 147–149]

Laser-assisted printing, also known as laser-induced forward transfer (LIFT), is an emerging 3D printing technique that is gaining attention in tissue engineering. The printer consists of three layers: an energy-absorbing layer, a ribbon layer containing the bio-ink, and a substrate layer. The laser pulse causes vaporization, generating a jet of liquid bio-ink that is deposited onto the collection substrate when a laser is applied to the energy-absorbing layer. There is no ejection process involved, allowing for a wide range of bio-ink viscosities (1–300 mPa s) and minimizing shear stress on the cell loaded bio-ink. Laser-assisted printing offers extremely high print resolution and can even print individual cells at a high speed (5 kHz). The heat generated by the laser, however, may result in lower cell viability and the cost of this method is relatively high due to

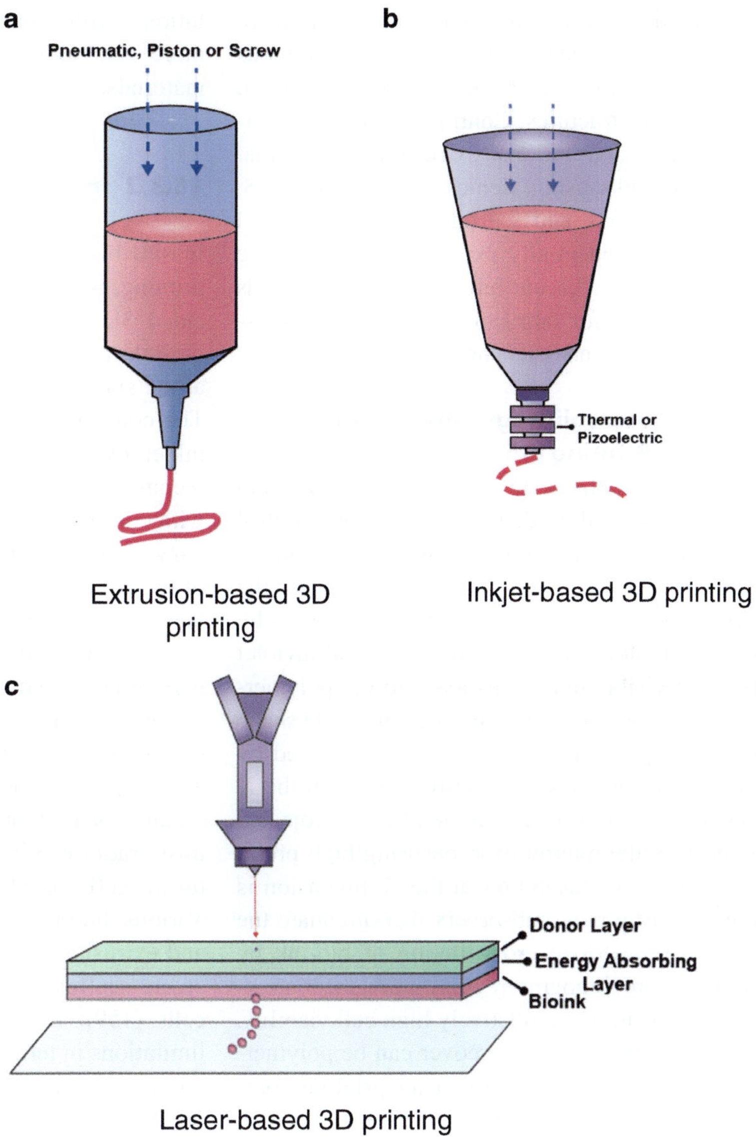

Fig. 16.5 Basic illustrations of the most common methods of 3D printing. (**a**) Extrusion-based 3D printing. (**b**) Inkjet-based 3D printing. (**c**) Laser-based 3D printing

the use of precision lasers, which limits its potential for widespread applications. Drop-on-demand 3D printing: uses a piezoelectric actuator to eject droplets of bio-ink on demand.

16.3.1.4 Digital Light Processing (DLP) 3D Printing [77, 90, 150–152]

Digital Light Processing 3D printing is a technique that offers significant advantages in fabricating complex stereoscopic objects. It allows for high printing speed (approximately 30 min, mm^3 s^−1) and high-resolution geometry (approximately 1 μm) without the need for a scaffold. DLP printing is based on the localized photopolymerization of liquid monomers/oligomers using UV light and photo-initiators. Another interesting 3D printing method is volumetric printing, which constructs entire 3D objects by irradiating a volume of photopolymer resins from multiple angles, rather than layer-by-layer polymerization. Recent advancements in volumetric printing enable the fabrication of cell-laden constructs of arbitrary size. The high cost and complexity of DLP systems, however, limit their applications in clinical translation. Additive manufacturing techniques such as continuous chaotic printing have been developed to create hierarchical structures. Continuous chaotic printing is an unconventional extrusion method that mixes bio-inks using Kenics static mixer [153, 154] printheads and extrudes defined internal lamellae, exponentially expanding the interface areas between adjacent bio-inks. These methods show promise for fabricating heterogeneous tissues like bone and osteochondral tissue.

16.3.1.5 Stereolithography-Based 3D Printing [155, 156]

Stereolithography is an emerging and appealing 3D printing method that enables precise control over the solidification of photosensitive resins to fabricate 3D structures. The process involves the generation of free radicals or reactive species by photo-initiators upon exposure to ultraviolet (UV) or visible light. This leads to the polymerization of the resin into a pre-designed 2D shape using a digital micromirror device, followed by layer-by-layer stacking. The resolution in the X and Y dimensions is determined by the projected light from the micromirror, ensuring high precision, while the resolution in the Z dimension is controlled by photo-absorbers that attenuate the light. The selective cross-linking of bio-ink by light in stereolithography minimizes shear stress on cells, resulting in relatively high cell viability. The entire resin layer moreover can be polymerized instantly, allowing for faster printing compared to other methods involving nozzles. There are, however, still challenges to overcome with stereolithography, such as the requirement for specific reactive groups in the resin, which limits its multi-material functionality. Resins additionally need to be transparent with minimal light scattering to ensure uniform light penetration. The cumulative UV exposure during cell-laden printing is also a concern that needs to be addressed.

Each technique has its advantages and disadvantages and the choice of technique depends on the specific application and requirements of the printed structure. For example, DLP has superior vertical structure fidelity and high printing resolution, while extrusion-based techniques are more versatile and can print a wider range of materials.

16.3.2 In Situ Bioprinting

In situ bioprinting, also known as in vivo bioprinting, is a promising alternative to computer-aided 3D printing. It involves directly printing bio-inks to create or repair living tissues or organs at the site of a defect in a clinical setting [125]. The concept was first introduced in 2007 using inkjet technology and aims to regenerate and reconstruct damaged tissues, especially those with complex geometries that are challenging for conventional 3D printing techniques [157]. One of the advantages of in situ bioprinting for cartilage regeneration is its ability to match the defect geometry without the need for specific preliminary image analysis. The bio-scaffold can be shaped within the defect, ensuring optimal contact between the bio-scaffold and the host tissue. This approach has shown great potential in the repair of skin, bone, and cartilage [158]. In contrast, traditional in vitro bioprinting involves culturing cells in 3D scaffolds outside the body. Various bioprinting techniques, such as inkjet and extrusion-based printing, have been used to create scaffolds with multiple biomaterials and cells [159]. In vitro bioprinting, however, has limitations in terms of its clinical applicability. It requires the development of functional tissue or organ in vitro, which is still a challenge. Handling and implanting fragile 3D constructs in the body pose difficulties, including disruption of the construct's structure, contamination risks and compatibility issues with native tissues. The created construct's shape may additionally differ from the actual defect size, leading to further adjustments during surgery [160].

In situ tissue engineering (TE) approaches have advantages over ex-vivo approaches because they eliminate the need for creating an artificial microenvironment for tissue development. In situ bioprinting involves using robotic arms or handheld devices to reconstruct damaged tissue within the body. The human body acts as an "in vivo bioreactor," facilitating the development and maturation of the printed construct. However, the immobilization of the recipient organ during the printing process is crucial [161]. Although in situ bioprinting is still in its early stages and primarily applied to superficial organs, its potential for clinical applications in skin, bone, and cartilage repair is promising. Cartilage regeneration is particularly challenging due to its avascular nature that prevents self-repair. Current treatments for chondral defects have limitations in reproducing normal hyaline cartilage and providing long-term solutions. Prefabricated constructs used in traditional TE approaches often result in a mismatch between the defect and the construct, requiring additional debridement steps. Early attempts to inject cells into damaged regions failed due to the lack of structural support and nutrients [162]. To overcome these limitations, researchers developed a handheld pneumatic extrusion device called the "Bio-Pen" for in vivo repair of osteochondral defects. The device allowed the printing of multiple inks in a collinear geometry. In vitro studies demonstrated high cell viability in post-printed hydrogels. Subsequent advancements in the Bio-pen design enabled single-session in vivo surgery in sheep's knee joints, where bio-scaffolds and cells were simultaneously extruded into the chondral defect. Co-axial printing, where different inks are extruded in a core-shell manner, protected the cells and resulted in the formation of hyaline-like cartilage [132, 163, 164]. Although in situ bioprinting is still in its early stages and has not been commercialized for clinical use, it shows great potential in complementing traditional TE approaches. In situ bioprinting offers a promising avenue for tissue and organ regeneration by addressing the limitations of in vitro bioprinting and providing a more suitable environment for tissue development (Table 16.5).

In conclusion, 3D bioprinting holds tremendous potential for advancing tissue engineering and regenerative medicine. The ongoing research and development efforts are focused on several future directions to further enhance the capabilities and applications of this technology. These

Table 16.5 Difference between in situ and ex vivo bioprinting

• **Location:** In situ bioprinting involves printing bio-inks directly at the site of a defect within the body, while ex vivo bioprinting refers to printing outside the body, typically in a laboratory or controlled environment
• **Clinical Setting:** In situ bioprinting is performed in a clinical setting, aiming to create or repair living tissues or organs, while ex vivo bioprinting is conducted in a laboratory or research setting for tissue engineering and regenerative medicine purposes
• **Complexity:** In situ bioprinting is suitable for complex geometries that are challenging for conventional 3D printing techniques, as it allows for matching the defect geometry without the need for specific preliminary image analysis. Ex vivo bioprinting involves culturing cells in 3D scaffolds and creating constructs outside the body
• **Preliminary Image Analysis:** In situ bioprinting does not require specific preliminary image analysis, as the bio-scaffold is shaped within the defect itself. In ex vivo bioprinting, preliminary image analysis may be required to determine the shape and size of the defect
• **Tissue Development:** In situ bioprinting utilizes the human body as an "in vivo bioreactor" for the development and maturation of the printed construct. Ex vivo bioprinting involves creating an artificial microenvironment for tissue development outside the body
• **Immobilization:** Immobilization of the recipient organ is crucial in in situ bioprinting to ensure the accuracy and stability of the printing process. Ex vivo bioprinting does not require organ immobilization
• **Clinical Applicability:** In situ bioprinting has the potential for clinical applications in skin, bone, and cartilage repair. Ex vivo bioprinting has limitations in terms of clinical applicability, as it involves handling and implanting fragile 3D constructs in the body
• **Structural Support:** In situ bioprinting provides structural support to the printed construct directly within the body. Ex vivo bioprinting requires the creation of scaffolds to provide structural support to the constructs outside the body
• **Nutrient Supply:** In situ bioprinting takes advantage of the natural nutrient supply within the body for tissue development. Ex vivo bioprinting requires the provision of nutrients to the constructs through culture media
• **Mismatch Between Defect and Construct:** In situ bioprinting minimizes the mismatch between the defect and the construct, as the bio-scaffold is shaped within the defect itself. Ex vivo bioprinting may require additional adjustments during surgery to ensure a proper fit between the defect and the construct

include the development of new bio-inks with improved properties, the advancement of multi-material printing for complex tissue construction, the exploration of in situ bioprinting for minimally invasive tissue repair, the integration of 3D bioprinting with other technologies to enhance its functionality, and the scaling up of production for mass manufacturing of tissue constructs. 3D bioprinting is poised to revolutionize healthcare by providing new possibilities for personalized medicine, organ transplantation, and drug discovery by addressing these challenges and exploring these opportunities.

References

1. Buckwalter JA. Articular cartilage: injuries and potential for healing. J Orthop Sports Phys Ther. 1998;28(4):192–202.
2. Koo S, Andriacchi TP. A comparison of the influence of global functional loads vs. local contact anatomy on articular cartilage thickness at the knee. J Biomech. 2007;40(13):2961–6.
3. Sophia Fox AJ, Bedi A, Rodeo SA. The basic science of articular cartilage: structure, composition, and function. Sports Health. 2009;1(6):461–8.
4. Kuettner KE, Aydelotte MB, Thonar EJ. Articular cartilage matrix and structure: a minireview. J Rheumatol Suppl. 1991;27:46–8.
5. Hunziker EB, Quinn TM, Hauselmann HJ. Quantitative structural organization of normal adult human articular cartilage. Osteoarthr Cartil. 2002;10(7):564–72.
6. Buckwalter JA, Mankin HJ. Articular cartilage: tissue design and chondrocyte-matrix interactions. Instr Course Lect. 1998;47:477–86.
7. Hwang HS, Kim HA. Chondrocyte apoptosis in the pathogenesis of osteoarthritis. Int J Mol Sci. 2015;16(11):26035–54.
8. Li W, et al. The Nrf2/HMGB1/NF-kappaB axis modulates chondrocyte apoptosis and extracellular matrix degradation in osteoarthritis. Acta Biochim Biophys Sin Shanghai. 2023;55(5):818–30.
9. Alford JW, Cole BJ. Cartilage restoration, part 1: basic science, historical perspective, patient evaluation, and treatment options. Am J Sports Med. 2005;33(2):295–306.
10. Mlynarik V, Trattnig S. Physicochemical properties of normal articular cartilage and its MR appearance. Investig Radiol. 2000;35(10):589–94.
11. Alcaide-Ruggiero L, et al. Main and minor types of collagens in the articular cartilage: the role of collagens in repair tissue evaluation in chondral defects. Int J Mol Sci. 2021;22(24)
12. Clark JM. The organisation of collagen fibrils in the superficial zones of articular cartilage. J Anat. 1990;171:117–30.
13. Hardingham TE, Fosang AJ. The structure of aggrecan and its turnover in cartilage. J Rheumatol Suppl. 1995;43:86–90.
14. O'Hara BP, Urban JP, Maroudas A. Influence of cyclic loading on the nutrition of articular cartilage. Ann Rheum Dis. 1990;49(7):536–9.
15. Petty RE, et al. Textbook of pediatric rheumatology. 8th ed. Philadelphia, PA, Ann Arbor, Michigan: Elsevier, Inc.; 2021. ProQuest Ebook Central
16. Roughley PJ. Articular cartilage and changes in arthritis: noncollagenous proteins and proteoglycans in the extracellular matrix of cartilage. Arthritis Res. 2001;3(6):342–7.
17. Muttigi MS, et al. Matrilin-3 role in cartilage development and osteoarthritis. Int J Mol Sci. 2016;17:4.
18. Posey KL, Coustry F, Hecht JT. Cartilage oligomeric matrix protein: COMPopathies and beyond. Matrix Biol. 2018;71-72:161–73.
19. Eggli PS, Hunziker EB, Schenk RK. Quantitation of structural features characterizing weight- and less-weight-bearing regions in articular cartilage: a stereological analysis of medial femoral condyles in young adult rabbits. Anat Rec. 1988;222(3):217–27.
20. Venn M, Maroudas A. Chemical composition and swelling of normal and osteoarthrotic femoral head cartilage. *I Chemical composition*. Ann Rheum Dis. 1977;36(2):121–9.
21. Eggli PS, et al. Matrix compartments in the growth plate of the proximal tibia of rats. Anat Rec. 1985;211(3):246–57.
22. Guilak F, Mow VC. The mechanical environment of the chondrocyte: a biphasic finite element model of cell-matrix interactions in articular cartilage. J Biomech. 2000;33(12):1663–73.
23. Poole CA, Flint MH, Beaumont BW. Chondrons in cartilage: ultrastructural analysis of the pericellular microenvironment in adult human articular cartilages. J Orthop Res. 1987;5(4):509–22.
24. Mow VC, Guo XE. Mechano-electrochemical properties of articular cartilage: their inhomogeneities and anisotropies. Annu Rev Biomed Eng. 2002;4:175–209.
25. Choi JB, et al. Zonal changes in the three-dimensional morphology of the chondron under compression: the relationship among cellular, pericellular, and extracellular deformation in articular cartilage. J Biomech. 2007;40(12):2596–603.
26. Edmonds EW, Shea KG. Osteochondritis dissecans: editorial comment. Clin Orthop Relat Res. 2013;471(4):1105–6.
27. Wall E, Von Stein D. Juvenile osteochondritis dissecans. Orthop Clin North Am. 2003;34(3):341–53.
28. Crawford DC, Safran MR. Osteochondritis dissecans of the knee. J Am Acad Orthop Surg. 2006;14(2):90–100.

29. Cahill BR. Osteochondritis Dissecans of the knee: treatment of juvenile and adult forms. J Am Acad Orthop Surg. 1995;3(4):237–47.
30. Weiss JM, et al. Incidence of osteochondritis Dissecans in adults. Am J Sports Med. 2018;46(7):1592–5.
31. Linden B. The incidence of osteochondritis dissecans in the condyles of the femur. Acta Orthop Scand. 1976;47(6):664–7.
32. Kessler JI, et al. Osteochondritis dissecans of the ankle in children and adolescents: demographics and epidemiology. Am J Sports Med. 2014;42(9):2165–71.
33. Kessler JI, et al. Demographics and epidemiology of osteochondritis Dissecans of the elbow among children and adolescents. Orthop J Sports Med. 2018;6(12):2325967118815846.
34. Wall EJ, et al. Trochlear groove osteochondritis dissecans of the knee patellofemoral joint. J Pediatr Orthop. 2014;34(6):625–30.
35. Kida Y, et al. Prevalence and clinical characteristics of osteochondritis Dissecans of the humeral Capitellum among adolescent baseball players. Am J Sports Med. 2014;42(8):1963–71.
36. Pareek A, et al. Incidence of symptomatic osteochondritis dissecans lesions of the knee: a population-based study in Olmsted County. Osteoarthr Cartil. 2017;25(10):1663–71.
37. Nissen CW. Osteochondritis dissecans of the elbow. Clin Sports Med. 2014;33(2):251–65.
38. Andriolo L, et al. Osteochondritis Dissecans of the knee: etiology and pathogenetic mechanisms. *A Systematic Review*. Cartilage. 2020;11(3):273–90.
39. Hefti F, et al. Osteochondritis dissecans: a multicenter study of the European pediatric orthopedic society. J Pediatr Orthop B. 1999;8(4):231–45.
40. Aichroth P. Osteochondritis dissecans of the knee. A clinical survey. J Bone Joint Surg Br. 1971;53(3):440–7.
41. McElroy MJ, et al. Catcher's knee: posterior femoral condyle juvenile osteochondritis Dissecans in children and adolescents. J Pediatr Orthop. 2018;38(8):410–7.
42. Chow RM, Guzman MS, Dao Q. Intercondylar notch width as a risk factor for medial femoral condyle osteochondritis Dissecans in skeletally immature patients. J Pediatr Orthop. 2016;36(6):640–4.
43. Wechter JF, et al. Proximal tibial morphology and its correlation with osteochondritis dissecans of the knee. Knee Surg Sports Traumatol Arthrosc. 2015;23(12):3717–22.
44. Nambu T, et al. Deformation of the distal femur: a contribution towards the pathogenesis of osteochondrosis dissecans in the knee joint. J Biomech. 1991;24(6):421–33.
45. Cavaignac E, et al. Relationship between tibial spine size and the occurrence of osteochondritis dissecans: an argument in favour of the impingement theory. Knee Surg Sports Traumatol Arthrosc. 2017;25(8):2442–6.
46. Ishikawa M, et al. Unique anatomic feature of the posterior cruciate ligament in knees associated with osteochondritis Dissecans. Orthop J Sports Med. 2016;4(5):2325967116648138.
47. Pestka JM, et al. Clinical outcome of autologous chondrocyte implantation for failed microfracture treatment of full-thickness cartilage defects of the knee joint. Am J Sports Med. 2012;40(2):325–31.
48. Bai L, et al. Clinical outcomes of osteochondral lesions of the talus with large subchondral cysts treated with osteotomy and autologous chondral grafts: minimum 2-year follow-up and second-look evaluation. Orthop J Sports Med. 2020;8(7):2325967120937798.
49. Goncalves AM, et al. Osteochondral tissue engineering: the potential of electrospinning and additive manufacturing. Pharmaceutics. 2021;13:7.
50. Steadman JR, et al. The microfracture technic in the management of complete cartilage defects in the knee joint. Orthopade. 1999;28(1):26–32.
51. Angermann P, Riegels-Nielsen P, Pedersen H. Osteochondritis dissecans of the femoral condyle treated with periosteal transplantation. Poor outcome in 14 patients followed for 6-9 years. Acta Orthop Scand. 1998;69(6):595–7.
52. Panics G, et al. Osteochondral autograft and mosaicplasty in the football (soccer) athlete. Cartilage. 2012;3(1 Suppl):25S–30S.
53. Harris JD, et al. Autologous chondrocyte implantation: a systematic review. J Bone Joint Surg Am. 2010;92(12):2220–33.
54. Basad E, et al. Matrix-induced autologous chondrocyte implantation (MACI) in the knee: clinical outcomes and challenges. Knee Surg Sports Traumatol Arthrosc. 2015;23(12):3729–35.
55. Matthews JR, et al. A systematic review of cartilage procedures for unstable osteochondritis dissecans. Phys Sportsmed. 2022:1–9.
56. Lach MS, et al. The induced pluripotent stem cells in articular cartilage regeneration and disease modelling: are we ready for their clinical use? Cells. 2022;11(3)
57. Wei W, et al. A one-Stone-two-birds strategy for osteochondral regeneration based on a 3D printable biomimetic scaffold with Kartogenin biochemical stimuli gradient. Adv Healthc Mater. 2023;12:e2300108.
58. Mandrycky C, et al. 3D bioprinting for engineering complex tissues. Biotechnol Adv. 2016;34(4):422–34.
59. Abdollahiyan P, et al. Hydrogel-based 3D bioprinting for bone and cartilage tissue engineering. Biotechnol J. 2020;15(12):e2000095.
60. Li M, et al. Application and development of 3D bioprinting in cartilage tissue engineering. Biomater Sci. 2022;10(19):5430–58.
61. Dufour A, et al. Integrating melt electrowriting and inkjet bioprinting for engineering structurally organized articular cartilage. Biomaterials. 2022;283:121405.

62. Jia L, et al. Bioprinting and regeneration of auricular cartilage using a bioactive bioink based on microporous photocrosslinkable acellular cartilage matrix. Bioact Mater. 2022;16:66–81.
63. Maharajan N, Cho GW, Jang CH. Application of mesenchymal stem cell for tympanic membrane regeneration by tissue engineering approach. Int J Pediatr Otorhinolaryngol. 2020;133:109969.
64. Bittner SM, et al. Fabrication and mechanical characterization of 3D printed vertical uniform and gradient scaffolds for bone and osteochondral tissue engineering. Acta Biomater. 2019;90:37–48.
65. Chakraborty J, et al. Development of a biomimetic arch-like 3D bioprinted construct for cartilage regeneration using gelatin methacryloyl and silk fibroin-gelatin bioinks. Biofabrication. 2023;15(3):035009.
66. Dutta SD, et al. Electrically stimulated 3D bioprinting of gelatin-polypyrrole hydrogel with dynamic semi-IPN network induces osteogenesis via collective signaling and immunopolarization. Biomaterials. 2023;294:121999.
67. Osi AR, et al. Three-dimensional-printable Thermo/photo-cross-linked Methacrylated chitosan-gelatin hydrogel composites for tissue engineering. ACS Appl Mater Interfaces. 2021;13(19):22902–13.
68. Kurian AG, et al. Multifunctional GelMA platforms with nanomaterials for advanced tissue therapeutics. Bioact Mater. 2022;8:267–95.
69. Daly AC, Kelly DJ. Biofabrication of spatially organised tissues by directing the growth of cellular spheroids within 3D printed polymeric microchambers. Biomaterials. 2019;197:194–206.
70. Kim SH, et al. 3D bioprinted silk fibroin hydrogels for tissue engineering. Nat Protoc. 2021;16(12):5484–532.
71. Rajput M, et al. Light-based 3D bioprinting of bone tissue scaffolds with tunable mechanical properties and architecture from photocurable silk fibroin. Int J Biol Macromol. 2022;202:644–56.
72. Cao H, et al. Current hydrogel advances in physicochemical and biological response-driven biomedical application diversity. Signal Transduct Target Ther. 2021;6(1):426.
73. Zhang C, et al. Cartilage 3D bioprinting for rhinoplasty using adipose-derived stem cells as seed cells: review and recent advances. Cell Prolif. 2023;56(4):e13417.
74. Tian A, Xue J, Sun N. Advantages of self-assembled Nano peptide hydrogels in biological tissue engineering. Curr Protein Pept Sci. 2022;23(6):395–401.
75. Chen C, Xi Y, Weng Y. Recent advances in cellulose-based hydrogels for tissue engineering applications. Polymers (Basel). 2022;14(16)
76. Kim SH, et al. 4D-bioprinted silk hydrogels for tissue engineering. Biomaterials. 2020;260:120281.
77. Sultan MT, et al. Three-dimensional digital light-processing bioprinting using silk fibroin-based bio-ink: recent advancements in biomedical applications. Biomedicine. 2022;10(12)
78. Jiang G, et al. A 3D-printed PRP-GelMA hydrogel promotes osteochondral regeneration through M2 macrophage polarization in a rabbit model. Acta Biomater. 2021;128:150–62.
79. Flegeau K, Puiggali-Jou A, Zenobi-Wong M. Cartilage tissue engineering by extrusion bioprinting utilizing porous hyaluronic acid microgel bioinks. Biofabrication. 2022;14(3):034105.
80. Wang T, et al. Intraarticularly injectable silk hydrogel microspheres with enhanced mechanical and structural stability to attenuate osteoarthritis. Biomaterials. 2022;286:121611.
81. Mohammadpour Z, Kharaziha M, Zarrabi A. 3D-printing of silk Nanofibrils reinforced alginate for soft tissue engineering. Pharmaceutics. 2023;15(3)
82. Shi W, et al. Dynamic hyaluronic acid hydrogel with covalent linked gelatin as an anti-oxidative bioink for cartilage tissue engineering. Biofabrication. 2021;14(1)
83. Carvalho T, et al. Injectable nanocomposite hydrogels of gelatin-hyaluronic acid reinforced with hybrid lysozyme nanofibrils-gold nanoparticles for the regeneration of damaged myocardium. ACS Appl Mater Interfaces. 2023;15(21):25860–72.
84. Sekar MP, et al. Hyaluronic acid as bioink and hydrogel scaffolds for tissue engineering applications. ACS Biomater Sci Eng. 2023;9(6):3134–59.
85. Murab S, et al. Alginate based hydrogel inks for 3D bioprinting of engineered orthopedic tissues. Carbohydr Polym. 2022;296:119964.
86. Elkhoury K, et al. Gelatin Methacryloyl (GelMA) nanocomposite hydrogels embedding bioactive naringin liposomes. Polymers (Basel). 2020;12(12)
87. Badhe RV, et al. Current advancements in bio-ink technology for cartilage and bone tissue engineering. Bone. 2023;171:116746.
88. Fani N, et al. Fabricating the cartilage: recent achievements. Cytotechnology. 2023;75(4):269–92.
89. Hu G, et al. Construction of 3D-bioprinted cartilage-mimicking substitute based on photo-crosslinkable Wharton's jelly bioinks for full-thickness articular cartilage defect repair. Mater Today Bio. 2023;21:100695.
90. Sun Y, et al. 3D bioprinting dual-factor releasing and gradient-structured constructs ready to implant for anisotropic cartilage regeneration. Sci Adv. 2020;6(37)
91. Pei Z, et al. Experimental study on repair of cartilage defects in the rabbits with GelMA-MSCs scaffold prepared by three-dimensional bioprinting. Int J Bioprint. 2023;9(2):662.

92. Khan IM, et al. Cartilage integration: evaluation of the reasons for failure of integration during cartilage repair. *A review*. Eur Cell Mater. 2008;16:26–39.
93. Trengove A, Di Bella C, O'Connor AJ. The challenge of cartilage integration: understanding a major barrier to chondral repair. Tissue Eng Part B Rev. 2022;28(1):114–28.
94. Allon AA, et al. Augmenting the articular cartilage-implant interface: functionalizing with a collagen adhesion protein. J Biomed Mater Res A. 2012;100(8):2168–75.
95. Horbert V, et al. In vitro analysis of cartilage regeneration using a collagen type I hydrogel (CaReS) in the bovine cartilage punch model. Cartilage. 2019;10(3):346–63.
96. Wu X, et al. Marginal sealing around integral bilayer scaffolds for repairing osteochondral defects based on photocurable silk hydrogels. Bioact Mater. 2021;6(11):3976–86.
97. Moro A, et al. Hyaluronic acid based next generation bioink for 3D bioprinting of human stem cell derived corneal stromal model with innervation. Biofabrication. 2022;15(1):015020.
98. Pereira I, et al. Hyaluronic acid-based bioink improves the differentiation and network formation of neural progenitor cells. Front Bioeng Biotechnol. 2023;11:1110547.
99. Prabhakaran P, et al. Prospect and retrospect of 3D bio-printing. Acta Histochem. 2022;124(7):151932.
100. Tsanaktsidou E, Kammona O, Kiparissides C. Recent developments in hyaluronic acid-based hydrogels for cartilage tissue engineering applications. Polymers (Basel). 2022;14(4)
101. Bhattacharyya A, et al. 3D bioprinting of complex tissue scaffolds with in situ homogeneously mixed alginate-chitosan-kaolin bioink using advanced portable biopen. Carbohydr Polym. 2023;317:121046.
102. Hafezi M, et al. Self-healing interpenetrating network hydrogel based on GelMA/alginate/nano-clay. Int J Biol Macromol. 2023;242(Pt 2):124962.
103. Kim J, et al. 142Development of an alginate-gelatin bioink enhancing osteogenic differentiation by gelatin release. Int J Bioprint. 2023;9(2):660.
104. Senturk E, et al. 3D bioprinting of tyramine modified hydrogels under visible light for osteochondral interface. Biofabrication. 2023;15(3):034102.
105. Shehzad A, et al. Dual-crosslinking of gelatin-based hydrogels: promising compositions for a 3D printed organotypic bone model. Bioengineering (Basel). 2023;10(6)
106. Guo K, et al. Bioprinting of light-crosslinkable neutral-dissolved collagen to build implantable connective tissue with programmable cellular orientation. Biofabrication. 2023;15(3):035007.
107. Karanth D, et al. Towards resorbable 3D-printed scaffolds for craniofacial bone regeneration. Orthod Craniofac Res. 2023;26:188.
108. Liang L, et al. Extrusion bioprinting of cellular aggregates improves mesenchymal stem cell proliferation and differentiation. Biomater Adv. 2023;149:213369.
109. Ravi S, et al. 3D bioprintable hypoxia-mimicking PEG-based Nano bioink for cartilage tissue engineering. ACS Appl Mater Interfaces. 2023;15(16):19921–36.
110. Bandyopadhyay A, Mandal BB. A three-dimensional printed silk-based biomimetic tri-layered meniscus for potential patient-specific implantation. Biofabrication. 2019;12(1):015003.
111. Beketov EE, et al. Bioprinting of cartilage with bioink based on high-concentration collagen and chondrocytes. Int J Mol Sci. 2021;22(21)
112. Betsch M, et al. Incorporating 4D into bioprinting: real-time magnetically directed collagen fiber alignment for generating complex multilayered tissues. Adv Healthc Mater. 2018;7(21):e1800894.
113. Kim SW, et al. Three-dimensional bioprinting of cell-laden constructs using polysaccharide-based self-healing hydrogels. Biomacromolecules. 2019;20(5):1860–6.
114. Naranda J, et al. Recent advancements in 3D printing of polysaccharide hydrogels in cartilage tissue engineering. Materials (Basel). 2021;14(14)
115. Singh YP, Bandyopadhyay A, Mandal BB. 3D bioprinting using cross-linker-free silk-gelatin bioink for cartilage tissue engineering. ACS Appl Mater Interfaces. 2019;11(37):33684–96.
116. Yang X, et al. Collagen-alginate as bioink for three-dimensional (3D) cell printing based cartilage tissue engineering. Mater Sci Eng C Mater Biol Appl. 2018;83:195–201.
117. Chakraborty J, et al. Recent advances in bioprinting using silk protein-based bioinks. Biomaterials. 2022;287:121672.
118. Deng C, et al. 3D bio-printed biphasic scaffolds with dual modification of silk fibroin for the integrated repair of osteochondral defects. Biomater Sci. 2021;9(14):4891–903.
119. Zhang X, et al. Crosslinker-free silk/decellularized extracellular matrix porous bioink for 3D bioprinting-based cartilage tissue engineering. Mater Sci Eng C Mater Biol Appl. 2021;118:111388.
120. Daly AC, et al. A comparison of different bioinks for 3D bioprinting of fibrocartilage and hyaline cartilage. Biofabrication. 2016;8(4):045002.
121. Lim KS, et al. Bio-resin for high resolution lithography-based biofabrication of complex cell-laden constructs. Biofabrication. 2018;10(3):034101.

122. Yang Z, et al. Microenvironmentally optimized 3D-printed TGFbeta-functionalized scaffolds facilitate endogenous cartilage regeneration in sheep. Acta Biomater. 2022;150:181–98.
123. Stone RN, Reeck JC, Oxford JT. Advances in cartilage tissue engineering using bioinks with decellularized cartilage and three-dimensional printing. Int J Mol Sci. 2023;24(6)
124. Volova LT, et al. 3D bioprinting of hyaline articular cartilage: biopolymers, hydrogels, and bioinks. Polymers (Basel). 2023;15(12)
125. Ozbolat IT. Bioprinting scale-up tissue and organ constructs for transplantation. Trends Biotechnol. 2015;33(7):395–400.
126. Cao B, et al. 3D-printed vascularized biofunctional scaffold for bone regeneration. Int J Bioprint. 2023;9(3):702.
127. Congress Z, Brovold M, Soker S. Cell viability assays for 3D cellular constructs. Methods Mol Biol. 2023;2644:387–402.
128. de Barros NR, et al. Gelatin methacryloyl and laponite bioink for 3D bioprinted organotypic tumor modeling. Biofabrication. 2023;15:045005.
129. Fadilah NIM, et al. Functionalised-biomatrix for wound healing and cutaneous regeneration: future impactful medical products in clinical translation and precision medicine. Front Bioeng Biotechnol. 2023;11:1160577.
130. Fan M, et al. 3D bioprinted hydrogel/polymer scaffold with factor delivery and mechanical support for growth plate injury repair. Front Bioeng Biotechnol. 2023;11:1210786.
131. Liu C, Tong YW. Interfacial polyelectrolyte complexation-inspired bioprinting of vascular constructs. ACS Appl Mater Interfaces. 2023;15(17):20712–25.
132. Duchi S, et al. Handheld co-axial bioprinting: application to in situ surgical cartilage repair. Sci Rep. 2017;7(1):5837.
133. Farsheed AC, et al. 3D printing of self-assembling nanofibrous multidomain peptide hydrogels. Adv Mater. 2023;35(11):e2210378.
134. Raja IS, et al. State-of-the-art techniques for promoting tissue regeneration: combination of three-dimensional bioprinting and carbon nanomaterials. Int J Bioprint. 2023;9(1):635.
135. Yuan N, et al. Chitosan, alginate, hyaluronic acid and other novel multifunctional hydrogel dressings for wound healing: a review. Int J Biol Macromol. 2023;240:124321.
136. Zhang X, et al. 3D printed reduced graphene oxide-GelMA hybrid hydrogel scaffolds for potential neuralized bone regeneration. J Mater Chem B. 2023;11(6):1288–301.
137. Placone JK, Engler AJ. Recent advances in extrusion-based 3D printing for biomedical applications. Adv Healthc Mater. 2018;7(8):e1701161.
138. Hassan K, et al. Functional inks and extrusion-based 3D printing of 2D materials: a review of current research and applications. Nanoscale. 2020;12(37):19007–42.
139. Yu C, et al. Photopolymerizable biomaterials and light-based 3D printing strategies for biomedical applications. Chem Rev. 2020;120(19):10695–743.
140. Verisqa F, et al. Digital light processing 3D printing of Gyroid scaffold with isosorbide-based photopolymer for bone tissue engineering. Biomolecules. 2022;12(11)
141. Idaszek J, et al. 3D bioprinting of hydrogel constructs with cell and material gradients for the regeneration of full-thickness chondral defect using a microfluidic printing head. Biofabrication. 2019;11(4):044101.
142. Messaoudi O, et al. Stem cells and extrusion 3D printing for hyaline cartilage engineering. Cells. 2020;10(1)
143. Negro A, Cherbuin T, Lutolf MP. 3D inkjet printing of complex, cell-laden hydrogel structures. Sci Rep. 2018;8(1):17099.
144. Sakai S, et al. Drop-on-drop multimaterial 3D bioprinting realized by peroxidase-mediated cross-linking. Macromol Rapid Commun. 2018;39(3)
145. Xiao X, et al. Experimental study of the jetting behavior of high-viscosity Nanosilver inks in inkjet-based 3D printing. Nanomaterials (Basel). 2022;12(17)
146. Li X, et al. Inkjet bioprinting of biomaterials. Chem Rev. 2020;120(19):10793–833.
147. Dong H, et al. Robotic-assisted automated in situ bioprinting. Int J Bioprint. 2023;9(1):629.
148. Ma K, et al. Application of robotic-assisted in situ 3D printing in cartilage regeneration with HAMA hydrogel: an in vivo study. J Adv Res. 2020;23:123–32.
149. Ho CMB, et al. Femtosecond-laser-based 3D printing for tissue engineering and cell biology applications. ACS Biomater Sci Eng. 2017;3(10):2198–214.
150. Kim SH, et al. Correction to: silk fibroin bioinks for digital light processing (DLP) 3D bioprinting. Adv Exp Med Biol. 2020;1249:C1.
151. Kim SH, et al. Silk fibroin bioinks for digital light processing (DLP) 3D bioprinting. Adv Exp Med Biol. 2020;1249:53–66.
152. Lee YJ, et al. Biocompatible fluorescent silk fibroin bioink for digital light processing 3D printing. Int J Biol Macromol. 2022;213:317–27.
153. Bolivar-Monsalve EJ, et al. One-step bioprinting of multi-channel hydrogel filaments using chaotic advection: fabrication of pre-vascularized muscle-like tissues. Adv Healthc Mater. 2022;11(24):e2200448.
154. Jokic A, et al. Kenics static mixer combined with gas sparging for the improvement of cross-flow microfiltration: modeling and optimization. Membranes (Basel). 2022;12(7)

155. Della Bona A, et al. 3D printing restorative materials using a stereolithographic technique: a systematic review. Dent Mater. 2021;37(2):336–50.
156. Aisenbrey EA, et al. A stereolithography-based 3D printed hybrid scaffold for in situ cartilage defect repair. Macromol Biosci. 2018;18(2)
157. Campbell PG, Weiss LE. Tissue engineering with the aid of inkjet printers. Expert Opin Biol Ther. 2007;7(8):1123–7.
158. Keriquel V, et al. In vivo bioprinting for computer- and robotic-assisted medical intervention: preliminary study in mice. Biofabrication. 2010;2(1):014101.
159. Guillemot F, et al. High-throughput laser printing of cells and biomaterials for tissue engineering. Acta Biomater. 2010;6(7):2494–500.
160. Hong S, et al. Cellular behavior in micropatterned hydrogels by bioprinting system depended on the cell types and cellular interaction. J Biosci Bioeng. 2013;116(2):224–30.
161. Murdock MH, Badylak SF. Biomaterials-based in situ tissue engineering. Curr Opin Biomed Eng. 2017;1:4–7.
162. Huang BJ, Hu JC, Athanasiou KA. Cell-based tissue engineering strategies used in the clinical repair of articular cartilage. Biomaterials. 2016;98:1–22.
163. O'Connell CD, et al. Development of the Biopen: a handheld device for surgical printing of adipose stem cells at a chondral wound site. Biofabrication. 2016;8(1):015019.
164. Onofrillo C, et al. Biofabrication of human articular cartilage: a path towards the development of a clinical treatment. Biofabrication. 2018;10(4):045006.

17 Differences in the Treatment of Cartilage Lesions According to Anatomic Localizations

Fatih Karaaslan, Turan Cihan Dülgeroğlu, and Yavuz Kocabey

Articular cartilage is the tissue that covers the end of bones in synovial joints. It is a connective tissue with an extracellular matrix containing highly organized chondrocyte cells. Approximately 10% of this cartilage tissue consists of chondrocytes, while the rest mainly comprises Type 2 collagen tissue with collagen, as well as extracellular matrix and water containing glucosaminoglycans and proteoglycans. Cartilage tissue provides a smooth surface for the movement of the articulating bones and is resistant to compressive and shearing forces. It lacks blood vessels, nerves, and lymphatic tissue. When left to heal on its own, articular cartilage does not have significant regenerative capacity [1, 2].

Hyaline cartilage is the cornerstone of almost all joints in the body, especially in synovial joints. Due to its avascular structure and lack of undifferentiated cells that can respond to damage, treating hyaline cartilage pathologies is quite challenging as it has limited regenerative capabilities. Superficial cartilage injuries that do not reach the bone do not heal spontaneously [3]. Injuries that reach the bone can partially heal with an intrinsic reparative response, but this healing does not result in hyaline cartilage and instead leads to the formation of fibrous cartilage. As a consequence, joint incongruity, pain, and degeneration are frequently encountered in the joint over the years [4].

Prevalence studies have shown that about 60% of active individuals undergoing arthroscopy have cartilage lesions [5]. While many cartilage lesions are asymptomatic, symptomatic ones, such as those in degenerative arthritis patients requiring arthroplasty, can be painful [6]. The goals of conservative and surgical treatments for cartilage lesions are to restore joint congruity, promote cartilage tissue regeneration, prevent the development of osteoarthritis, and thereby avoid joint degeneration [7].

Cartilage defects can manifest in various forms, ranging from small, unilateral, focal chondral, or osteochondral lesions to large, unipolar, or bipolar defects [6]. When planning the repair and treatment of cartilage damage, factors such as the patient's age, weight, anatomical localization of the cartilage lesion, size and depth of the lesion, ligament and ligament damage, alignment deformity, and the presence of comorbidities within the joint should be taken into account. Despite the static, avascular nature and limited self-renewal capacity of joint cartilage, in the last

F. Karaaslan (✉)
Department of Orthopedics and Traumatology, Memorial Hospital, Kayseri, Turkey

T. C. Dülgeroğlu
Department of Orthopedics and Traumatology, Kütahya Health Sciences University Faculty of Medicine, Kütahya, Turkey

Y. Kocabey
Department of Orthopedics and Traumatology, Kocabey Clinic, Istanbul, Turkey

M. E. Erdil et al. (eds.), *Current Concept in Cartilage Treatment*,
https://doi.org/10.1007/978-3-032-27099-3_17

40 years, many new methods have emerged in the treatment of joint cartilage injuries, considering its dynamic and remodelization capacity [8]. Basic surgical intervention techniques have been developed and applied for osteochondral lesions, such as cartilage fragment fixation, surface abrasion, debridement, microfracture, and nanofracture, among others. Surgical treatment options for focal cartilage lesions in the knee include debridement/chondroplasty, bone marrow stimulation, autologous chondrocyte implantation (ACI), matrix-assisted chondrocyte implantation (MACI), osteochondral autograft transplantation (OAT), osteochondral allograft transplantation (OCA), and newer techniques such as particulated cartilage implantation procedures (autograft and juvenile allograft) [9]. In cases of irreversible degeneration and osteoarthritis, arthroplasty becomes an essential treatment method. Surgical treatment selection depends on morphological factors such as the location of the chondral lesion. Decisions are made based on the location within the joint, the position on the joint surface (inferior or superior), size, depth (involvement of subchondral bone), contained or uncontained, age, body mass index (BMI), limb and extensor mechanism strength, alignment, and the individual's activity level [10].

The variations in cartilage structure and thickness in different anatomical locations, chondrocyte count, group distribution, exposure to mechanical loads, and matrix distribution lead to changes in the diagnosis and treatment modalities of joint cartilage pathologies. Although diagnostic and treatment modalities for local cartilage lesions are seemingly similar due to their different structures in different anatomical locations, the ranking of treatment options and response to treatment can vary, especially across different anatomical localizations [11].

17.1 Tibiofemoral Joint

The management of articular cartilage defects remains one of the most challenging clinical problems for orthopedic surgeons. First and foremost, as with all examination methods, a detailed patient history should be taken. The mechanism of injury, time since the injury, severity of symptoms, any previous surgeries, and previously applied treatments should be thoroughly discussed. Diagnosing tibiofemoral cartilage defects through physical examination is quite difficult. Focal chondral lesions typically present with pain, stiffness, a feeling of joint giving way, locking, and limited range of motion if there is effusion. When there is a displaced osteochondral fragment, locking, catching, and triggering become more pronounced [12].

Cartilage lesions cannot be visualized on X-rays unless there is bone loss or joint space narrowing. Magnetic resonance imaging (MRI) is the gold standard method for diagnosing cartilage lesions [13]. T2-weighted fat-suppressed sequences are very useful in imaging degenerative cartilage lesions. Computed tomography (CT) is helpful in diagnosing pathologies that involve the bone beneath the cartilage and in visualizing the size and depth of the defect [14].

After physical examination and radiological imaging, other pathologies should be investigated and diagnoses established through examination under anesthesia. Subsequently, diagnostic arthroscopy is performed to determine the location, structure, surface area, depth, presence of fissuring, and the existence of a flap-style cartilage lesion, as well as the structure of the adjacent cartilage tissue and the presence of any other cartilage lesions. Surgical treatment decisions are made accordingly.

Cartilage defects are most commonly seen in the femoral condyles (43–58%), followed by the patella, and less commonly in the trochlea (6–16%). 68% of the defects are focal chondral defects, 3% are osteochondritis dissecans (OCD), and 29% are degenerative defects. 90% of the defects are smaller than 4 cm^2 [15].

The most commonly used classifications for tibiofemoral joint cartilage pathologies are the ICRS (International Cartilage Repair Society) and Outbridge classifications [16, 17]. For ICRS I-II lesions, supportive and pharmacological treatment methods, such as basic cartilage matrix reinforcement, collagen and glucosamine supplementation, and viscosupplementation, are recommended. ICRS III lesions are considered more repairable lesions. The treatment choice for ICRS III/IV lesions is mainly based on the structure, size of the defect, and the extent of bony involvement [18, 19].

After cartilage lesion repair, several factors such as age, smoking, and obesity influence the treatment outcome. Generally, we observe a more positive response to treatment at a younger age and a less successful treatment response in older age groups [20].

Currently, the treatment strategy for tibiofemoral joint cartilage lesions includes palliative joint debridement and lavage, bone marrow stimulation techniques that promote intrinsic repair such as microfracture and nanofracture, and finally, reconstructive biological treatment techniques such as osteochondral autograft/allograft, autologous chondrocyte implantation, and matrix-based autologous chondrocyte implantation [21–24].

17.1.1 Microfracture

Bone marrow stimulation techniques such as microfracture and nanofracture are the most commonly used methods for treating small symptomatic cartilage lesions in the knee joint. These procedures are technically simple and cost-effective compared to other treatments. In the bone marrow stimulation technique, subchondral bone is perforated to allow mesenchymal stem cells from the bone marrow to migrate to the lesion site [25–30]. Mesenchymal stem cells can differentiate into fibrochondrocytes, which contribute to fibrocartilage repair. The concentration of mesenchymal stem cells in the bone marrow is relatively low and decreases further with advancing age. The formation of a stable blood clot that fills the defect is crucial for the success of cartilage defect repair and bone marrow stimulation procedures. Unstable fibrin clots can lead to unsuccessful repairs [31–34]. Microfracture is more suitable for lesions with a surface area of 2–4 cm^2 and has been shown to be successful in 60–80% of cases. However, it may result in fibrocartilage rather than hyaline cartilage, making it less preferable for larger lesions. Some studies have explored the use of additional substances such as chitosan, platelet-derived growth factor, and insulin-like growth factor to enhance fibrin clot stabilization. Hyaluronic acid supplementation has also been observed to promote cartilage repair that more closely resembles hyaline cartilage. Platelet-rich plasma has shown to improve cartilage repair in many studies [35–38].

17.1.2 Osteochondral Autograft Transfer System (OATS)

Osteochondral autograft transfer system (OATS) is another method for treating focal chondral defects ranging from 2 to 4 cm^2. It involves transplanting one or multiple small cylindrical autologous osteochondral grafts collected from less weight-bearing areas of the femoral joint surface. These grafts are transferred to the defect area with an appropriate fit to create a compatible and durable surface. OATS can be more successful in younger patients (under 30 years old), and Hangody recommends it for patients under 50 years old. This technique allows for mature hyaline cartilage transfer but should be used for smaller focal chondral defects due to limited donor site availability. OATS offers several advantages over other repair techniques, such as a relatively short rehabilitation period and the ability to perform the procedure in a single operation. However, donor site morbidity is a significant drawback. Other potential limitations include differences in direction, thickness, and mechanical properties between the donor and recipient sites and gaps between grafts. Problems such as cartilage collapse and insufficient stabilization of the underlying bone may occur with postoperative weight-bearing. The choice of treatment depends on the surgeon's experience and the patient's expectations. OATS has shown better results in high-demand athletes, and it should be preferred for smaller lesions with higher expectations. Hangody reported a success rate of 92% on the femoral side, 87% on the tibial side, and 79% on the patellar side in 831 cases of mosaicplasty. He also reported a donor site morbidity rate of 3% in the same series [39, 40].

17.1.3 Autologous Chondrocyte Implantation (ACI) for Tibiofemoral Large Defects

For lesions larger than 4 cm^2, autologous chondrocyte implantation (ACI) or osteochondral allograft transplantation is more successful than microfracture and OATS. The size of the defect does not affect the outcome of autologous chondrocyte implantation. ACI was originally described in 1994 [41, 42]. Its primary theoretical advantage is the development of hyaline-like cartilage instead of fibrocartilage in the defect, which may lead to long-lasting and durable results. However, the technique involves two surgical procedures, periosteal morbidity at the harvest site, delamination, graft failure, graft hypertrophy, and high costs [43]. It is also a technically demanding procedure. Although it is commonly used for larger defects, studies have shown better outcomes with microfracture-like basic procedures for small focal lesions. To apply this technique, the condition of the subchondral bone is crucial. Generally, intact subchondral bone is required for ACI application. However, it cannot be said that it cannot be used in the presence of bone defects. ACI can be successfully applied after the defect area is filled with bone grafting. ACI results have been reported to be superior to mosaicplasty and microfracture in clinical studies [44–46].

17.1.4 Matrix-Based Autologous Chondrocyte Implantation (MOKİ)

Although cell-based treatments inducing cartilage regeneration, such as autologous chondrocyte implantation, have been described, the results have not been highly predictable or reproducible [47]. Second-generation techniques have been developed to support cells during preimplantation, culture, and postoperative healing stages with the use of matrix-associated chondrocyte implantation [48]. Even though chondrocytes are harvested in the same way, matrix-associated chondrocyte implantation for autologous chondrocyte implantation procedures prevents the deterioration and differentiation of chondrocytes during the process, including periosteal morbidity and implantation. Moreover, this procedure can be applied arthroscopically in selected cases, which is an advantage [49]. It can be used for large chondral lesions and requires only the attachment of the scaffold to the lesion surface using a fibrin adhesive. Bartlett et al. reported good results with the sandwich technique in 8 mm deep lesions [50].

17.1.5 Hyaluronan-Based Scaffolds

Hyaluronan-based scaffolds are another approach for cartilage repair, utilizing a three-dimensional structure that supports cell proliferation and provides structural support for matrix accumulation and cell adhesion. It prevents the breakdown and differentiation of chondrocytes and gradually allows chondrocytes to produce extracellular matrix as the scaffold structure wears off and is replaced by the extracellular matrix [51, 52].

17.1.6 Osteochondral Allograft Transplantation

Osteochondral allograft transplantation involves the transplantation of an intact, live articular cartilage and subchondral bone graft from a cadaver to repair a cartilage surface [53]. The size and depth of the lesion are crucial factors in choosing the graft site. The advantage is that it allows for immediate placement of live hyaline cartilage in the defective area without donor site morbidity. Limitations of osteochondral allograft transplantation include limited graft availability, high cost, risk of immune rejection, potential graft integration issues, potential disease transmission, and technical challenges related to graft processing and sizing. Osteochondral allograft transplantation is more suitable for larger chondral lesions where bone defects are the primary concern [54]. Based on this, for lesions limited to the articular cartilage, autologous chondrocyte implantation (ACI) should be preferred, while for larger lesions involving extensive bone tissue or with deep subchondral bone edema where intralesional osteophyte is predominant, osteochondral allograft transplantation should be preferred. Moreover, in revision cartilage repairs, ACI and superficial cartilage tissue repairs, osteochondral allograft transplantation is more suitable. For lesions involving bone tissue, matrix-based autologous chondrocyte implantation (MACI) can be combined with grafting [55].

17.1.7 Patellofemoral Cartilage Lesions

The patellofemoral joint is a complex structure, and the patella is the largest sesamoid bone in the body, with morphologically the thickest hyaline cartilage in the anatomical region, distinguishing it from other chondral structures [56]. Moreover, there is no cartilage tissue in the distal one-fourth of the patella. The patellofemoral joint (PFJ) is a common site for symptomatic cartilage lesions of the knee. In recent years, an MRI-based study examining cartilage lesions of the knee joint showed that approximately 52% of knees with symptomatic pain and osteoarthritis had patellofemoral joint issues [57, 58]. The etiology of patellofemoral OA involves extensor mechanism insufficiency related to alignment, chronic repetitive microtrauma, and, most commonly, patellar dislocations, including about 95% of chondral defects, and several factors play a role in its etiology. Approximately 20–40% of knee problems are attributed to the patellofemoral joint. Another issue is that this problem is more prevalent in young, active individuals and athletes [59]. In the patellofemoral joint, the basic movement is sliding rather than rolling, resulting in increased load on the joint. Due to its complex biomechanical structure and the forces acting on it, cartilage lesions can occur, leading to problems such as knee pain, even without any trauma. The unique structure of the patellofemoral joint exposes it to forces, which can result in various problems, ranging from chondral lesions to osteoarthritis. To resolve this problem, a thorough medical history, physical examination, and precise radiological imaging are necessary [60, 61].

The goal of treatment is to achieve a pain-free and functionally improved extremity. In treatment planning, accurately establishing the pathology is crucial. Conservative treatment is generally preferred initially, which may include nonsteroidal anti-inflammatory drugs, knee braces, and intra-articular viscosupplementation. In addition to strengthening the muscles to reduce the absorption of physiological loads along the knee, weight loss and activity modification can help alleviate worsening pain and functional limitations. Conservative treatment can be applied to patients with knee pain at least 3 months before considering surgical intervention [62].

Patellofemoral joint problems are more common in cases of unstable patellofemoral joint and valgus knees. Therefore, various ligament repairs and osteotomies have been defined for joint stabilization and alignment. It is important to be aware that the knee, especially the patellofemoral joint, does not tolerate multiple surgeries well when planning for surgical interventions [63].

17.1.8 Chondroplasty

Chondroplasty is one of the most commonly performed surgical procedures for cartilage lesions. It is mostly indicated for typical partial or full-thickness cartilage lesions and can be performed for lesions smaller than 1–2 cm^2, but also for larger lesions, with the purpose of preparing the area for subsequent cartilage repair processes. Creating a stable vertical-walled surface is of utmost importance, and aggressive debridement for cartilage viability is recommended [64–66]. Several studies evaluating preoperative and postoperative outcomes have reported positive results for chondroplasty. However, these studies have not explained any observable relationship between anatomical location and the extent and depth of the lesion [67, 68].

17.1.9 Bone Marrow Stimulation Technique (Microfracture)

In this technique, fibrocartilage tissue healing is observed, where pluripotent mesenchymal stem cells migrate from the subchondral tissue toward the defective cartilage lesion area. The most popular techniques are the Kirschner wire with the pridie drilling technique and the angled and straight awls described by Steadman [69, 70]. This technique can be used effectively for lesions up to 4 cm^2 in the tibiofemoral joint, while it is suitable for lesions up to 2 cm^2 in the patellofemoral joint. The reason for this is that the durability of the formed fibrocartilage is affected by the distinctive biomechanics and high stresses in this joint. Additionally, if microfracture is preferred, it should be used in patients with a body mass index (BMI) below 30, under the age of 40, and contained lesions. The procedure begins with clearly defining the edges of the lesion using curettage to obtain a stable and contained lesion wall. Following the removal of the cartilage layer, perpendicular holes are drilled with a depth of 3 mm and a 3–4 mm gap between them in the lesion area. If the lesion is in the trochlear region, arthroscopic intervention is easier, but if it is in the patella, arthroscopic intervention is more challenging [45].

In patellofemoral joint problems, studies have shown that the failure rate of the microfracture technique increases after the first 2 years and in 5-year follow-ups, especially senior surgeons have found it more suitable for lesions smaller than 2 cm^2. Furthermore, it is more likely to be preferred in trochlear lesions of the patellofemoral joint as it reduces the need for subsequent surgeries [55, 71].

In recent years, bone marrow aspirate concentrate (BMAC) application has shown promising results, but these studies are still in the research stage. High-density pluripotent bone marrow cells obtained from the bone marrow are placed in the defective area with a protective membrane. It can be used as a biological integrator with osteochondral autograft transplantation (OAT) and osteochondral allograft (OCA), and with further studies in cartilage lesions, it may become an alternative treatment [72].

17.1.10 Autologous Chondrocyte Implantation (ACI)

ACI is one of the preferred methods by experienced surgeons for patellofemoral joint problems. This technique is highly beneficial in resolving complex and challenging chondral lesions in the patellofemoral region. This technique has been used for chondral lesions for approximately 30 years, and three different generations of ACI have been reported [73].

Initially, about 100–300 mg of full-thickness cartilage tissue is obtained arthroscopically from the non-weight-bearing femoral condyle or the superolateral intercondylar notch surface. In vitro, the cartilage matrix is processed, and chondrocytes are cultured for at least 2 weeks. In the second stage, the chondral lesion is debrided, and the cartilage matrix is placed in this lesion. It is important to avoid damaging the subchondral plate during debridement and to obtain a stable vertical wall. Then, the membrane containing the embedded chondrocytes is fixed to the surface using 6–0 Vicryl sutures and fibrin glue. In the original technique, a periosteal flap from the anterior tibia surface was used, but due to donor site morbidity and excessive overgrowth of cartilage tissue and unsatisfactory outcomes, this led surgeons to use a second-generation collagen matrix and a two-layer synthetic scaffold containing enlarged chondrocytes for ACI [74].

The third-generation ACI, also known as Matrix-Induced Autologous Chondrocyte Implantation (MACI), involves multiplying chondrocytes in a three-dimensional structural scaffold membrane. ACI application allows surgical treatment for large full-thickness lesions of 3–4 cm^2 and athletes. Preoperative MRI evaluation is crucial for ACI application. Subchondral bone loss may require bone grafting and sandwich application or necessitate allograft. ACI should be avoided in patients with previous microfracture surgery and subchondral cystic lesions with degenerative changes and extensive subchondral edema [75–78].

However, the ACI method contains challenges due to the unique topographical structure of the patellar cartilage surface. It can be performed in conjunction with osteochondral autograft transfer. Smoking, obesity, and inflammatory arthritis are contraindications for ACI treatment.

17.1.11 Osteochondral Autograft Transfer (OAT)

As mentioned earlier, with this method, approximately 10–15 mm deep osteochondral cylindrical pieces are harvested from the non-weight-bearing medial or lateral trochlear origin, posterior femoral condyle, or intercondylar notch region of the knee and transferred to the lesion area of the same side. OAT has advantages such as being non-immunogenic, applicable in the same session, and providing hyaline cartilage transfer, but donor site morbidity remains a significant concern. Due to this limitation, it is a method that can be used for treating small lesions of 2–3 cm^2 in size. If multiple osteochondral graft transfers are to be performed, it is called mosaicplasty. Although the occurrence of immunogenicity problems is not common, the removal of bone marrow cells from the transferred block through pulsatile lavage can be beneficial [79, 80].

In a biomechanical study, Garretson et al. found that cylindrical grafts for PFJ can be obtained from the medial trochlea and distal lateral trochlea due to their low contact loads [81]. When performing the OAT method, obtaining a smooth and congruent surface in the PFJ can be challenging [82, 83]. Graft prominence above 1 mm has been reported to result in catching and continuation of symptoms in patients. The unique anatomy of the patellar and trochlear surfaces makes it difficult to create a smooth joint surface; each donor graft will have a thinner cartilage layer than the surrounding patella, leading to an incongruity at the local cartilage-bone interface. While some authors report a 92% success rate for OAT application in the femoral condyle of the knee, they have reported a success rate of 79% for the patellofemoral joint due to its unique structural problems. However, other studies have indicated that with meticulous graft selection and placement, better results can be achieved [84–86].

17.1.12 Osteochondral Allograft Transplantation (OCA)

Osteochondral Allograft Transplantation (OCA) is perhaps the most challenging cartilage procedure in the PFJ. The same challenges that apply to OAT surgery, regarding graft surface congruency and smoothness, also apply to OCA. However, the complexity and variability of the PFJ necessitate planning for donor graft matching. While no imaging studies have been conducted for preoperative imaging and planning, the FDA's careful and cautious approach to obtaining and storing tissue and organ transplants encourages the wider use and even consideration of OCA as a salvage surgical procedure in chondral lesions [87, 88].

Fresh osteochondral allografts are collected within 24 h after the donor's death and stored at 4 °C. The graft has a shelf life of 28 days. Through an open arthrotomy, the lesion area is reached, and the anesthetized donor graft is press-fit into the defect site according to the prepared defect. The graft volume is related to immunogenicity, so the bone piece volume is kept as thin as possible while ensuring that the cartilage surface is smooth. Additionally, washing with pulse lavage is performed to remove bone marrow products [89–91]. OCA is primarily indicated for large full-thickness lesions greater than 2 cm^2 with abnormal subchondral bone surface. It is also becoming the primary treatment procedure for all cartilage lesions [92]. Relative contraindications include smoking and obesity. The advantages of OCA include its ability to be applied in a single session, overcoming the potential donor site morbidity problem of OAT, being an optional primary treatment procedure in bipolar lesions, and treating uncontained chondral lesions and large chondral lesions as a salvage procedure [93, 94]. However, in the literature, the failure rate in patellar chondral lesions, particularly patellar chondral lesions, has been reported to be higher compared to tibiofemoral joint problems. For patellofemoral chondral lesions, OCA is especially recommended as a revision salvage procedure for failed chondral surgery, while on the trochlear side, it is suggested as the primary treatment for chondral lesions larger than 2 cm^2 and as a revision salvage surgery [95, 96].

17.2 Hip Joint Cartilage Lesions

Diagnosis and treatment of hip chondral lesions continue to pose a challenge for orthopedic surgeons. As the understanding of hip joint structure improves, effective treatment modalities emerge [97]. Conditions such as femoroacetabular impingement (FAI), acetabular dysplasia, trauma, and avascular necrosis (AVN) commonly lead to chondral surface damage and subsequent clinical symptoms in young adults [98]. Factors such as athletic history, previous trauma, childhood hip pathologies, past surgical interventions, and treatments can also play a role. Over the past decade, advancements in imaging techniques, hip education programs, and data from basic sciences and clinical research have resulted in an increase in hip arthroscopy procedures, leading to a rise in the diagnosis of hip cartilage lesions. The evaluation of chondral lesions in the hip includes a thorough patient history, comprehensive physical examination, and the use of complementary imaging methods. Clinical manifestations of hip joint cartilage lesions include pain, catching, locking, and a sense of giving way. However, these symptoms may be encountered in various hip intra-articular pathologies, not limited to chondral lesions. A comprehensive physical examination includes the evaluation of joint range of motion in standing, supine, prone, and lateral positions, assessment of passive and active joint motion ranges, and identification of positions that provoke pain and sensitivity to palpation, which are often informative. Clicking, catching, and trigger points may be noted during the examination [99].

The acetabulum is the most common location for hip chondral lesions, and a study has shown that 88% of chondral defects are located in the anterior superior acetabulum [100].

Chondral lesions are often associated with labral tears, with anterior superior labrum being the most common location in correlation with chondral lesions [101].

Several classification methods have been proposed for classifying cartilage pathologies, including Outerbridge, Beck, International Cartilage Repair Society (ICRS), and Ilizaliturri's extended classification system, which is defined by six acetabular regions for FAI pathology [17, 102–104].

17.3 Treatment Methods

Apart from arthroplasty, surgical treatment methods used for hip joint cartilage lesions resemble those used in other joints. The lesion should be focal and not overlapping, and the joint space should be adequate. Repair methods should not be used in inflammatory arthritis. Treatment options for hip chondral lesions include local measures such as debridement (chondroplasty), microfracture, cartilage transplantations such as osteochondral autograft transfer (OAT), mosaicplasty, osteochondral allograft (OCA) transplantation, and the inclusion of orthobiologics (autologous chondrocyte implantation [ACI], autologous matrix-induced chondrogenesis [AMIC], mononuclear concentrate in platelet-rich plasma [PRP] matrix [MCC], expanded mesenchymal stem cells [MSCs]).

Chondroplasty is a debridement procedure mainly used for partial chondral lesions. It is employed to remove loose bodies and eliminate lesions causing mechanical blockage, especially to create well-defined lesions. In a large database study, chondroplasty was preferred in approximately 49% of hip arthroscopy cases. However, it has been observed that young patients who underwent chondroplasty had a considerable incidence of hip degenerative arthritis, close to 50% [105]. Additionally, Yen and Kocher demonstrated that chondroplasty is successful in low-grade, partial thickness lesions. The use of radiofrequency ablation devices should be avoided in chondral tissue due to the potential harm to chondrocytes [106].

17.3.1 Microfracture

Microfracture is used to initiate the body's healing potential and promote cartilage healing by introducing pluripotent mesenchymal stem cells from the bone marrow. Microfracture procedures are the most commonly used in hip and other joint cartilage injuries [107]. It can be applied to any region of the femur and acetabulum. During the procedure, the cartilage and underlying calcified cartilage are debrided, and holes are created at 3 mm depth and 3 mm apart to allow pluripotent mesenchymal stem cells from the bone marrow to come in. It is recommended that the lesion size for microfracture in the hip joint should not exceed 3–4 cm^2. After surgery, partial weight-bearing is advised. The best response is seen in lesions not exceeding 2–4 cm^2. Microfracture is not a suitable choice for lesions with a partial cartilage defect but a bone defect underneath it [108].

Advantages of microfracture include its low cost and relatively straightforward technique [105].

17.3.2 Autologous Chondrocyte Implantation (ACI)

Autologous chondrocyte implantation is preferred for large hip cartilage defects that are too extensive for microfracture. Hip joint applications are mostly performed on the acetabular surface. Autologous chondrocyte implantation, whether unassisted or supported by a matrix scaffold, is mainly used for lesions between 3–10 cm^2 in patients under 45 years of age. As described in other chondral injuries, ACI is a two-step method. In the first step, cartilage biopsy is taken, and laboratory procedures are applied. In the second step, the chondrocytes are multiplied and embedded in the matrix or placed in a gel-like structure into the defect. For gels prepared, a natural tissue such as periosteum or a synthetic tissue may be required, and after placement in the defect, it is sutured to the cartilage. Fibrin glue may be used. This treatment method requires an open surgical procedure. The matrix-supported method requires either an open or arthroscopic surgery. In the medium and long term, ACI has shown superiority over microfracture [105].

Risks of ACI include nerve injury due to traction during the procedure, fragile cartilage formation, and the development of hip instability, subluxation, or dislocation [109].

17.3.3 Autologous Matrix-Induced Chondrogenesis (AMIC)

AMIC treatment is a one-step procedure that can be applied to grade 3 and 4 acetabular chondral defects with a width of 2–4 cm^2 in patients between 18–55 years of age. Developed considering the combined two-step application and open surgical intervention of ACI and MACI, AMIC involves covering the defective surface with a chondral implant combined with microfracture procedure [110]. Roof implants may contain collagen, hyaluronan, or polyglycolic acid. The matrix is placed arthroscopically and contributes to the coverage and stabilization of the fibrin clot obtained with microfracture. A proper chondrectomy creates sufficient stability due to the concavity of the acetabulum and the pressure applied by the femoral head to the implant. In a recent publication, AMIC treatment was shown to yield better results than microfracture in 5-year follow-ups. In Fontana and Mancini's 5-year follow-up studies, there was no significant difference in acetabular cartilage healing between ACI and AMIC in FAI patients [111].

17.3.4 Mosaicplasty

Osteochondral autograft transplantation (OAT) and mosaicplasty are procedures that involve using osteochondral plugs. These plugs are obtained from a weight-bearing surface and prepared by creating a hole similar to the size of the lesion, which is then implanted into the chondral defect. This method has been applied in hip joint patients based on other experiences. For the application of this method in the hip joint, patient selection under the age of 45 and lesions smaller than 3 cm^2 are necessary. This procedure requires open surgical intervention. The graft source can be from the femur lateral anterior surface with minimal weight-bearing in the knee joint, posterior condylar surface, or femoral head inferolateral surface [112].

The difference between OAT and mosaicplasty lies in the size and number of treated lesions. Mosaicplasty addresses multiple small lesions and is typically applied with hip joint dislocation. OAT, on the other hand, is used for large lesions with subchondral damage, and in cases where microfracture or wear chondroplasty has failed [105].

OAT can be performed with an arthroscopic approach depending on the lesion. A review by Logan and others found that mosaicplasty is routinely used to treat femoral head defects and has not been previously used in acetabular cartilage [113, 114].

Both mosaicplasty and OAT are low-cost, one-step surgeries that utilize the patient's natural hyaline cartilage. The most important morbidity is donor site morbidity. Additionally, the contour of the harvested cartilage may not match that of the lesion [105].

Various studies have looked into PRP treatments for various pathologies, and although different results have been obtained, the common conclusion is that PRP has anti-inflammatory properties and a procoagulant effect. In a study using a sheep model with PRP clot, it was shown that chondral lesions were completely filled with normal hyaline cartilage [115].

To demonstrate the effectiveness of this treatment in hip cartilage lesions, larger numbers of data and longer follow-up periods are needed.

17.3.5 OCA Transplantation

OCA transplantation is a surgical procedure that involves using an allograft. Bone blocks are taken from a cadaver and, after the donor site is inspected and debrided until smooth edges are achieved, are transferred to the recipient's cartilage-defective area. The depth and width of the defect are measured, and the graft is later fixed to the recipient site using various fixation methods [116].

OCA transfer is advantageous due to the absence of donor site morbidity and involving the transplantation of hyaline cartilage. Measurements of the donor and recipient sites are made under CT guidance, and the transfer should take place within 28 days from the donor to the recipient [117].

The suitability of the donor site to the recipient site, disease transmission, donor rejection, and high cost are seen as disadvantages of the procedure. However, its advantage lies in its use for large osteochondral defects and its potential as a rescue chondral surgical procedure in failed cartilage procedures [118].

17.4 Ankle Cartilage Lesions

Ankle joint cartilage lesions are more common in the young population and often occur due to trauma-related reasons. The difficulty in accessing and the challenging nature of cartilage healing in the ankle joint make the treatment of ankle cartilage lesions more challenging [119].

The knee and ankle joints are hinge-type joints, with the ankle joint having better compatibility compared to the knee joint. The ankle joint has higher levels of glucosamine and lower water content, making it more dynamically rigid and more resistant to compressive forces. Additionally, the high level of proteoglycan in the ankle provides higher resistance to compressive forces compared to the knee joint. Moreover, after trauma, chondrocytes in the ankle are less sensitive to IL-1, and they have a higher capacity to synthesize proteoglycan, which contributes to a higher repair capacity [120].

Ankle sprains and rotational injuries are often associated with talus osteochondral injuries. Medial talar lesions are more common than lateral ones, but lateral injuries are more frequently associated with trauma, whereas approximately 64% of medial talar lesions develop secondary to trauma [121]. Medial lesions tend to be deeper and have a higher likelihood of turning into cystic lesions, while lateral lesions are shallower and more likely to be associated with cartilage fractures [122].

Due to the scarcity of long-term follow-up studies, the natural course of talus osteochondral lesions remains uncertain [123]. Typically, conservative treatment methods are applied first, which can include rest, activity modification, and immobilization with a cast. The goal of conservative treatment is to reduce or eliminate the load on the injured cartilage, thereby reducing bone edema and the chance of necrosis. It also aims to allow the detached cartilage fragment to adhere to the underlying bone tissue, increasing the chances of healing [124, 125].

However, based on the available literature, there is no specific outcome regarding the duration of non-operative immobilization, weight-bearing status, use of non-steroidal anti-inflammatory drugs (NSAIDs), and physical therapy protocol. Surgical management involves the use of ankle arthroscopy techniques to support the healing of TOLs that do not respond to conservative treatment, as well as new applications of biological stimulation and allograft techniques (excision, excision with curettage, excision with curette and drilling/microfracture, excision with curette and autogenous grafting, excision with curetted and particulated juvenile cartilage, retrograde drilling, autogenous chondrocyte implantation, osteochondral autograft transplantation, and osteochondral allograft transplantation) [126, 127].

17.5 Surgical Treatment

The principle of operative treatment is to restore the function of the ankle joint by removing chondral tissue or debriding and stabilizing the osteochondral fragment, cartilage edge, and subchondral bone, stimulating healing in damaged cartilage and eliminating pain. Curettage and microfracture methods are recommended for repairing TOL lesions larger than 15 mm and not deeper than 7 mm [128, 129].

For deeper and larger lesions, other options such as autologous chondrocyte implantation (ACI), osteochondral autograft transplantation (OATS), allograft transplantation, and metal implants should be considered [130].

Indications for operative treatment include failure of conservative treatment for at least 6 weeks to 6 months and acute osteochondral fragment Berndt and Harty grade III and IV osteochondral lesions. The exact timing of surgery indicated in the literature is not yet established. O'Farrell et al. recommend surgical treatment within the first 12 months after injury [131].

However, Alexander et al. showed that delayed surgical treatment did not negatively affect outcomes after injury [132–134].

Postoperative protocols vary depending on specific treatment methods but generally include early mobilization followed by protected movements. Weight-bearing with boots and a gradual return to sports activities are recommended.

17.5.1 Position

Treatment of lesions in the anterior and middle parts of the talus involves the supine position, while lateral lesions require the lateral decubitus position, and posterior talus lesions are treated in the prone position [135–137].

17.5.2 Open Surgical Technique

Anterolateral and mid-lateral lesions can be treated using either open or arthroscopic techniques. Anterolateral chondral lesions can be addressed through an open anterior arthrotomy or fibular osteotomy [138]. Posterolateral lesions can be managed with posterior open arthrotomy or arthroscopic approaches. Anteromedial and midmedial lesions can be treated through anterior arthroscopy or anterior arthrotomy with medial malleolus osteotomy. Posteriomedial lesions are addressed with posterior arthroscopic intervention [139, 140].

17.5.3 Excision, Curette, and Microfracture/Drilling

The excision of the osteochondral fragment helps alleviate ankle pain by preventing joint irritation and minimizing further damage to the loose osteochondral fragment [141]. The microfracture technique induces fibrocartilaginous repair of the cartilage damage, resulting in favorable functional outcomes. Multiple small subchondral holes, spaced 3–4 mm apart, are made to stimulate the release of mesenchymal stem cells and growth factors, promoting the formation of fibrocartilaginous repair tissue [142]. This microfracture technique has been proven effective for both chondral and cartilage treatment of osteochondral lesions of the talus, especially for lesions smaller than 1.5 cm^2, making it a recommended first-line treatment [143].

17.5.4 Retrograde Drilling (RD)

Retrograde drilling (RD) is employed as a non-transarticular procedure in patients with intact cartilage to prevent injury to undamaged cartilage. Taranow et al. first described this technique in 1999, using anterolateral and posterolateral approaches [144]. However, due to a potential failure rate of around 20%, new methods have been developed in recent years to shorten surgical time and enhance technical success. Kerimaa et al. achieved a 100% accuracy with MRI guidance, while Hoffmann et al. demonstrated higher accuracy compared to standard fluoroscopy using an electromagnetic navigation system, along with reduced surgery duration [145, 146].

17.5.5 Fixation of the Osteochondral Fragment

Previous studies have reported successful internal fixation of large osteochondral lesions. The lesion is commonly located in the anterolateral part of the talus and is often associated with trauma. In young patients, the size of the lesion is of significant importance when planning osteochondral fragment fixation [147]. Stone et al. recommend fixation for lesions larger than 7.5 mm [148]. Additionally, Chandran et al. reported excellent outcomes after fixation using three absorbable pins in 2008 [149].

17.5.6 Autologous Chondrocyte Implantation (ACI)

Autologous Chondrocyte Implantation (ACI) involves the use of cultured chondrocytes with a periosteal patch. The cartilage cells can be obtained from separated cartilage, the edges of the lesion, or the knee joint. The area surrounding the lesion is debrided until the cartilage tissue becomes stable, and no necrotic bone remains at the base of the lesion. After obtaining approximately 200–300 mg of cartilage, it is collected to yield at least ten times and produce around 12 million cells. After being cultured for 6–8 weeks, the chondrocytes are applied to the lesion in the second stage [150, 151]. While anterolateral lesions can be treated arthroscopically, medial malleolus osteotomy is required for posteromedial lesions. The chondrocyte implantation is placed beneath the periosteal flap taken from the tibia using a fibrin adhesive. ACI is generally used for the surgical treatment of lesions larger than 1–1.5 cm^2 with complete and well-defined borders [152, 153].

Recently, matrix-assisted ACI (MACI) has emerged as a more straightforward and time-saving alternative to periosteal flaps. Ander et al. reported their results with MACI in 22 patients with an average follow-up period of 63.5 weeks. They observed improvements in AOFAS score from 70.1 to 95.3, VAS score from 5.7/10 to 0.9/10, and Tegner activity level from 2.4 to 4.7, with no major complications during the 60-month follow-up period [154]. Although promising results have been reported with ACI techniques, donor site morbidity and high costs remain potential barriers.

17.5.7 Osteochondral Autograft Transplantation

Osteochondral Autograft Transplantation is a reconstructive bone grafting technique using one or more cylindrical osteochondral grafts harvested from the less weight-bearing periphery of the same knee or talus. The goal of osteochondral autograft transplantation is to transfer the mechanical, structural, and biochemical properties of the damaged and injured original hyaline joint cartilage from the non-weight-bearing donor site to the weight-bearing prepared area. Indications for this technique include the treatment of osteochondral lesions larger than 10–15 mm and previously failed chondral lesions. Technically, it is applied as OATS for small lesions and as mosaicplasty for larger lesions. However, due to donor site morbidity, it is more commonly preferred for isolated lesions smaller than 1.5 cm^2 [155–157].

17.5.8 Osteochondral Allograft Transplantation

Osteochondral allograft transplantation is an effective procedure used to treat large osteochondral lesions. An anatomically suitable osteochondral allograft, obtained from a cadaver, is placed at the lesion site to repair the hyaline cartilage and bone defect [158, 159]. This technique is applied in cases where autogenous bone graft placement is difficult or not feasible. Osteochondral allograft transplantation prevents the complications of both the OATS procedure, which is associated with donor site morbidity, and mosaicplasty, where fibrocartilage growth can be observed between grafts. It serves as a salvage surgical modality for large, deep osteochondral lesions and previously failed surgical interventions. Although it is a salvage surgical procedure, it comes with challenges in surgical technique, disease transmission, and high surgical costs [160, 161].

17.6 Shoulder Joint

Cartilage lesions in non-weight-bearing shoulder joints are not very common. They usually occur as a result of trauma, previous shoulder surgery, focal osteonecrosis, septic arthritis, osteochondritis dissecans, full-thickness rotator cuff tears, or secondary to instability [162]. Diagnosis can be challenging, especially when they are incidentally found during open or arthroscopic surgeries. Glenohumeral joint chondral defects are often asymptomatic and well-tolerated. Initial treatment is conservative management. Surgical strategies include arthroscopic debridement, microfracture, osteochondral autograft or allograft transplantation, autologous chondrocyte implantation, and particulated juvenile allograft chondral implantation. These surgical procedures have reported good results in anatomical locations where cartilage lesions are more commonly observed, such as the knee and ankle [163].

Patients typically present with painful and stiff joints. Radiographic findings show narrowing of the joint space and subchondral cystic changes [164]. Shoulder instability is the most common underlying pathology leading to such lesions. Additionally, recurrent shoulder dislocations can lead to shoulder cartilage lesions. Superior labrum anterior to posterior (SLAP) tears are frequently associated with superior cartilage lesions of the shoulder head and anterior glenoid lesions [165]. Iatrogenic chondral lesions, reported at a rate of 13%, can occur due to the use of non-absorbable suture materials, thermal injury, or postoperative bupivacaine injection. Being aware of postoperative chondrolysis is crucial, as this pathology can present as a widespread lesion involving the glenoid and humeral head, making it important to differentiate it from focal chondral defects [166].

Osteochondritis dissecans is less common in the shoulder joint compared to knee and ankle joints. This lesion typically occurs in the glenoid fossa of young adults [167, 168].

17.6.1 Conservative Treatment

Non-surgical treatment includes NSAIDs, physical therapy, corticosteroid injections, and viscosupplementation. Non-surgical treatments are applied to some symptomatic patients as they cause less damage to the joint. However, there are not many long-term publications available on the non-surgical treatment of focal chondral defects of the glenohumeral joint [169].

17.6.2 Surgical

Surgery can be considered in patients who have received conservative treatment but have not experienced improvement in their symptoms. Several surgical procedures have been described for the treatment of these lesions, including microfracture, osteochondral autograft transplantation, fresh osteochondral allograft transplantation, and autologous chondrocyte implantation [170, 171].

17.6.3 Arthroscopic Debridement

Arthroscopic debridement involves the removal of loose cartilage pieces during shoulder arthroscopy. Among the other cartilage treatments discussed, arthroscopic debridement is not a preferred surgical option for cases with full-thickness shoulder cartilage lesions [172].

17.6.4 Microfracture

This technique is similar to the surgical technique applied in other joints. After arthroscopic debridement, vertical holes are drilled from the periphery to the center, and bone marrow products are expected to fill these microfracture holes. Typically, each microfracture hole is spaced 3–4 mm apart and should reach a depth of 2 to 4 mm [173].

Positive data reported in several series of shoulder cartilage lesions have led to the application of arthroscopic microfracture surgical procedures. However, it has been shown to be more successful in lesions smaller than 1.5 cm^2 [174, 175].

17.6.5 Osteochondral Autograft Transplantation (OAT)

Osteochondral autograft transplantation (OAT) is used for small lesions that do not respond to initial treatment. OAT typically involves transferring an osteochondral autograft from any weight-bearing region of the knee to the area with cartilage defects in the shoulder [176]. The advantage is the transplantation of hyaline cartilage and filling the defective area with bone stock, but it should be noted that it is more suitable for smaller lesions rather than large cartilage defects to prevent donor site morbidity. Additionally, there is a requirement for open surgery, and the formation of hyaline cartilage in the gaps between graft plugs is not possible in mosaicplasty. While successful results have been reported in other anatomical locations (knee, ankle), it cannot be said that it is highly successful in the shoulder joint, especially on the glenoid surface [177, 178].

17.6.6 Fresh Osteochondral Allograft Transplantation

Allograft transplantation has become a preferred method for the treatment of many musculoskeletal disorders. The technique is similar to autologous osteochondral transfer. Fresh osteochondral allograft transplantation uses the same concepts as autologous osteochondral graft transfer. It can be used in glenoid, humeral head, and bipolar lesions. The advantages of allografts are shorter surgical time and less donor site morbidity associated with autologous osteochondral grafts. However, disease transmission potential and cost are considered as disadvantages [179].

17.6.7 Autologous Chondrocyte Implantation (ACI)

Autologous chondrocyte implantation (ACI) is a two-stage technique. Chondrocytes are cultured for several weeks from a cartilage biopsy taken from the lesion edge or from the knee joint. In the second stage, an arthrotomy procedure is required. The arthrotomy is usually performed with a deltopectoral incision. A portion of the subscapularis muscle tendon insertion is detached, and after the arthrotomy procedure, the prepared graft material is placed under the subperiosteal or defect-specific membrane and sutured or fixed with fibrin adhesive. The current method is widely used in other anatomical locations, but there are limited publications regarding its use in the shoulder joint. Therefore, it has not yet become a routine procedure [180].

References

1. Steinwachs MR, Guggi T, Kreuz PC. Marrow stimulation techniques. Injury. 2008;39(Suppl 1):S26–31.
2. Pearle AD, Warren RF, Rodeo SA. Basic science of articular cartilage and osteoarthritis. Clin Sports Med. 2005;24:1–12.
3. Shah MR, Kaplan KM, Meislin RJ, Bosco JA 3rd. Articular cartilage restoration of the knee. Bull NYU Hosp Jt Dis. 2007;65(1):51–60.
4. Theodorides AA, Williams A, Guthrie H, Church S. Diagnosis and management of chondral delamination injuries of the knee. Knee. 2019;26(3):647–52.
5. Mats B, Andreas HG, José AC, Jack F, Martin L, James H. Cartilage repair in the degenerative ageing knee. Acta Orthopaedica. 2016;87(sup363):26–38.
6. Heir S, Nerhus TK, Røtterud JH, Løken S, Ekeland A, Engebretsen L, Arøen A. Focal cartilage defects in the knee impair quality of life as much as severe osteoarthritis: a comparison of knee injury and osteoarthritis outcome score in 4 patient categories scheduled for knee surgery. Am J Sports Med. 2010;38(2):231–7. https://doi.org/10.1177/0363546509352157. Epub 2009 Dec 30.
7. Davies-Tuck ML, Wluka AE, Wang Y, Teichtahl AJ, Jones G, Ding C, et al. The natural history of cartilage defects in people with knee osteoarthritis. Osteoarthritis Cartil. 2008;16(3):337–42.
8. Stanish WD, McCormack R, Forriol F, Mohtadi N, Pelet S, Desnoyers J, et al. Novel scafold-based BST–CarGel treatment results in superior cartilage repair compared with microfracture in a randomized controlled trial. J Bone Joint Surg Am. 2013;95(18):1640–50.
9. Knutsen G, Drogset JO, Engebretsen L, Grøntvedt T, Isaksen V, Ludvigsen TC, et al. A randomized trial comparing autologous chondrocyte implantation with microfracture. Findings at five years. J Bone Joint Surg Am. 2007;89(10):2105–12.
10. Gomoll AH, Farr J, Gillogly SD, Kercher JS, Minas T. Surgical management of articular cartilage defects of the knee. Instr Course Lect. 2011;60:461–83.
11. Buckwalter JA, Mankin HJ, Grodzinsky AJ. Articular cartilage and osteoarthritis. Instr Course Lect. 2005;54:465–80.
12. Mandelbaum BR, Browne JE, Fu F, Micheli L, Mosely JB, Erggelet C, Minas T, Peterson L. Articular cartilage lesions of the knee. Am J Sports Med. 1998;26:853–61.
13. Potter HG, le Chong R, Sneag DB. Magnetic resonance imaging of cartilage repair. Sports Med Arthrosc Rev. 2008;16(4):236–45.
14. Welsch GH, Mamisch TC, Quirbach S, Zak L, Marlovits S, Trattnig S. Evaluation and comparison of cartilage repair tissue of the patella and medial femoral condyle by using morphological MRI and biochemical zonal T2 mapping. Eur Radiol. 2009 May;19(5):1253–62.
15. Widuchowski W, Widuchowski J, Trzaska T. Articular cartilage defects: study of 25,124 knee arthroscopies. Knee. 2007;14(3):177–82.
16. Slattery C, Kweon CY. Classifications in brief: outer bridge classification of chondral lesions. Clin Orthop Relat Res. 2018;476(10):2101–4.
17. ICRS Cartilage injury evaluation package 2000. https://cartilage.org/content/uploads/2014/10/ICRS_evaluation.pdf
18. Ronga M, Stissi P, Barbera LAG, Valoroso M, Angeretti G, Genovese E, Cherubino P. Treatment of unstable osteochondritis dissecans in adults with autogenous osteochondral grafts (Mosaicplasty): long-term results. Joints. 2016;3(4):173–8.
19. Mithoefer K, Saris DB, Farr J, Kon E, Zaslav K, Cole BJ, Ranstam J, Yao J, Shive M, Levine D, Dalemans W, Brittberg M. Guidelines for the design and conduct of clinical studies in knee articular cartilage repair: international cartilage repair society recommendations based on current scientific evidence and standards of clinical care. Cartilage. 2011;2(2):100–21.
20. Bedi A, Feeley BT, Williams RJ. Management of articular cartilage defects of the knee. J Bone Joint Surg Am. 2010;92(4):994–1009.
21. Brittberg M, Lindahl A, Nilsson A, Ohlsson C, Isaksson O, Peterson L. Treatment of deep cartilage defects in the knee with autologous chondrocyte transplantation. N Engl J Med. 1994;331:889–95.
22. Jones KJ, Kelley B, Arshi A, McAllister DR, Fabricant PD. Comparative effectiveness of cartilage repair with respect to the minimal clinically important difference. Am J Sports Med. 2019;47:3284–93.

23. Vonk LA, Roël G, Hernigou J, Kaps C, Hernigou P. Role of matrix-associated autologous chondrocyte implantation with spheroids in the treatment of large chondral defects in the knee: a systematic review. Int J Mol Sci. 2021;22(13):7149.
24. Aşık M, Bozkurt M, Tandoğan NR, Elmalı N, Aktekin CN. Kıkırdak Tusyad Eğitici Kitap Serisi. İstanbul Tıp Kitap Evleri; 2016.
25. Williams RJ 3rd, Harnly HW. Microfracture: indications, technique, and results. Instr Course Lect. 2007;56:419–28.
26. Frisbie DD, Oxford JT, Southwood L, Trotter GW, Rodkey WG, Steadman JR, Goodnight JL, McIlwraith CW. Early events in cartilage repair after subchondral bone microfracture. Clin Orthop Relat Res. 2003;407:215–27.
27. Frisbie DD, Trotter GW, Powers BE, Rodkey WG, Steadman JR, Howard RD, Park RD, McIlwraith CW. Arthroscopic subchondral bone plate microfracture technique augment shealing of large chondral defects in the radial carpal bone and medial femoral condyle of horses. Vet Surg. 1999;28:242–55.
28. Frisbie DD, Morisset S, Ho CP, Rodkey WG, Steadman JR, McIlwraith CW. Effects of calcified cartilage on healing of chondral defects treated with microfracture in horses. Am J Sports Med. 2006;34:1824–31.
29. Stafford GH, Bunn JR, Villar RN. Arthroscopic repair of delaminated acetabular articular cartilage using fibrin adhesive. Results at one to three years. Hip Int. 2011;21(6):744–50.
30. Hoemann CD, Hurtig M, Rossomacha E, Sun J, Chevrier A, Shive MS, Buschmann MD. Chitosan-glycerol phosphate/blood implants improve hyaline cartilage repair in ovine microfracture defects. J Bone Joint Surg Am. 2005;87:2671–86.
31. Fortier LA, Nixon AJ, Lust G. Phenotypic expression of equine articular chondrocytes grown in three-dimensional cultures supplemented with supra physiologic concentrations of insulin-like growth factor-1. Am J Vet Res. 2002;63:301–5.
32. Nixon AJ, Haupt JL, Frisbie DD, Morisset SS, McIlwraith CW, Robbins PD, Evans CH, Ghivizzani S. Gene-mediated restoration of cartilagematrix bycombinationinsulin-likegrowthfactor-I/interleukin-1 receptor antagonist therapy. Gene Ther. 2005;12:177–86.
33. Kieswetter K, Schwartz Z, Alderete M, Dean DD, Boyan BD. Platelet derived growth factor stimulate schondrocyte proliferation but prevents endochondral maturation. Endocrine. 1997;6:257–64.
34. Lohmann CH, Schwartz Z, Niederauer GG, Carnes DL Jr, Dean DD, Boyan BD. Pretreatment with platelet derived growth factor-BB modulates the ability of costochondral resting zone chondrocytes incorporated into PLA/PGA scaffolds to form new cartilage in vivo. Biomaterials. 2000;21:49–61.
35. Strauss E, Schachter A, Frenkel S, Rosen J. The efficacy of intra-articular hyaluronan injection after the microfracture technique for the treatment of articular cartilage lesions. Am J Sports Med. 2009;37:720–6.
36. Sun Y, Feng Y, Zhang CQ, Chen SB, Cheng XG. The regenerative effect of platelet-rich plasma on healing in large osteochondral defects. Int Orthop. 2009;34:589.
37. Mishra A, Tummala P, King A, Lee B, Kraus M, Tse V, Jacobs CR. Buffered platelet-rich plasma enhances mesenchymal stem cell proliferation and chondrogenic differentiation. Tissue Eng Part C Methods. 2009;15:431–5.
38. Akeda K, An HS, Okuma M, Attawia M, Miyamoto K, Thonar EJ, Lenz ME, Sah RL, Masuda K. Platelet-richplasmastimulatesporcinearticularchondrocyteproliferation and matrix biosynthesis. Osteoarthritis Cartilage. 2006;14:1272–80.
39. Rose T, Craatz S, Hepp P, Raczynski C, Weiss J, Josten C, Lill H. The autologous osteochondral transplantation of the knee: clinical results, radiographic findings and histological aspects. Arch Orthop Trauma Surg. 2005;125:628–37.
40. Hangody L, Vásárhelyi G, Hangody LR, Sükösd Z, Tibay G, Bartha L, Bodó G. Autologous osteochondral grafting—technique and long-term results. Injury. 2008;39(Suppl 1):S32–9.
41. Brittberg M, Lindahl A, Nillson A, Ohlsson C, Isaksson O, Peterson L. Treatment of deep cartilage defects in the knee with autologous chondrocyte transplantation. N Engl J Med. 1994;331:889–95.
42. Kish G, Hangody L. A prospective, randomised comparison of autologouschondrocyteimplantationversusmosaicplastyforosteochondraldefects in the knee. J Bone Joint Surg Br. 2004;86:619.
43. Gikas PD, Aston WJ, Briggs TW. Autologous chondrocyte implantation: where do west and now? J Orthop Sci. 2008;13:283–92.
44. Anderson AF, Fu F, Mandelbaum B. A controlled study of autologous chondrocyte implantation vs microfracture for articular cartilage lesions of the femur. In: Read at the 69th Annual Meeting of the American Academy of Orthopaedic Surgeons 13–17, Dallas, TX; 2002.
45. Mithoefer K, McAdams T, Williams RJ, Kreuz PC, Mandelbaum BR. Clinical efficacy of the microfracture technique for articular cartilage repair in the knee: an evidence-based systematic analysis. Am J Sports Med. 2009;37:2053–63.
46. Bentley G, Biant LC, Carrington RW, Akmal M, Goldberg A, Williams AM, SkinnerJA, Pringle J. A prospective, randomised comparison of autologous chondrocyte implantation versus mosaicplasty for osteochondral defects in the knee. J Bone Joint Surg Br. 2003;85:223–30.
47. Peterson L, Minas T, Brittberg M, Nilsson A, Sjogren-Jansson E, LindahlA. Two-to 9-year outcome after autologous chondrocyte transplantation of the knee. Clin Orthop Relat Res. 2000;374:212–34.
48. Minas T. Autologous chondrocyte implantation for focal chondral defects of the knee. Clin Orthop Relat Res. 2001;391(Suppl):S349–61.

49. Kreuz PC, Steinwachs, Erggelet C, Krause SJ, Ossendorf C, Maier D, Ghanem N, Uhl M, Haag M. Classification of graft hypertrophy after autologous chondrocyte implantation of full-thickness chondral defects in the knee. Osteoarthr Cartil. 2007;15:1339–47.
50. Bartlett W, Gooding CR, Carrington RW, Skinner JA, Briggs TW, Bentley G. Autologous chondrocyte implantation at the knee using a bilayer collagen membrane with bone graft. A preliminary report. J Bone Joint Surg Br. 2005;87:330–2.
51. Filova E, Jelínek F, Handl M, Lytvynets A, Rampichová M, Varga F, Cinátl J, Soukup T, Trc T, Amler E. Novel composite hyaluronan/type I collagen/fibrin scaffold enhances repair of osteochondral defect in rabbit knee. J Biomed Mater Res B Appl Biomater. 2008;87:415–24.
52. Schlegel W, Nurnberger S, Hombauer M, Albrecht C, Vecsei V, Marlovits S. Scaffold-dependent differentiation of human articularchondrocytes. Int J Mol Med. 2008;22:691–9.
53. Bugbee WD. Fresh osteochondral allografts. J Knee Surg. 2002;15:191–5. Bakay A, Cs¨onge L, Papp G, Fekete L. Osteochondralresurfacing of thekneejointwithallograft. Clinicalanalysis of 33 cases. IntOrthop 1998;22:277–81.
54. Beaver RJ, Mahomed M, Backstein D, Davis A, Zukor DJ, Gross AE. Fresh osteochondral allografts for post-traumatic defects in the knee. A survivorship analysis. J Bone Joint Surg Br. 1992;74:105–10.
55. Minas T, Gomoll AH, Rosenberger R, Royce RO, Bryant T. Increased failure rate of autologous chondrocyte implantation after previous treatment with marrow stimulation techniques. Am J Sports Med. 2009;37(5):902–8.
56. Duncan RC, Hay EM, Saklatvala J, Croft PR. Prevalence of radiographic osteoarthritis—it all depends on your point of view. Rheumatology (Oxford). 2006;45(6):757–60.
57. Hart HF, Stefanik JJ, Wyndow N, Machotka Z, Crossley KM. The prevalence of radiographic and MRI-defined patellofemoral osteoarthritis and structural pathology: a systematic review and meta-analysis. Br J Sports Med. 2017;51(16):1195–208.
58. Nomura E, Inoue M, Kurimura M. Chondral and osteochondral injuries associated with acute patellar dislocation. Arthroscopy. 2003;19(7):717–21.
59. Gomoll AH, Gillogly SD, Cole BJ, Farr J, Arnold R, Hussey K, et al. Autologous chondrocyte implantation in the patella: a multi center experience. Am J Sports Med. 2014;42(5):1074–81. This is a multi center study showing good ACI outcomes for the PFJ and its applicability on bipolar lesions.
60. Strauss EJ, Galos DK. The evaluation and management of cartilage lesions affecting the patellofemoral joint. Curr Rev Musculoskelet Med. 2013;6:141.
61. Flanigan DC, Harris JD, Trinh TQ, Siston RA, Brophy RH. Prevalence of chondral defects in athletes' knees: a systematic review. Med Sci Sports Exerc. 2010;42(10):1795–801.
62. Werner S. Anterior knee pain: an update of physical therapy. Knee Surg Sports Traumatol Arthrosc. 2014;22(10):2286–94.
63. Mosier BA, Arendt EA, Dahm DL, Dejour D, Gomoll AH. Management of patellofemoral arthritis: from cartilage restoration to arthroplasty. Instr Course Lect. 2017;66:531–42.
64. Montgomery SR, Foster BD, Ngo SS, Terrell RD, Wang JC, Petrigliano FA, et al. Trends in the surgical treatment of articular cartilage defects of the knee in the United States. Knee Surg Sports Traumatol Arthrosc. 2014;22(9):2070–5.
65. Grieshober JA, Stanton M, Gambardella R. Debridement of articular cartilage: the natural course. Sports Med Arthrosc. 2016;24(2):56–62.
66. Kaplan LD, Chu CR, Bradley JP, Fu FH, Studer RK. Recovery of chondrocyte metabolic activity after thermal exposure. Am J Sports Med. 2003;31(3):392–8.
67. Anderson DE, Rose MB, Wille AJ, Wiedrick J, Crawford DC. Arthroscopic mechanical chondroplasty of the knee is beneficial for treatment of focal cartilage lesions in the absence of concurrent pathology. Orthop J Sports Med. 2017;5(5):2325967117707213.
68. Federico DJ, Reider B. Results of isolated patellar debridement for patellofemoral pain in patients with normal patellar alignment. Am J Sports Med. 1997;25(5):663–9.
69. Steadman JR, Rodkey WG, Rodrigo JJ. Microfracture: surgical technique and rehabilitation to treat chondral defects. Clin Orthop Relat Res. 2001;391(Suppl):S362–9.
70. Steadman JR, Rodkey WG, Briggs KK. Microfracture to treat full thickness chondral defects: surgical technique, rehabilitation, and outcomes. J Knee Surg. 2002;15(3):170–6.
71. Kreuz PC, Steinwachs MR, Erggelet C, Krause SJ, Konrad G, UhlM, et al. Results after microfracture of full-thickness chondral defects in different compartments in the knee. Osteoarthr Cartil. 2006;14(11):1119–25.
72. Moatshe G, Morris ER, Cinque ME, Pascual-Garrido C, Chahla J, Engebretsen L, et al. Biological treatment of the knee with platelet-rich plasma or bone marrow aspirate concentrates. Acta Orthop. 2017;88:1–5.
73. Welch T, Mandelbaum B, Tom M. Autologous chondrocyte implantation: past, present, and future. Sports Med Arthrosc. 2016;24(2):85–91.
74. Niemeyer P, Lenz P, Kreuz PC, Salzmann GM, Sudkamp NP, Schmal H, et al. Chondrocyte-seeded type I/III collagen membrane for autologous chondrocyte transplantation: prospective 2-year results in patients with cartilage defects of the knee joint. Arthroscopy. 2010;26(8):1074–82.
75. Gille J, Behrens P, Schulz AP, Oheim R, Kienast B. Matrix associated autologous chondrocyte implantation: a clinical follow-up at 15 years. Cartilage. 2016;7(4):309–15.

76. Gomoll AH, Ambra LF, Phan A, Mastrocola M, Shah N. Cell seeded autologous chondrocyte implantation: a simplified implantation technique that maintains high clinical outcomes. Am J Sports Med. 2017;45(5):1028–36.
77. Minas T, Gomoll AH, Solhpour S, Rosenberger R, ProbstC, Bryant T. Autologous chondrocyte implantation for joint preservation in patients with early osteoarthritis. Clin Orthop Relat Res. 2010;468(1):147–57.
78. Minas T, VonKeudell A, Bryant T, Gomoll AH. The John Insall award: a minimum 10-year out come study of autologous chondrocyte implantation. Clin Orthop Relat Ress. 2014;472(1):41–51. Study with a large 198 Curr Rev Musculoskelet Med (2018) 11:188–200.
79. Ossendorf C, Steinwachs MR, Kreuz PC, Osterhoff G, LahmA, Ducommun PP, et al. Autologous chondrocyte implantation (ACI) for the treatment of large and complex cartilage lesions of the knee. Sports Med Arthrosc Rehabil Ther Technol. 2011;3:11.
80. Ambra LF, de Girolamo L, Mosier B, Gomoll AH. Review: interventions for cartilage disease: current state-of-the-art and emerging technologies. Arthritis Rheumatol. 2017;69(7):1363–73.
81. Garretson RB 3rd, Katolik LI, Verma N, Beck PR, Bach BR, Cole BJ. Contact pressure at osteochondral donor sites in the patellofemoral joint. Am J Sports Med. 2004;32(4):967–74.
82. McCoy B, Miniaci A. Osteochondral autograft transplantation/mosaicplasty. J Knee Surg. 2012;25(2):99–108.
83. Nakagawa Y, Suzuki T, Kuroki H, Kobayashi M, Okamoto Y, Nakamura T. The effect of surface incongruity of grafted plugs in osteochondral grafting: a report of five cases. Knee Surg Sports Traumatol Arthrosc. 2007;15(5):591–6.
84. Hangody L, Rathonyi GK, Duska Z, Vasarhelyi G, Fules P, Modis L. Autologous osteochondral mosaicplasty. Surgical technique. J Bone Joint Surg Am. 2004;86-A(Suppl 1):65–72.
85. Yabumoto H, Nakagawa Y, Mukai S, Saji T. Osteochondral autograft transplantation for isolated patello femoral osteoarthritis. Knee. 2017;24:1498–503.
86. Zouzias IC, Bugbee WD. Osteochondral allograft transplantation in the knee. Sports Med Arthrosc. 2016;24(2):79–84.
87. Determann JR, Fleischli JE, D'Alessandro DF, Piasecki DP. Patello femoral osteochondral allografts: can we improve the matching process? J Knee Surg. 2017;30(8):835–41.
88. McCormick F, Harris JD, Abrams GD, Frank R, Gupta A, Hussey K, et al. Trends in the surgical treatment of articular cartilage lesions in the United States: an analysis of a large private-payer database over a period of 8 years. Arthroscopy. 2014;30(2):222–6.
89. Hunt HE, Sadr K, Deyoung AJ, Gortz S, Bugbee WD. The role of immunologic response in fresh osteochondral allografting of the knee. Am J Sports Med. 2014;42(4):886–91.
90. Meyer MA, MA MC, Gitelis ME, Poland SG, Urita A, Chubinskaya S, et al. Effectiveness of lavage techniques in removing immunogenic elements from osteochondral allografts. Cartilage. 2017;8(4):369–73.
91. Sun Y, Jiang W, Cory E, Caffrey JP, Hsu FH, Chen AC, et al. Pulsed lavage cleansing of osteochondral grafts depends on lavage duration, flow intensity, and graft storage condition. PLoS One. 2017;12(5):e0176934.
92. Oladeji LO, Stannard JP, Cook CR, Kfuri M, Crist BD, Smith MJ, et al. Effects of autogenous bone marrow aspirate concentrate on radiographic integration of femoral condylar osteochondral allografts. Am J Sports Med. 2017;45(12):2797–803.
93. Gracitelli GC, Moraes VY, Franciozi CE, Luzo MV, Belloti JC. Surgical interventions (microfracture, drilling, mosaicplasty, and allograft transplantation) for treating isolated cartilage defects of the knee in adults. Cochrane Database Syst Rev. 2016;9:CD010675.
94. Jamali AA, Emmerson BC, Chung C, Convery FR, Bugbee WD. Fresh osteochondral allografts: results in the patello femoral joint. Clin Orthop Relat Res. 2005;437:176–85.
95. TorgaSpak R, Teitge RA. Fresh osteochondral allografts for patello femoralarthritis: long-term follow up. Clin Orthop Relat Res. 2006;444:193–200.
96. Assenmacher AT, Pareek A, Reardon PJ, Macalena JA, Stuart MJ, Krych AJ. Long-term outcomes after osteochondral allograft: a systematic review at long-term follow-up of 12.3 years. Arthroscopy. 2016;32(10):2160–8.
97. Bedard NA, Pugely AJ, Duchman KR, et al. When hip scopes fail, they do so quickly. J Arthroplast. 2016;31:1183–7.
98. Kemp JL, Makdissi M, Schache AG, et al. Hip chondropathy at arthroscopy: prevalence and relationship to labral pathology, femoro acetabular impingement and patient-reported outcomes. Br J Sports Med. 2014;48:1102–7.
99. Sing DC, Feeley BT, Tay B, et al. Age-related trends in hip arthroscopy: a large cross-sectional analysis. Arthroscopy. 2015;31:2307–13.
100. Schmid MR, Notzli HP, Zanetti M, et al. Cartilage lesions in the hip: diagnostic effectiveness of MR arthrography. Radiology. 2003;226:382–6.
101. McCarthy JC, Noble PC, Schuck MR, et al. The Otto E. Aufranc award: the role of labral lesions to development of early degenerative hip disease. Clin Orthop Relat Res. 2001;393:25–37.
102. Beck M, Kalhor M, Leunig M, Ganz R. Hip morphology influences the pattern of damage to the acetabular cartilage: femoro acetabular impingement as a cause of early osteoarthritis of the hip. J Bone Joint Surg Br. 2005;87:1012–8.
103. Outerbridge RE. The etiology of chondromalacia patellae. J Bone Joint Surg Br. 1961;43-B:752–7.

104. Ilizaliturri VM Jr, Byrd JW, Sampson TG, et al. A geographic zone method to describe intra-articular pathology in hip arthroscopy: cadaveric study and preliminary report. Arthroscopy. 2008;24:534–9.
105. Fortun CM, Streit J, Patel SH, Salata MJ. Cartilage defects in the hip. Oper Tech Sports Med. 2012;20:287–94.
106. Yen YM, Kocher MS. Chondral lesions of the hip: microfracture and chondroplasty. Sports Med Arthrosc. 2010;18:83–9.
107. Mardones R, Larrain C. Cartilage restoration technique of the hip. J Hip Preserv Surg. 2016;3:30–6.
108. McGill KC, Bush-Joseph CA, Nho SJ. Hip microfracture: indications, technique, and outcomes. Cartilage. 2010;1:127–36.
109. Al-Qarni A, Lewington MR, Wong IH. Reconstruction of focal femoral head cartilage defects with a chitin-based scaffold. Arthrosc Tech. 2016;5:e257–62.
110. Fontana A, de Girolamo L. Sustained five-year benefit of autologous matrix-induced chondrogenesis for femoral acetabular impingement-induced chondral lesions compared with microfracture treatment. Bone Joint J. 2015;97-B:628–35.
111. Mancini D, Fontana A. Five-year results of arthroscopic techniques for the treatment of acetabular chondral lesions in femoroacetabular impingement. Int Orthop. 2014;38:2057–64.
112. Petit CJ, Philippon MJ. Arthroscopic management of osteochondral defects of the hip. Oper Tech Sports Med. 2008;16:194–200.
113. Logan ZS, Redmond JM, Spelsberg SC, et al. Chondral lesions of the hip. Clin Sports Med. 2016;35:361–72.
114. Cetinkaya S, Toker B, Taser O. Arthroscopic retrograde osteochondral autologous transplantation to chondral lesion in femoral head. Orthopedics. 2014;37:e600–4.
115. Milano G, SannaPassino E, Deriu L, et al. The effect of platelet rich plasma combined with microfractures on the treatment of chondral defects: an experimental study in a sheep model. Osteoarthritis Cartilage. 2010;18:971–80.
116. Stuhlman CR, Krych AJ, Levy BA, Kelly BT. Cartilage restoration of the hip. Oper Tech Sports Med. 2015;23:175–83.
117. Krych AJ, Lorich DG, Kelly BT. Treatment of focal osteochondral defects of the acetabulum with osteochondral allograft transplantation. Orthopedics. 2011;34:e307–11.
118. Oladeji LO, Cook JL, Stannard JP, Crist BD. Large fresh osteochondral allografts for the hip: growing the evidence. Hip Int. 2018;28:284–90.
119. Boraiah S, Paul O, Parker RJ, Miller AN, Hentel KD, Lorich DG. Osteochondral lesions of talus associated with ankle fractures. Foot Ankle Int. 2009;30(6):481–5.
120. Kuettner KE, Cole AA. Cartilage degeneration in different human joints. Osteoarthritis Cartilage. 2005;13(2):93–103.
121. Canale ST, Belding RH. Osteochondral lesions of the talus. J Bone Joint Surg Am. 1980;62(1):97–102.
122. Elias I, Zoga AC, Morrison WB, Besser MP, Schweitzer ME, Raikin SM. Osteochondral lesions of the talus: localization and morphologic data from 424 patients using a novel anatomical grid scheme. Foot Ankle Int. 2007;28(2):154–61.
123. Schachter AK, Chen AL, Reddy PD, Tejwani NC. Osteochondral lesions of the talus. J Am Acad Orthop Surg. 2005;13(3):152–8.
124. Verhagen RA, Struijs PA, Bossuyt PM, van Dijk CN. Systematic review of treatment strategies for osteochondral defects of the talar dome. Foot Ankle Clin. 2003;8(2):233–42.
125. Hannon CP, Smyth NA, Murawski CD, Savage-Elliott I, Deyer TW, Calder JD, et al. Osteochondral lesions of the talus: aspects of current management. Bone Joint J. 2014;96:164.
126. Zengerink M, Struijs PA, Tol JL, van Dijk CN. Treatment of osteochondral lesions of the talus: a systematic review. Knee Surg Sports Traumatol Arthrosc. 2010;18(2):238–46.
127. McGahan PJ, Pinney SJ. Current concept review: osteochondral lesions of the talus. Foot Ankle Int. 2010;31(1):90–101.
128. Cuttica DJ, Smith WB, Hyer CF, Philbin TM, Berlet GC. Osteochondral lesions of the talus: predictors of clinical outcome. Foot Ankle Int. 2011;32(11):1045–51.
129. Deol PP, Cuttica DJ, Smith WB, Berlet GC. Osteochondral lesions of the talus: size, age, and predictors of outcomes. Foot Ankle Clin. 2013;18(1):13–34.
130. Gilbert JE. Current treatment options for the restoration of articular cartilage. Am J Knee Surg. 1998;11(1):42–6.
131. O Farrell TA, Costello BG. Osteochondritis dissecans of the talus. The late results of surgical treatment. J Bone Joint Surg Br. 1982;64(4):494–7.
132. Alexander AH, Lichtman DM. Surgical treatment of trans chondral talar-dome fractures (osteochondritis dissecans). Long-term follow-up. J Bone Joint Surg Am. 1980;62(4):646–52.
133. Huylebroek JF, Martens M, Simon JP. Transchondral Talar Dome fracture. Arch Orthop Trauma Surg. 1985;104(4):238–41.
134. Chuckpaiwong B, Berkson EM, Theodore GH. Microfracture for osteochondral lesions of the ankle: outcome analysis and outcome predictors of 105 cases. Arthroscopy. 2008;24(1):106–12.
135. Nickisch F, Barg A, Saltzman CL, et al. Post operative complications of posterior ankle and hindfoot arthroscopy. J Bone Joint Surg Am. 2012;94(5):439–46.
136. Lui TH. Arthroscopic bone grafting of talar bone cyst using posterior ankle arthroscopy. J Foot Ankle Surg. 2013;52(4):529–32.
137. Kim HN, Kim GL, Park JY, Woo KJ, Park YW. Fixation of a posteromedial osteochondral lesion of the talus using a three-portal poste-

rior arthroscopic technique. J Foot Ankle Surg. 2013;52(3):402–5.
138. Kreuz PC, Steinwachs M, Erggelet C, Lahm A, Henle P, Niemeyer P. Mosaicplasty with autogenous talar autograft for osteochondral lesions of the talus after failed primary arthroscopic management: a prospective study with a 4-year follow-up. Am J Sports Med. 2006;34(1):55–63.
139. G. J. The juxtoretroperoneal route in the operative treatment of fracture of the malleolus with posterior margin fragment. Surg Gynecol Obstet. 1931;52:67–70.
140. Loomer R, Fisher C, Lloyd-Smith R, Sisler J, Cooney T. Osteochondral lesions of the talus. Am J Sports Med. 1993;21(1):13–9.
141. Becher C, Driessen A, Hess T, Longo UG, Maffulli N, Thermann H. Microfracture for chondral defects of the talus: maintenance of early results at midterm follow-up. Knee Surg Sports Traumatol Arthrosc. 2010;18(5):656–63.
142. Park HW, Lee KB. Comparison of chondral versus osteochondral lesions of the talus after arthroscopic microfracture. Knee Surg Sports Traumatol Arthrosc. 2015;23(3):860–7.
143. Gobbi A, Francisco RA, Lubowitz JH, Allegra F, Canata G. Osteochondral lesions of the talus: randomized controlled trial comparing chondroplasty, microfracture, and osteochondral autograft transplantation. Arthroscopy. 2006;22(10):1085–92.
144. Taranow WS, Bisignani GA, Towers JD, Conti SF. Retrograde drilling of osteochondral lesions of the medial talar dome. Foot Ankle Int. 1999;20(8):474–80.
145. Kerimaa P, Ojala R, Sinikumpu JJ, et al. MRI-guided percutaneous retro grade drilling of osteochondritis dissecans of the talus: a feasibility study. Eur Radiol. 2014;24(7):1572–6.
146. Hoffmann M, Schroeder M, Rueger JM. A novel computer navigation system for retro grade drilling of osteochondral lesions. Sports Med Arthrosc Rev. 2014;22(4):215–8.
147. Fractures JCD. Fractures and dislocations of the foot. (ed 1991.150) Stone JW. Osteochondral lesions of the Talar Dome. J Am Acad Orthop Surg. 1996;4(2):63–73.
148. Stone JW. Osteochondral lesions of the Talar Dome. J Am Acad Orthop Surg. 1996;4(2):63–73.
149. Chandran PKR, Nihal A. Osteochondral fracture of talus treated with bio absorbable pins. Foot. 2008;18:56.
150. Giannini S, Buda R, Vannini F, DiCaprio F, Grigolo B. Arthroscopic autologous chondrocyte implantation in osteochondral lesions of the talus: surgical technique and results. Am J Sports Med. 2008;36(5):873–80.
151. Mitchell ME, Giza E, Sullivan MR. Cartilage transplantation techniques for talar cartilage lesions. J Am Acad Orthop Surg. 2009;17(7):407–14.
152. Botchwey EA, Dupree MA, Pollack SR, Levine EM, Laurencin CT. Tissue engineered bone: measurement of nutrient transport in three dimensional matrices. J Biomed Mater Res A. 2003;67(1):357–67.
153. Whittaker JP, Smith G, Makwana N, et al. Early results of autologous chondrocyte implantation in the talus. J Bone Joint Surg Br. 2005;87(2):179–83.
154. Anders S, Goetz J, Schubert T, Grifka J, Schaumburger J. Treatment of deep particular talus lesions by matrix associated autologous chondrocyte implantation results at five years. Int Orthop. 2012;36(11):2279–85.
155. Scranton PE Jr, McDermott JE. Treatment of type V osteochondral lesions of the talus with ipsilateral knee osteochondral autografts. Foot Ankle Int. 2001;22(5):380–4.
156. Hangody L, Kish G, Kárpáti Z, Szerb I, Eberhardt R. Treatment of osteochondritis dissecans of the talus: use of themosaicplasty technique a preliminary report. Foot Ankle Int. 1997;18(10):628–34.
157. Sammarco GJ, Makwana NK. Treatment of talar osteochondral lesions usinglocalosteochondral graft. Foot Ankle Int. 2002;23(8):693–8.
158. Gross AE, Agnidis Z, Hutchison CR. Osteochondral defects of the talus treated with fresh osteochondral allograft transplantation. Foot Ankle Int. 2001;22(5):385–91.
159. Chang E, Lenczner E. Osteochondritis dissecans of the talar dome treated with an osteochondral autograft. Can J Surg J can Chirurgie. 2000;43(3):217. Jun Central PMCID: 3695165
160. Irwin TA, Kou JX, Fortin PT. Classification and treatment of severe ankle articular segment deficits: osteochondral allograft reconstruction. Foot Ankle Clin. 2007;12(1):41–55.
161. Berlet GC, Hyer CF, Philbin TM, Hartman JF, Wright ML. Does fresh osteochondral allograft transplantation of talar osteochondral defects improve function? Clin Orthop Relat Res. 2011;469(8):2356–66.
162. Cole BJ, Yanke A, Provencher MT. Non arthroplasty alternatives for the treatment of glenohumeral arthritis. J Shoulder Elbow Surg. 2007;16(5 Suppl):S231–40.
163. Richter DL, Schenck RC Jr, Wascher DC, Treme G. Knee articular cartilage repair and restoration techniques: a review of the literature. Sports Health. 2016;8(2):153–60.
164. Serrato JA Jr, Fleckenstein CM, Hasan SS. Glenohumeral chondrolysis associated with use of an intra-articular pain pump delivering local anesthetics following manipulation under anesthesia: a report of four cases. J Bone Joint Surg Am. 2011;93(17):e99(1–8).
165. Bailie DS, Ellenbecker TS. Severe chondrolysis after shoulder arthroscopy: a case series. J Shoulder Elbow Surg. 2009;18(5):742–7.
166. McNickle AG, L'Heureux DR, Provencher MT, Romeo AA, Cole BJ. Postsurgical glenohumeral arthritis in young adults. Am J Sports Med. 2009;37(9):1784–91.

167. Lunden JB, Legrand AB. Osteochondritis dissecans of the humeral head. J Orthop Sports PhysTher. 2012;42(10):886.
168. Mima Y, Matsumura N, Ogawa K, et al. Osteochondritis dissecans on the medial aspect of the humeral head. Int J Shoulder Surg. 2016;10(2):89–91.
169. McCarty LP III, Cole BJ. Nonarthroplasty treatment of glenohumeral cartilage lesions. Arthroscopy. 2005;21(9):1131–42.
170. Riboh JC, Cole BJ, Farr J. Particulated articular cartilage for symptomatic chondral defects of the knee. Curr Rev Musculoskelet Med. 2015;8(4):429–35.
171. Saltzman BM, Lin J, Lee S. Particulated juvenile articular cartilage allograft transplantation for osteochondral talar lesions. Cartilage. 2017;8(1):61–72.
172. Kerr BJ, McCarty EC. Outcome of arthroscopic débridement is worse for patients with glenohumeral arthritis of both sides of the joint. Clin Orthop Relat Res. 2008;466(3):634–8.
173. Frank RM, Van Thiel GS, Slabaugh MA, Romeo AA, Cole BJ, Verma NN. Clinical outcomes after microfracture of the glenohumeral joint. Am J Sports Med. 2010;38(4):772–81.
174. Millett PJ, Huffard BH, Horan MP, Hawkins RJ, Steadman JR. Outcomes of full-thickness articular cartilage injuries of the shoulder treated with microfracture. Arthroscopy. 2009;25(8):856–63.
175. Snow M, Funk L. Microfracture of chondral lesions of the glenohumeral joint. Int J Shoulder Surg. 2008;2(4):72–6.
176. Scheibel M, Bartl C, Magosch P, Lichtenberg S, Habermeyer P. Osteochondral autologous transplantation for the treatment of full-thickness articular cartilage defects of the shoulder. J Bone Joint Surg Br. 2004;86(7):991–7.
177. Kircher J, Patzer T, Magosch P, Lichtenberg S, Habermeyer P. Osteochondral autologous transplantation for the treatment of full-thickness cartilage defect soft he shoulder: results at nine years. J Bone Joint Surg Br. 2009;91(4):499–503.
178. Samilson RL, Prieto V. Dislocation arthropathy of the shoulder. J Bone Joint Surg Am. 1983;65(4):456–60.
179. Black LO, Ko JK, Quilici SM, Crawford DC. Fresh osteochondral allograft to the humeral head for treatment of an engaging reverse Hill-Sachs lesion: technical case report and literature review. Orthop J Sports Med. 2016;4(11):2325967116670376.
180. Buchmann S, Salzmann GM, Glanzmann MC, Wörtler K, Vogt S, Imhoff AB. Early clinical and structural results after autologous chondrocyte transplantation at the glenohumeral joint. J Shoulder Elbow Surg. 2012;21(9):1213–21.

Cell and Gene Therapy for Cartilage Regeneration

18

Sevil Köse, Çağla Zübeyde Köprü, and Petek Korkusuz

18.1 Introduction: Why Is Cartilage Repair a Problem

Cartilage is an avascular specialized connective tissue that supports critical parts of the musculoskeletal, respiratory, and auditory systems in our body. It consists of mesoderm derived chondrocytes that differentiate from chondroblasts and a resilient extracellular matrix (ECM) with collagen and elastic fibers and also glycosaminoglycan (GAG), proteoglycan, glycoproteins [1]. The proportion and subclassification of the cellular and extracellular content may vary in hyaline, elastic, and fibrous cartilages. Although it is known for its flexible features due to the high level of hyaluronic acid-bound water in its ECM, lack of vascular network makes the repair challenging when the tissue is damaged mechanically. The joint cartilages are especially vulnerable to mechanical stresses and the lack of perichondrium struggles with the healing process. The synovial layer that replaces perichondrium within the knee joint is open to metabolic stresses that cause acute or chronic inflammation which may induce degenerative changes. Various joint pathologies such as rheumatoid arthritis (RA), osteonecrosis, osteochondritis dissecans, and hemarthrosis, which occur after trauma or following hemophilia, can damage the joint structures as well as damage the articular cartilage, and cause minor local injuries that lead to progressive joint degeneration [1].

One of the most common degenerative cartilage damages occurs in osteoarthritis (OA), which is a chronic, debilitating, painful, and incurable degenerative condition that causes high morbidity and mortality in a significant percentage of the human population [2]. As the most common form of arthritis, OA affects approximately 30 million individuals and causes $186 billion in economic losses each year in the USA alone [3, 4]. Knee joint OA was detected in 654.1 million people over the age of 40 in 2022 and its incidence was reported to be 203 out of 10,000 people [5]. And also in 2016, Osteoarthritis Research Society International (OARSI) defined

Sevil Köse and Çağla Zübeyde Köprü contributed equally with all other contributors.

S. Köse
Department of Plastic, Reconstructive, and Aesthetic Surgery and Advanced Research Center, Faculty of Medicine, Akdeniz University, Antalya, Turkey
e-mail: sevilkose@akdeniz.edu.tr

Ç. Z. Köprü
Department of Histology and Embryology, Faculty of Medicine, Yüksek İhtisas University, Ankara, Turkey
e-mail: caglakopru@yiu.edu.tr

P. Korkusuz (✉)
Department of Histology and Embryology, Faculty of Medicine, Hacettepe University, Ankara, Turkey

METU MEMS Center, Ankara, Türkiye
e-mail: petek@hacettepe.edu.tr

M. E. Erdil et al. (eds.), *Current Concept in Cartilage Treatment*,
https://doi.org/10.1007/978-3-032-27099-3_18

OA as a serious global disease in 9.6% of men and 18.0% of women over the age of 60 [6].

Early treatment of articular cartilage defects is crucial to prevent or delay the pathogenesis of acute and chronic arthritis. Pharmacological options used to relieve pain for most RA and OA patients include analgesics such as paracetamol, non-steroidal anti-inflammatory drugs (NSAIDs) such as ibuprofen tablets, and topical treatments such as NSAIDs capsaicin, as also immune suppressive medications [7]. However, these drugs generally do not cure the disease and their long-term use for arthritis produces adverse side effects on the renal, cardiovascular, and gastrointestinal systems [8]. A review of recent treatment guidelines shows that acetaminophen (pain reliever) is weakly recommended by European Society for Clinical and Economic Aspects of Osteoporosis (ESCEO) [9] and is not recommended by American College of Rheumatology (ACR) [10] and OARSI [11]. Recent repair strategies based on invasive surgical approaches like microfracture, osteochondral transplantation, and autologous chondrocyte implantation have several serious drawbacks like delaying cartilage degeneration only in the short-term, need several operations, and long recovery times [3, 4]. These issues underline the acute necessity for the development of newer and safer treatments for OA, placing greater emphasis on the need to understand their underlying molecular endotypes, disease phenotypes and target their associated molecules and pathways with individual differences [12] (Fig. 18.1).

Currently, cell-based therapies and gene therapies have led to significant advances in cartilage regeneration [5]. Using gene therapies to transduce therapeutic genes directly or indirectly to the site of injury has quickly become an approach to cartilage regeneration with promising results that are being tried and reflected in the clinic [13]. The purpose of this chapter is to clarify the cellular and genetic basis of chondral lesions and to provide an overview of the different approaches of the latest systems used in therapeutic cell and gene-mediated repair of cartilage tissue.

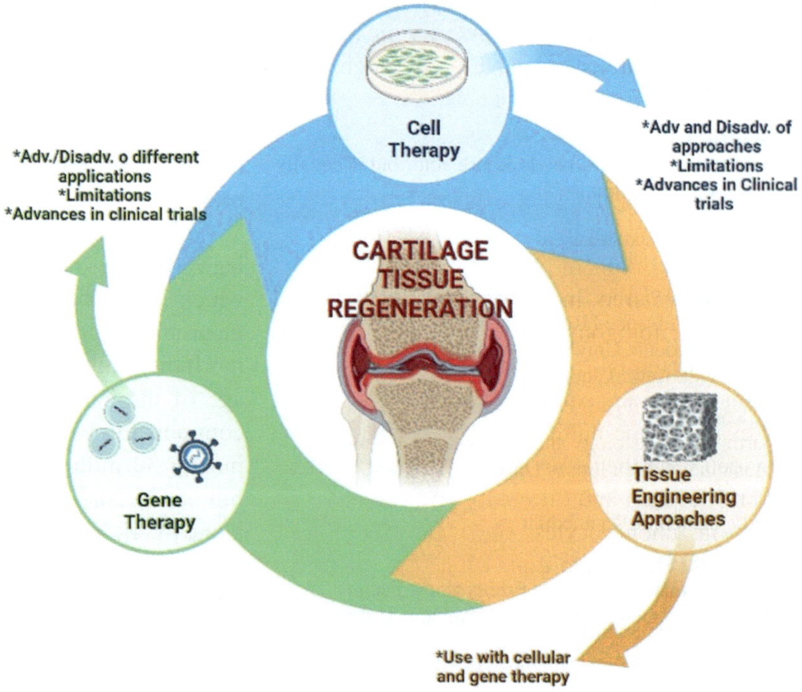

Fig. 18.1 Current therapeutic strategies for cartilage tissue regeneration

18.2 Cell Therapies for Cartilage

18.2.1 Cell Therapy Procedures in Cartilage Regeneration

Cell therapy is the name given to an approach based on the regeneration of damaged tissue using autologous or allogeneic cells. When we look at cartilage tissue regeneration specifically, we can examine cellular therapy methods under three subheadings: (1) Autologous chondrocytes, (2) Mesenchymal stem cells, and (3) Pluripotent stem cells.

18.2.1.1 Autologous Chondrocyte Implantation

Autologous chondrocyte implantation (ACI) has been performed in the clinic for about 30 years [1]. In this technique, it is important to arthroscopically collect cartilage from a low-weight area of the joint. Cartilage is enzymatically broken down to release chondrocytes, and the cells are cultured before implantation [1]. Since the joint cartilage treatment first performed by Brittber et al. in 1994, three generations of applications have been made [14]. In the first-generation practice, the autologous periosteum was sewn to the edge of the cartilage defect and chondrocytes were injected into the defective lacunae. In the second-generation application, periosteal tissue has been replaced with type I/III collagen membrane. Matrix-stimulated ACI has been performed in the third-generation application [15]. In this application, the condition of hypertrophy of chondrocytes encountered in ACI is eliminated [16]. Although autologous chondrocytes are considered as a potential treatment for cartilage regeneration, there are some limitations in practice. For example, the number of chondrocytes to be provided from the donor is limited. The potential for proliferation and differentiation is low, especially in chondrocytes obtained from elder patients [15]. In addition, ACI is a preferred option for the treatment of chondral defects larger than 2 cm^2. The culture of chondrocytes in clinical use is expensive. It also needs a good manufacturing practice (GMP) facility that can culture cells for a period of 3–6 weeks [1]. In order to overcome the limitations of ACI, an alternative strategy called minced cartilage implantation (MCI) has been developed [15]. In this application, cartilage fragments are collected during arthroscopy, broken down, and mixed. The advantage of MCI is the application of undifferentiated autologous chondrocytes without the need for cell culture or cytoskeleton when compared to ACI [17]. It is known that MCI is not effective in large defects, that is, it is a technique limited to the defect area. It is also not a technique that can be followed up for a long time. As there is an age restriction in areas such as the talus, at the same time, the defective area is not fully filled [18, 19].

18.2.1.2 Mesenchymal Stem Cells

Mesenchymal stem cells (MSCs) are multipotent stromal cells that are resident adult organs with the capacity of differentiating into mesoderm derived tissues [20]. These cells have the ability to adhere to the culture plate and can be differentiated into cartilage, bone, and adipose tissue cells under appropriate conditions [21–23]. According to the identification criteria of International Society For Cell and Gene Therapy (ISCT), cultured MSCs are CD90, CD105, and CD73 positive, while CD14, CD31, CD45, CD34, CD11b, CD79α, CD19, and HLA-DR negative [22]. The anti-inflammatory [24] and immunomodulatory [25] properties of MSCs and their potential to transform into musculoskeletal and vascular cells are increasing their field of use in the orthopedic and traumatology clinic [21, 26–29]. The autologous and allogeneic MSCs may induce regeneration by their secretomes consisting of various growth factors (transforming growth factor-β1 (TGF-β1), tumor necrosis factor-α (TNF-α), prostaglandin E2 (PGE2), interferon gamma (IFN-γ), hepatocyte growth factor (HGF), fibroblast growth factor (FGF) [30–32] and cytokines (IL-4, IL-6, IL-8, IL-10, Ang-1, CXCL5, CXCL6, and CXCL7) that mediate immunomodulation [33]. A local anti-inflammatory response in the damaged area by preventing T lymphocyte maturation and reducing macrophage activation induces/improves secretion of immunomodulatory factors [1, 34]. MSCs also promote angiogenesis and regulate the immune response [35] by secreting extracellular vesicles (EV) [36]. Preclinical studies in which EV is investigated instead of MSCs in the treatment of OA have increased in the last decade [37]. Thus, the EVs released from MSCs are also known to increase osteoblastic cell viability [38], proliferation [39], migration, vascularization, and extracellular matrix formation that contribute to rat, mouse, and pig models cartilage repair [40]. From the point of view of cartilage regeneration, MSCs are used a lot and are promising for reasons such as their ability to differentiate into chondrocytes and their ease of production. The MSCs, when used in cartilage repair, can be obtained from various autologous sources, including bone marrow (BM), adipose tissue and peripheral blood, synovium, and umbilical cord [21]. Depending on the condition of the damaged cartilage, MSCs can either be implanted after surgical incision or injected into the joint [41]. However, compared to MSCs implantation, intra-articular injections are more likely to go to non-target tissues [41] (Fig. 18.2).

Bone Marrow-Derived Mesenchymal Stem Cells

Bone marrow-derived stem cells (BM-MSCs) are found in BM cavities, and these cells are applied with cell engineering strategies in combination with BM stimulation [15, 42–47]. In this way, in situ cartilage regeneration can be achieved in one step without the need for more than one operation. For this reason, it is often used in articular cartilage in knee joints for regeneration [15]. The multipotential character of BM-MSCs is useful for tissue engineering and cartilage regeneration. At the same time, it is also an important advantage that it can be reproduced more easily than autologous chondrocytes. From a clinical point of view, there are two completed studies on BM-MSCs (Table 18.1). Also, there are quite a lot of studies on the in vitro chondrogenic differentiation of BM-MSCs [48]. Although BM-MSC transplantation is more effective than autologous chondrocyte transplantation or non-autologous chondrocyte transplantation, clinical studies have been limited due to reasons such as excessive cell requirement in the studies to be conducted with BM-MSCs and decreasing differentiation capacity with age [49].

In an ongoing study at the clinic, autologous BM-MSCs (8 out of 16 patients with knee OA, 8 with focal chondral defect in the knee) are being investigated for the reliability of intra-articular injection (ClinicalTrials.gov Id: NCT03477942). Again, another ongoing clinical study is investigating which one will be more effective when cultured MSCs or chondrocytes (alone or in combination) are applied in the treatment of cartilage damage (https://www.isrctn.com: ISRCTN98997175). BM-MSCs-derived EVs have been increasingly used in cartilage regeneration studies and showed higher EV production and secretion capacity for BM-MSCs when compared to adipose tissue-derived MSCs [50]. In a study, OA chondrocytes cultured in fibrin structures, treatment with BM-MSC EVs also increased the synthesis of type II collagen and aggrecan [40].

Adipose Tissue-Derived Stem Cells

Adipose tissue-derived stem cells (ASCs) are obtained by isolating the stromal vascular fraction (SVF) of adipose tissue [51]. Although ASCs have less chondrogenic potentials than BM-MSCs, they can be used in cartilage tissue regeneration [21]. SVF is a cell pellet that is a waste product of liposuction surgery digested by enzymes such as collagenase [51]. After a series of passaging, the adhering cells are obtained as ASCs. Both SVFs and ASCs have therapeutic potential; thus considered as an alternative to BM-MSCs because they can be obtained by a less invasive culture method and in higher quantities when compared to BM-MSC aspirates [48]. A total of 1×10^7–5×10^8 ASC is obtained routinely from 300 mL of lipoaspirate, and the viability rates are >90% [48]. In addition, ASC expansion in culture is easier than that of the BM-MSCs since their proliferation rate is higher [48]. Therefore ASCs can be cultured for long periods before aging [48]. The co-administration of ASCs with platelet rich plasma (PRP) in animal models with OA has improved knee joint function [49]. ASCs' secretory profile on cyto-

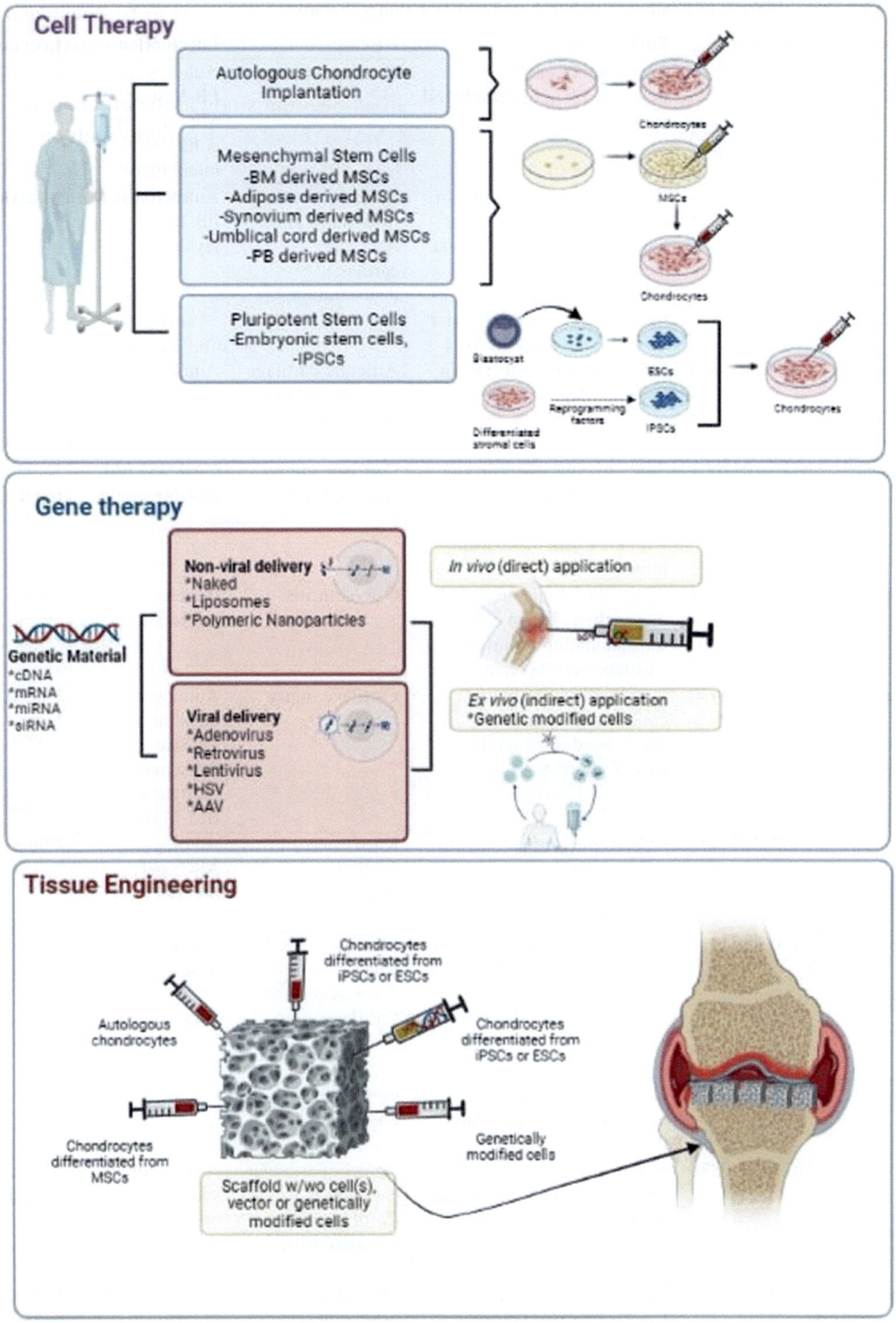

Fig. 18.2 Current tissue engineering strategies for treating cartilage lesions

Table 18.1 Clinical trials evaluating stem cell-based cartilage injury therapy

Status	Study number	Study name	Disease	Intervention	Location
Not yet recruiting	NCT04953572	Treatment of cartilage defects with peripheral blood stem cells	Cartilage injury	Autologous PB-MSCs Microfracture + collagen membrane	China
Completed	NCT03101163	Efficacy and safety study of intra-articular injections of autologous peripheral blood stem cells following subchondral drilling surgery for the treatment of articular cartilage injury in the knee	Articular cartilage disorder of knee Articular cartilage; degeneration	Autologous PB-MSCs Hyaluronic acid	Malaysia
Completed	NCT02118519	Mesenchymal stem cells in knee cartilage injuries	Articular cartilage disorder of knee Osteoarthritis, knee	Autologous MSCs	Jordan
Completed	NCT01041001	Study to compare efficacy and safety of Cartistem and microfracture in patients with knee articular cartilage injury	Cartilage injury Osteoarthritis	CARTISTEM Microfracture	Korea, republic of (and 5 more...)
Completed	NCT01895413	Autologous bone marrow mesenchymal stem cells transplantation for articular cartilage defects repair	Osteoarthritis	Bone marrow aspiration	Brazil
Completed	NCT04739930	Autologous bone marrow concentrate in knee osteochondral allograft transplantation	Cartilage injury	Autologous bone marrow aspirate Bone marrow aspirate + BM-MSCs	United States
Unknown	NCT03955497	Effectiveness of autologous adipose-derived stem cells in the treatment of knee cartilage injury	Knee osteoarthritis Cartilage degeneration	Autologous ASCs gel Sodium hyaluronate	China
Recruiting	NCT03477942	Impact of mesenchymal stem cells in knee osteoarthritis	Musculoskeletal pain Knee osteoarthritis Cartilage injury Cartilage degeneration	Autologous MSCs	United States
Recruiting	NCT05016011	Efficacy of allogeneic UCMSCs for treating large defects knee injury	Osteoarthritis, knee	UC-MSCs	Malaysia
Recruiting	NCT02696876	Synovium brushing to augmented microfracture for improved cartilage repair	Defect of articular cartilage Cartilage injury Osteoarthritis, knee	Arthroscopic synovial brushing Microfracture	United Kingdom
Completed	NCT01626677	Follow-up study of CARTISTEM® versus microfracture for the treatment of knee articular cartilage injury or defect	Degenerative osteoarthritis Defect of articular cartilage	CARTISTEM Microfracture	Korea, republic of (and 7 more...)

(continued)

Table 18.1 (continued)

Status	Study number	Study name	Disease	Intervention	Location
Recruiting	NCT03497780	Longitudinal assessment of cartilage injury and remodeling after anterior cruciate ligament rupture and reconstruction	ACL—Anterior cruciate ligament rupture ACL injury Healthy	Anterior cruciate ligament reconstruction	United States
Not yet recruiting	NCT05120700	Synovial tissue and fat pad stromal vascular fraction bioengineering in patients with knee articular cartilage injury	Cell- and tissue-based therapy Cartilage injury Knee injuries	Synovial tissue Fat pad SVF	
Completed	NCT02993510	A randomized controlled trial comparing Chondro-Gide® to microfracture alone for treatment of knee cartilage defects.	Cartilage injury Osteochondritis Dissecans	Microfracture Chondro-Gide sutured Chondro-Gide glued	Germany (and 4 more...)
Active, not recruiting	NCT01458782	ACI-C versus AMIC. A randomized trial comparing two methods for repair of cartilage defects in the knee	Osteochondritis Dissecans Osteoarthritis Cartilage injury Osteonecrosis	Treatment of cartilage defects in the knee	Norway
Completed	NCT01227694	Adult stem cell therapy for repairing articular cartilage in Gonarthrosis	Osteoarthritis, knee Knee injuries Joint diseases (and 2 more...)	Autologous MSC knee implantation	Spain
Recruiting	NCT02090140	Microfracture versus adipose derived stem cells for the treatment of articular cartilage defects	Degenerative lesion of articular cartilage of knee	ASC application Microfracture	United States

kines, chemokines, growth factors, and EVs are different from other MSC sources. For example, some markers' expression like CD34 is different in ASCs when we compared to other MSC sources. CD40d is also expressed by ASCs but not by BM-MSCs. However, CD45, CD106, CD133, and CD144 markers are expressed by BM-MSC, but not by ASCs. Also, Stro-1 expression is higher in BM-MSCs than ASCs [52]. Taken together these two mechanisms may play a role in cartilage regeneration of musculoskeletal system [51]. In a study currently underway in the clinic, ASCs are applied to patients with degenerative arthritis through arthroscopy for the purpose of cartilage regeneration (ClinicalTrials.gov Id: NCT04821102).

Synovium-Derived Stem Cells

Synovium is a thin membrane under the joint capsule replacing the perichondrium for the knee cartilage. It consists of a multilayered lining layer made up of type A macrophage like a type B fibroblast-like synoviocytes with type C reserve cells that is underlined by an areolar loose subsynovial connective tissue rich in fenestrated capillaries [53]. Synovium covers the inner cavity of the synovial joints. It provides nutrition to the cartilage with the synovial fluid it produces and the debris it phagocytoses. Synovial tissue is infiltrated by acute and chronic inflammatory cells during arthritis such as RA [54] and OA [53]. Synovium-derived MSCs (Sy-MSCs) show negative or low expression of CD34, CD45, CD14, and HLA-DR, while CD44, CD105, CD73, CD166, CD90, CD106, STRO-1 are positive [21]. Sy-MSCs show an advantage in chondrogenic differentiation compared to BM-MSCs and ASCs [20]. This superiority may be due to the fact that the gene expression profiles of Sy-MSCs and articular cartilage chondrocytes are similar [41]. They maintain their proliferation capacity even at the end of ten passages, regardless of the donor's age or place of assembly [21]. These characteristics make Sy-MSCs a suitable option in cartilage regeneration. The combination of dexamethasone, TGF-β and bone morphogenetic protein-2 (BMP-2) is suitable for the stimulation of Sy-MSCs for chondrogenesis purposes [21].

Not all cells obtained from the synovium carry the character of stem cells [55]. Whether inflammatory activity in the synovium can lead to changes in the functional characteristics of the stem cell population also requires further research [55]. For this reason, the mechanism of action of diseases such as OA is important in clarifying the character of Sy-MSCs [55]. The disadvantage of Sy-MSCs in cartilage regeneration is that these cells maintain their fibroblastic properties after implantation [56]. This limits their chondrogenic regenerative capacity. On the other hand, EVs obtained from Sy-MSCs are also becoming increasingly important in clinical applications [37]. EVs obtained from Sy-MSCs transfected with miR-140-5p have been shown to protect against OA [57]. In a mouse model of collagenase-induced OA, exosomes obtained from iPSC-MSCs show greater therapeutic effect than exosomes obtained from Sy-MSCs [58].

Umbilical Cord-Derived Stem Cells

Umbilical cord-derived stem cells (UC-MSCs) are cells in a group of multipotent stem cells that can be obtained from the umbilical cord to be discarded or from umbilical cord blood banks [49]. The surface markers are the same as BM-MSCs and ASCs but the intensity of CD105 and CD90 expression is lower than BM-MSCs and ASCs [21]. Although their isolation rate is low compared to other MSC sources, their proliferation capacity is higher when compared to BM-MSCs and ASCs [21]. In recent years, allogeneic UC-MSCs have become commercially available [21]. UC-MSCs have no risks for the donor compared to adult MSCs. And they have an ability to produce an ECM-like cartilage tissue. These features make them good candidates for chondropathies [59]. There are both preclinical [59–63] and clinical [25, 64–68] studies that uses UC-MSCs. In in vitro studies, researchers investigated the chondrogenic differentiation potential of UC-MSCs. They have demonstrated their ability to show fibrous, elastic, and hyaline cartilage phenotypes. In vivo studies in different animal models (mice, horse, etc.) confirmed the in vitro studies showing that the applicability of using UC-MSCs for the treatment of RA, OA, and cartilage defects. In clinical trials for the treatment of OA showed significant recovery of pain. No severe adverse effects were reported. Also in RA, markers have decreased and joint function has improved in patients with RA [59].

The fetal mucous connective tissue that constitutes Wharton's jelly (WJ) part of the umbilical cord contains an excessive amount of type II collagen and proteoglycans with MSCs that reflect similarity to the content of articular cartilage [15]. For this reason, Wharton's jelly-derived MSCs (WJ-MSCs) have also become of interest in joint cartilage regeneration [15]. In WJ-MSCs, HLA-I expression is low, so they are less immunogenic and they have no host immune rejection [69]. And also, WJ-MSCs do not undergo malignant transformation [69]. A clinical study that is recruiting investigates the use of WJ-MSCs for knee OA. They evaluated the efficacy of the treatment by magnetic resonance imaging (MRI) at 12 months (ClinicalTrials.gov Id: NCT0296–3727).

Peripheral Blood-Derived Stem Cells

Circulating MSCs are called peripheral blood-MSCs (PB-MSCs) and their quantity is low. BM-MSCs and PB-MSCs share several similar characteristics in terms of proliferation and multipotential differentiation characteristics. CD73 is an important marker for distinguishing between BM-MSCs and PB-MSCs [21]. PB-MSCs have the advantage to be obtained with minimal invasive procedures from autologous or allogeneic sources. Thus freshly isolated PB-MSCs are ready to be used for cartilage repair and regeneration without being expanded in culture [70]. Granulocyte colony-stimulating factor (G-CSF) as a blood mobilizing agent may induce the number of PB-MSCs within the circulation. The number of MSCs, hematopoietic stem cells (HSCs) also increase simultaneously. For this reason, it is necessary to make sure that the PB-MSCs are differentiated from other cell groups by being placed in a chondrogenic differentiation environment and differentiating in the direction of cartilage [21, 71].

18.2.1.3 Pluripotent Stem Cells

Pluripotent stem cells (PSCs) have a high differentiation potential and can differentiate to three germ layers that are ectoderm, endoderm, and mesoderm; thus, make all of the body systems including musculoskeletal system with its cartilage. The origin of pluripotent embryonic stem cells (ESCs) is the inner cell mass of the blastocyst stage embryo. Induced pluripotent stem cells (iPSCs), on the other hand, are cells that can be produced using reprogramming from differentiated cells that present similar properties with ESCs [21].

Embryonic Stem Cells

Inner cell mass derived pluripotent ESCs of the blastocyst have the capacity of self-renewal and the ability to differentiate in many ways [15]. In theory, ESCs are ideal cells for regenerative medicine. However, there are ethical restrictions in terms of isolation and culture of embryo derived ESCs into functional chondrocytes and safety of undifferentiated cells with tumorigenic potential in clinic [21]. In addition, the experimental differentiation of ESCs into chondrocytes and regeneration of cartilage is complicated as it requires a complex microenvironment along with 3-dimensional (3D) structure and specific mechanotransduction signaling [72]. The ESC-derived MSCs showed protective and regenerative effects in the injured cartilage of mice OA models in studies with EVs isolated from the culture medium [73]. However, translation of these cells into clinic for cartilage matrix regeneration is strictly prohibited due to ethical problems. For this reason, although animal studies have been conducted, no clinical studies have been reported on repair of human articular cartilage by ESCs [15].

Induced Pluripotent Stem Cells

In 2007, human somatic cells were reprogrammed to undifferentiated pluripotent cells with similar properties to ESCs [74]. Four transcription factors (Oct4, Sox2, c-Myc, and Klf4) were added to the human fibroblasts used in this reprogramming process via viral vectors [74]. Those cells obtained using reprogramming techniques are called as iPSCs. Although ESCs and iPSCs share similar characteristics in terms of morphology, several surface markers and gene expression profiles are different [75]. The autologously obtained iPSCs are not controversial unlike ESCs from the ethical point of view, which makes them perfect sources for cell therapeutics [21].

In patients with articular cartilage damage, dermal fibroblast culture is obtained by removing some skin fragments from the patient and subjecting them to enzymatic decomposition. Then, transcription factors are added to obtain iPSCs, and cells are differentiated into chondrocytes. These chondrocytes are given to the damaged one [76]. Alternatively, chondrocytes of iPSC origin can be replicated in three-dimensional culture or cultured with a scaffold to form cartilage tissue in vitro using tissue engineering techniques before transplantation [76]. Therefore, iPSCs are considered as an alternative to MSCs. Other reason for their superiority is that after in vitro chondrogenesis, iPSCs express hypertrophic markers less than MSCs [77]. At the same time, the aging problem of MSCs due to age or passage is eliminated with iPSCs [76]. Another advantage of using iPSCs is that the risk of cross-reactivity and immunogenicity are reduced because patient-specific cells are used [72]. On the other hand, the potential of iPSCs to turn into all three germ layers, unlike MSCs, brings the risk of teratoma formation [77]. Teratoma formation in iPSCs can be prevented by using cell depletion agents from a cell culture after differentiation [77]. On the other hand, some limitations are encountered in clinical use due to the requirements of being able to produce iPSCs on a large scale and with an economically suitable model [72]. Studies on EVs of iPSCs are also making progress. For example, the iPSC EVs can delay progression of OA more effectively when compared to synovium derived EVs in an OA animal model [78]. The most important contribution of using iPSC technology for cartilage regeneration is its use in disease modeling studies. Chondrogenically differentiated iPSCs produced from patients will contribute to drug research in order to understand cartilage pathology and the mechanism here [76].

As of July 2023, the ClinicalTrials.gov database shows a total of nine clinical trials using the keywords "cartilage regeneration" and/or "stem cells." Of these studies, five are still in the recruiting phase, eight have been completed, three trials have not yet been recruited, and one is reported as unknown. Clinical trials using various stem cells to treat cartilage defects are summarized in Table 18.1.

18.3 Gene Therapy in Cartilage Repair

Since the skeletal cartilage carries a specific mechanical function, it is predominantly composed of collagen and proteoglycan-made ECM in which a low number of cells are embedded with limited vascular supply [56]. Therefore, healing is slow and often results in repair tissues with chronic inflammation, low composition, and mechanical properties [56]. Thanks to advances in molecular biology, numerous gene products (proteins and different types of RNA) have been identified with a great potential to prevent degenerative disease [79]. However, the use of these molecules has not been able to develop an effective treatment, due to the general lack of methods for safe and effective delivery and their short in vivo lifespan [80]. For this reason, the necessity of regulating gene expressions in a permanent and controlled manner has come to the fore. Changes in the expression of genes encoding structural components of regulatory enzymes and cartilage and their role in osteochondral pathologies are still unknown [80]. However, understanding the genetic basis of cartilage damage will contribute to the identification of early and specific diagnostic biomarkers, predicting and monitoring the prognosis of the disease, implementing preventive strategies, and most importantly, developing personalized therapeutic protocols. In general, gene therapies for cartilage damage have focused on reducing joint inflammation, preventing cartilage matrix degradation, and increasing cartilage matrix synthesis to promote healing [13, 81].

Gene therapy consists of a molecular technique that supplements, repairs, or replaces defective genes to treat, prevent, or cure a disease for life [82]. Gene therapies can be administered by a variety of mechanisms; replacing a disease-causing gene with a healthy copy of that gene [83], silencing a disease-causing gene [82], and/or introducing a new or altered gene [82] or cells containing that gene [83] to help treat a disease [84]. Gene therapies can be categorized in terms of the vectors used (viral and non-viral) and delivery methods (in vivo and ex vivo) [82, 84]. In addition, the use of different cells and/or different methods in gene therapy and the help of biomaterials have helped to eliminate the problems related to the reliability, vector efficiency, biodistribution, safety, and immunogenicity of this treatment method [13, 85].

18.3.1 Vectors for Gene Therapy

Since DNA molecules cannot pass through the mammalian cell membrane due to their charge, a vector is required to transfer the desired gene to the cells. Vectors are basically divided into two classes as viral and non-viral vectors [86, 87]. The biggest advantage of gene transfer using viruses is the high efficiency of transferring genetic materials to target cells [82]. It is also obtained in long-term expression. However, the possibility of mutations despite the curative modifications applied by genetic engineering causes this method to create safety problems [83]. The viruses used for gene therapy are generally adenoviruses, recombinant adeno-associated viral (rAAV), retroviruses, lentiviruses, and Herpes Simplex Viruses (HSV) [13, 81]. The rAAV vectors are mostly preferred in gene therapy studies for cartilage pathologies in recent years. Currently there are about 50 adenovirus serotypes available for gene therapy, but Serotype 5 (Ad5) is the most used serotype of all types of in vitro and in vivo studies [86, 87].

As an alternative to gene transfer using viruses [87], physical [88] and chemical [80, 88] methods have been developed to transfer genetic material into cells. Non-viral vectors can be classified as lipid-based vectors (liposomes), peptide and protein vectors, and polymeric vectors [89]. They provide short-term expression with non-viral vectors and are transferred into cells with lower efficiency than viral vectors. However, their efficiency has been increased in recent years with technological developments and, due to the low risk of mutation formation, their transfer to the clinic is easier than viral vectors [86–88]. Although both transfer methods have advantages and disadvantages, the method suitable for the pathogenesis of the disease can be selected (Table 18.2).

18.3.2 Application Method

In general, gene therapy is classified as in vivo (direct gene delivery to the host tissue within the lesion site or to the microenvironment that will provide regeneration) or ex vivo (regeneration through genetically modified cells) [82, 91]. Although the ex vivo gene therapy method is longer and multi-step, it is more reliable because genetic manipulation is performed outside the body, in a controlled laboratory environment [13, 85]. In addition, it is aimed to increase the efficiency of cellular treatments using healthy cells mentioned in the previous section, together with ex vivo gene therapy [83].

In vivo gene therapy applications for cartilage repair target cartilage tissue [92] and synovium [91]. Due to the dense ECM content of cartilage and the presence of low density of cells, the efficiency of the integration of the given vectors into the genetic material of chondrocyte cells could not be achieved at the desired level [91–94]. The synovium, which is a specialized connective tissue, is suitable for the distribution of the given vector due to its large surface area [91, 95]. Especially in the treatment of RA, high efficiency was found in terms of the uptake of vectors into cells and their distribution in the tissue [95]. In the treatment of OA, successful results have been obtained in animal models with the in vivo (directly to the synovium) application of adeno-

Table 18.2 Advantages and disadvantages of vectors used in gene therapy approaches [80, 84, 87, 90]

Type	Advantages	Disadvantages
Adenovirus	High efficiency Independent from cell cycle Approved for use in clinical trials	Immunogenic Cytotoxic Short-run expression Risk of replication competence Short-term transgene expression
Retrovirus	High efficiency Prolonged transgene expression Dependent from cell cycle	Insertional mutations Replication competence Risk of replication competence
Lentivirus	High efficiency Prolonged transgene expression	Insertional mutagenesis Replication competence
HSV	High efficiency High loading capacity Independent from cell cycle Large capacity	Cytotoxic Immunogenic Short-term transgene expression
AAV	High efficiency Prolonged transgene expression Low immunogenic Independent from cell cycle	Difficult to manufacture Small capacity
Non-viral vectors	Not toxic Noninfectious Easy to manufacture High loading capacity Independent from cell cycle Large capacity	Low and cell-specific efficiency Short-term transgene expression

viruses carrying the genetic material that provides the expression of insulin-like growth factor-1 (IGF-1) or IL-1Ra [92, 96]. However, undesirable effects such as fibrosis, swelling, cartilage degeneration have been observed after adenoviral-mediated delivery of BMP-2 and TGF-β1 to the synovium [97–99].

Various biomaterials are used to ensure that the vectors applied in vivo remain in the damaged tissue [100]. After the vectors are impregnated with these materials (genetically activated implants), local release is provided only from the material applied to the damaged area [101–103]. In another method, vector seeded BM clot were implanted into the osteochondral defects, allowing genetically modified BM cells to express chondrogenic transgene products (BMP-2, Indian hedgehog protein (IHH) and TGF-1 [104]. This method can be classified as both in vivo and ex vivo gene therapy methods [104].

In ex vivo gene therapy applications, mostly chondrocytes [105, 106] and MSCs [107, 108] are used as cell sources. Efficiency could be increased by improving gene transfer protocols via lipid-based gene transfer to articular chondrocytes [109]. ECM synthesis was stimulated by the application of growth factors such as TGF-β1, IGF-1, BMP-2 and BMP-7 or chondrocytes expressing transcription factors such as SOX9 and Runx2 using viral vectors [105, 110–114]. Gene-transfected chondrocytes can be administered directly to the damaged area or applied together with carrier materials [115, 116]. Chondrocytes expressing growth factors such as BMP-7, IGF-1, −2 and FGF-2 via adenovirus or liposomes were studied in horse and rabbit cartilage damage models using fibrin and alginate as carriers [105, 106, 117, 118].

The limited regenerative properties of chondrocytes due to both being differentiated cells and being used as autologous have highlighted the use of MSCs, which are frequently used in regenerative medicine, in cartilage repair [109]. As mentioned before, MSCs are known to contribute to the repair of damaged cartilage tissue by both repairing the ECM [20, 21], differentiating into cartilage cells [21, 22] and modulating inflammation [24]. However, studies have reported that cartilage repair is increased by transfecting growth factors such as TGF-β1, BMP-2, BMP-4, BMP-13, IGF-1 [107], which are prominent in cartilage repair, to MSCs with recombinant adenoviral, retroviral, lentiviral, AAV, and liposomal vectors [107–109, 119].

18.3.3 Gene Therapy Applications in Cartilage Treatment

In recent years, factors that increase cartilage tissue repair by targeting different cells/tissues and/or different mechanisms (such as proliferation, inhibition of apoptosis) have been well defined and good results have been obtained in studies in animal models [72, 95, 120]. However, during clinical practice, there are problems related to the application protocols [95, 121] of these substances and the short in vivo half-lives [90] of these substances, the inability to ensure a sustained and sufficient release [84] in the damaged area or their spread to unrelated tissues [84]. For this reason, direct application/delivery of therapeutic genes encoding regenerative gene products or cells carrying these genes to this area can overcome the mentioned problems.

Gene transfer to joint tissues with cartilage damage due to RA was first described and performed as a method by Evans et al. in 1996 [85]. After the success of retroviral-mediated gene transfer, which was first tried on animal models, clinical trials on humans were started. Expression was detected in the joint of nine patients who were treated with a vector containing the anti-arthritic cytokine gene, and no complications developed. In subsequent studies, various growth factors [80, 97, 99, 106], transcription factors [105, 108, 113], and genetic materials [88, 89, 98, 101, 102] of molecules were tested in gene therapy in vivo [106] or ex vivo [107] in order to increase chondrogenic differentiation and ECM production, inhibit osteogenesis, inflammation, senescence, and apoptosis [85].

When the Cochrane Library and ClinicalTrials.gov Database are searched for gene therapy studies (as of July 2023) for the treatment of cartilage damage, several clinical studies are carried out in the treatment of OA and degenerative arthritis with some gene therapy product. TissueGene C (TG-C, Invossa™) contains allogeneic primary chondrocytes and GP2–293 cells transfected with TGF-β1 by retroviruses (ClinicalTrials.gov Id: NCT03203330). Fibroblasts were irradiated with gamma or X-rays to prevent uncontrolled proliferation. This mixture was injected into the knee joint of a rabbit model of OA and demonstrated significant cartilage repair in damaged tissue [122, 123]. This approach has been shown to be an effective and safe procedure in Phase I, II, and III clinical trials and has been approved for the treatment of patients with moderate knee osteoarthritis in Korea [120, 121, 124]. The other products are FX201 (ClinicalTrials.gov Id: NCT04119687) and sc-rAAV2.5 IL-1Ra (ClinicalTrials.gov Id: NCT02790723). They are both in vivo, intra-articular (IA), IL-1 receptor antagonist (IL-1Ra) gene therapy in development for the treatment of OA and their Phase I studies were started in 2019 and still continue. Vector (Helper-Dependent Adenovirus (HDAd)-ratIL-1Ra) efficacy for the FX201 was evaluated in the anterior cruciate ligament transection (ACLT) rat OA model. The last product on the ClinicalTrials.gov, XT-150 is a plasmid DNA with a variant of IL-10. Its phase I studies have been completed but not published yet (ClinicalTrials.gov Id: NCT03769662).

18.4 Conclusion

Cartilage is a highly specialized connective tissue presenting a unique problem once articular cartilage is degenerated or injured due to a very limited capacity for self-repair and regeneration. By overexpressing or silencing the desired gene using gene transfer techniques, limitations of current treatments for articular cartilage lesions can be overcome. Various approaches have been developed and clinical studies have yielded positive results in order to efficiently transfer exogenous cDNAs to cartilage lesions in vivo in the presence of biomaterial or ex vivo together with cellular treatments, and to ensure continuous expression of related gene products. Currently, there are 17 cellular and 4 gene therapy studies in clinical trials. However, the application of gene therapies, whose safety is still debated, causes controversy in cartilage damage that produces a decrease in the quality of life but is not life-threatening at an acute level. Consequently, the administration of these technologies for clinical use is highly dependent on the use of efficient and safe delivery systems of transgenes and vectors, and therefore efforts to increase the safety of these vectors are as important as studies of cartilage repair. Although there are animal models of OA and other cartilage disorders in particular, none of them permit to predict equivalent disease in humans. Cell line disease models made with iPSCs are of great importance for in vitro studies in this sense. Therefore, more detailed studies are needed to determine the role of stem cells and gene therapy practices for cartilage repair.

References

1. Hulme CH, Perry J, McCarthy HS, Wright KT, Snow M, Mennan C, et al. Cell therapy for cartilage repair. Emerg Top Life Sci. 2021;5(4):575–89.
2. Mendy A, Park J, Vieira ER. Osteoarthritis and risk of mortality in the USA: a population-based cohort study. Int J Epidemiol. 2018;47(6):1821–9.
3. Kotlarz H, Gunnarsson CL, Fang H, Rizzo JA. Insurer and out-of-pocket costs of osteoarthritis in the US: evidence from national survey data. Arthritis Rheum. 2009;60(12):3546–53.
4. Cisternas MG, Murphy L, Sacks JJ, Solomon DH, Pasta DJ, Helmick CG. Alternative methods for defining osteoarthritis and the impact on estimating prevalence in a US population-based survey. Arthritis Care Res (Hoboken). 2016;68(5):574–80.
5. Cui A, Li H, Wang D, Zhong J, Chen Y, Lu H. Global, regional prevalence, incidence and risk factors of knee osteoarthritis in population-based studies. EClinicalMedicine. 2020;29–30:100587.
6. Jaiswal A, Goswami K, Haldar P, Salve HR, Singh U. Prevalence of knee osteoarthritis, its determinants, and impact on the quality of life in elderly persons in rural Ballabgarh. Haryana J Family Med Prim Care. 2021;10(1):354–60.
7. McAlindon TE, Bannuru RR, Sullivan MC, Arden NK, Berenbaum F, Bierma-Zeinstra SM, et al. OARSI guidelines for the non-surgical management of knee osteoarthritis. Osteoarthr Cartil. 2014;22(3):363–88.
8. McCrae JC, Morrison EE, MacIntyre IM, Dear JW, Webb DJ. Long-term adverse effects of

paracetamol—a review. Br J Clin Pharmacol. 2018;84(10):2218–30.
9. Bruyere O, Honvo G, Veronese N, Arden NK, Branco J, Curtis EM, et al. An updated algorithm recommendation for the management of knee osteoarthritis from the European Society for Clinical and Economic Aspects of osteoporosis, osteoarthritis and musculoskeletal diseases (ESCEO). Semin Arthritis Rheum. 2019;49(3):337–50.
10. Kolasinski SL, Neogi T, Hochberg MC, Oatis C, Guyatt G, Block J, et al. 2019 American College of Rheumatology/Arthritis Foundation guideline for the Management of Osteoarthritis of the hand, hip, and knee. Arthritis Rheumatol. 2020;72(2):220–33.
11. Bannuru RR, Osani MC, Vaysbrot EE, Arden NK, Bennell K, Bierma-Zeinstra SMA, et al. OARSI guidelines for the non-surgical management of knee, hip, and polyarticular osteoarthritis. Osteoarthr Cartil. 2019;27(11):1578–89.
12. Mobasheri A, van Spil WE, Budd E, Uzieliene I, Bernotiene E, Bay-Jensen AC, et al. Molecular taxonomy of osteoarthritis for patient stratification, disease management and drug development: biochemical markers associated with emerging clinical phenotypes and molecular endotypes. Curr Opin Rheumatol. 2019;31(1):80–9.
13. Evans CH, Ghivizzani SC, Robbins PD. Osteoarthritis gene therapy in 2022. Curr Opin Rheumatol. 2023;35(1):37–43.
14. Brittberg M, Lindahl A, Nilsson A, Ohlsson C, Isaksson O, Peterson L. Treatment of deep cartilage defects in the knee with autologous chondrocyte transplantation. N Engl J Med. 1994;331(14):889–95.
15. Jiang S, Guo W, Tian G, Luo X, Peng L, Liu S, et al. Clinical application status of articular cartilage regeneration techniques: tissue-engineered cartilage brings new Hope. Stem Cells Int. 2020;2020:5690252.
16. Angele P, Docheva D, Pattappa G, Zellner J. Cell-based treatment options facilitate regeneration of cartilage, ligaments and meniscus in demanding conditions of the knee by a whole joint approach. Knee Surg Sports Traumatol Arthrosc. 2022;30(4):1138–50.
17. Massen FK, Inauen CR, Harder LP, Runer A, Preiss S, Salzmann GM. One-step autologous minced cartilage procedure for the treatment of knee joint chondral and osteochondral lesions: a series of 27 patients with 2-year follow-up. Orthop J Sports Med. 2019;7(6):2325967119853773.
18. Roth KE, Ossendorff R, Klos K, Simons P, Drees P, Salzmann GM. Arthroscopic minced cartilage implantation for chondral lesions at the talus: a technical note. Arthrosc Tech. 2021;10(4):e1149–e54.
19. Schneider S, Ossendorff R, Holz J, Salzmann GM. Arthroscopic minced cartilage implantation (MCI): a technical note. Arthrosc Tech. 2021;10(1):e97–e101.
20. Sun L, Reagan MR, Kaplan DL. Role of cartilage forming cells in regenerative medicine for cartilage repair. Orthop Res Rev. 2010;2010(2):85–94.
21. Urlic I, Ivkovic A. Cell sources for cartilage repair-biological and clinical perspective. Cells. 2021;10(9):2496.
22. Dominici M, Le Blanc K, Mueller I, Slaper-Cortenbach I, Marini F, Krause D, et al. Minimal criteria for defining multipotent mesenchymal stromal cells. The International Society for Cellular Therapy position statement. Cytotherapy. 2006;8(4):315–7.
23. Kose S, Aerts Kaya F, Kuskonmaz B, Uckan CD. Characterization of mesenchymal stem cells in mucolipidosis type II (I-cell disease). Turk J Biol. 2019;43(3):171–8.
24. Muller L, Tunger A, Wobus M, von Bonin M, Towers R, Bornhauser M, et al. Immunomodulatory properties of mesenchymal stromal cells: an update. Front Cell Dev Biol. 2021;9:637725.
25. Wang L, Huang S, Li S, Li M, Shi J, Bai W, et al. Efficacy and safety of umbilical cord mesenchymal stem cell therapy for rheumatoid arthritis patients: a prospective phase I/II study. Drug Des Devel Ther. 2019;13:4331–40.
26. Onen S, Kose S, Yersal N, Korkusuz P. Mesenchymal stem cells promote spermatogonial stem/progenitor cell pool and spermatogenesis in neonatal mice in vitro. Sci Rep. 2022;12(1):11494.
27. Bal E, Hanalioglu S, Kopru CZ, Kose S, Basak AT, Pehlivan SB, et al. Effect of mesenchymal stem cells therapy in experimental kaolin induced syringomyelia model. J Neurosurg Sci. 2022;66(1):40–8.
28. Ozdogan H, Gur Dedeoglu B, Oztemur Islakoglu Y, Aydos A, Kose S, Atalay A, et al. DICER1 gene and miRNA dysregulation in mesenchymal stem cells of patients with myelodysplastic syndrome and acute myeloblastic leukemia. Leuk Res. 2017;63:62–71.
29. Onen S, Atik AC, Gizer M, Kose S, Yaman O, Kulah H, et al. A pumpless monolayer microfluidic device based on mesenchymal stem cell-conditioned medium promotes neonatal mouse in vitro spermatogenesis. Stem Cell Res Ther. 2023;14(1):127.
30. Li N, Hua J. Interactions between mesenchymal stem cells and the immune system. Cell Mol Life Sci. 2017;74(13):2345–60.
31. Song N, Scholtemeijer M, Shah K. Mesenchymal stem cell immunomodulation: mechanisms and therapeutic potential. Trends Pharmacol Sci. 2020;41(9):653–64.
32. Kopru CZ, Cagnan I, Akar I, Esendagli G, Korkusuz P, Gunel-Ozcan A. Dual effect of glucocorticoid-induced tumor necrosis factor-related receptor ligand carrying mesenchymal stromal cells on small cell lung cancer: a preliminary in vitro study. Cytotherapy. 2018;20(7):930–40.
33. Liang W, Chen X, Zhang S, Fang J, Chen M, Xu Y, et al. Mesenchymal stem cells as a double-edged sword in tumor growth: focusing on MSC-derived cytokines. Cell Mol Biol Lett. 2021;26(1):3.

34. Wyles CC, Houdek MT, Behfar A, Sierra RJ. Mesenchymal stem cell therapy for osteoarthritis: current perspectives. Stem Cells Cloning. 2015;8:117–24.
35. Ge L, Xun C, Li W, Jin S, Liu Z, Zhuo Y, et al. Extracellular vesicles derived from hypoxia-preconditioned olfactory mucosa mesenchymal stem cells enhance angiogenesis via miR-612. J Nanobiotechnol. 2021;19(1):380.
36. Ciftci E, Bozbeyoglu N, Gursel I, Korkusuz F, Bakan Misirlioglu F, Korkusuz P. Comparative analysis of magnetically activated cell sorting and ultracentrifugation methods for exosome isolation. PLoS One. 2023;18(2):e0282238.
37. Kodama J, Wilkinson KJ, Otsuru S. MSC-EV therapy for bone/cartilage diseases. Bone Rep. 2022;17:101636.
38. Arslan F, Lai RC, Smeets MB, Akeroyd L, Choo A, Aguor EN, et al. Mesenchymal stem cell-derived exosomes increase ATP levels, decrease oxidative stress and activate PI3K/Akt pathway to enhance myocardial viability and prevent adverse remodeling after myocardial ischemia/reperfusion injury. Stem Cell Res. 2013;10(3):301–12.
39. Qin Y, Wang L, Gao Z, Chen G, Zhang C. Bone marrow stromal/stem cell-derived extracellular vesicles regulate osteoblast activity and differentiation in vitro and promote bone regeneration in vivo. Sci Rep. 2016;6:21961.
40. Alcaraz MJ, Compan A, Guillen MI. Extracellular vesicles from mesenchymal stem cells as novel treatments for musculoskeletal diseases. Cells. 2019;9(1):98.
41. Liu Y, Shah KM, Luo J. Strategies for articular cartilage repair and regeneration. Front Bioeng Biotechnol. 2021;9:770655.
42. Kose S, Kankilic B, Gizer M, Ciftci Dede E, Bayramli E, Korkusuz P, et al. Stem cell and advanced Nano bioceramic interactions. Adv Exp Med Biol. 2018;1077:317–42.
43. Köse SAKF, Denkbas EB, Korkusuz P, Cetinkaya FD. Evaluation of biocompatibility of random or aligned electrospun polyhydroxybutyrate scaffolds combined with human mesenchymal stem cells. Turk J Biol. 2016;40:410–9.
44. Kankilic B, Kose S, Korkusuz P, Timucin M, Korkusuz F. Mesenchymal stem cells and Nano-bioceramics for bone regeneration. Curr Stem Cell Res Ther. 2016;11(6):487–93.
45. Sakar M, Korkusuz P, Demirbilek M, Cetinkaya DU, Arslan S, Denkbas EB, et al. The effect of poly(3-hydroxybutyrate-co-3-hydroxyhexanoate) (PHBHHx) and human mesenchymal stem cell (hMSC) on axonal regeneration in experimental sciatic nerve damage. Int J Neurosci. 2014;124(9):685–96.
46. Kose S, Yersal N, Onen S, Korkusuz P. Comparison of hematopoietic and Spermatogonial stem cell niches from the regenerative medicine aspect. Adv Exp Med Biol. 2018;1107:15–40.
47. Kose S, Aerts-Kaya F, Kopru CZ, Nemutlu E, Kuskonmaz B, Karaosmanoglu B, et al. Human bone marrow mesenchymal stem cells secrete endocannabinoids that stimulate in vitro hematopoietic stem cell migration effectively comparable to beta-adrenergic stimulation. Exp Hematol. 2018;57(30–41):e1.
48. Nam Y, Rim YA, Lee J, Ju JH. Current therapeutic strategies for stem cell-based cartilage regeneration. Stem Cells Int. 2018;2018:8490489.
49. Wang AT, Feng Y, Jia HH, Zhao M, Yu H. Application of mesenchymal stem cell therapy for the treatment of osteoarthritis of the knee: a concise review. World J Stem Cells. 2019;11(4):222–35.
50. Maumus M, Rozier P, Boulestreau J, Jorgensen C, Noel D. Mesenchymal stem cell-derived extracellular vesicles: opportunities and challenges for clinical translation. Front Bioeng Biotechnol. 2020;8:997.
51. Pak J, Lee JH, Kartolo WA, Lee SH. Cartilage regeneration in human with adipose tissue-derived stem cells: current status in clinical implications. Biomed Res Int. 2016;2016:4702674.
52. Czerwiec K, Zawrzykraj M, Deptula M, Skoniecka A, Tyminska A, Zielinski J, et al. Adipose-derived mesenchymal stromal cells in basic research and clinical applications. Int J Mol Sci. 2023;24(4):3888.
53. Korkusuz P, Dagdeviren A, Eksioglu F, Ors U. Immunohistological analysis of normal and osteoarthritic human synovial tissue. Bull Hosp Jt Dis. 2005;63(1–2):63–9.
54. Falconer J, Murphy AN, Young SP, Clark AR, Tiziani S, Guma M, et al. Review: synovial cell metabolism and chronic inflammation in rheumatoid arthritis. Arthritis Rheumatol. 2018;70(7):984–99.
55. Li N, Gao J, Mi L, Zhang G, Zhang L, Zhang N, et al. Synovial membrane mesenchymal stem cells: past life, current situation, and application in bone and joint diseases. Stem Cell Res Ther. 2020;11(1):381.
56. Tuan RS, Chen AF, Klatt BA. Cartilage regeneration. J Am Acad Orthop Surg. 2013;21(5):303–11.
57. Tao SC, Yuan T, Zhang YL, Yin WJ, Guo SC, Zhang CQ. Exosomes derived from miR-140-5p-overexpressing human synovial mesenchymal stem cells enhance cartilage tissue regeneration and prevent osteoarthritis of the knee in a rat model. Theranostics. 2017;7(1):180–95.
58. Zhu Y, Wang Y, Zhao B, Niu X, Hu B, Li Q, et al. Comparison of exosomes secreted by induced pluripotent stem cell-derived mesenchymal stem cells and synovial membrane-derived mesenchymal stem cells for the treatment of osteoarthritis. Stem Cell Res Ther. 2017;8(1):64.
59. Russo E, Caprnda M, Kruzliak P, Conaldi PG, Borlongan CV, La Rocca G. Umbilical cord mesenchymal stromal cells for cartilage regeneration applications. Stem Cells Int. 2022;2022:2454168.
60. Li Z, Bi Y, Wu Q, Chen C, Zhou L, Qi J, et al. A composite scaffold of Wharton's jelly and chondroitin sulphate loaded with human umbilical cord mesen-

chymal stem cells repairs articular cartilage defects in rat knee. J Mater Sci Mater Med. 2021;32(4):36.
61. Tong W, Zhang X, Zhang Q, Fang J, Liu Y, Shao Z, et al. Multiple umbilical cord-derived MSCs administrations attenuate rat osteoarthritis progression via preserving articular cartilage superficial layer cells and inhibiting synovitis. J Orthop Translat. 2020;23:21–8.
62. Xu K, Ma D, Zhang G, Gao J, Su Y, Liu S, et al. Human umbilical cord mesenchymal stem cell-derived small extracellular vesicles ameliorate collagen-induced arthritis via immunomodulatory T lymphocytes. Mol Immunol. 2021;135:36–44.
63. Vohra M, Sharma A, Bagga R, Arora SK. Human umbilical cord-derived mesenchymal stem cells induce tissue repair and regeneration in collagen-induced arthritis in rats. J Clin Transl Res. 2020;6(6):203–16.
64. He X, Yang Y, Yao M, Yang L, Ao L, Hu X, et al. Combination of human umbilical cord mesenchymal stem (stromal) cell transplantation with IFN-gamma treatment synergistically improves the clinical outcomes of patients with rheumatoid arthritis. Ann Rheum Dis. 2020;79(10):1298–304.
65. Qi T, Gao H, Dang Y, Huang S, Peng M. Cervus and cucumis peptides combined umbilical cord mesenchymal stem cells therapy for rheumatoid arthritis. Medicine (Baltimore). 2020;99(28):e21222.
66. Mead OG, Mead LP. Intra-articular injection of amniotic membrane and umbilical cord particulate for the Management of Moderate to severe knee osteoarthritis. Orthop Res Rev. 2020;12:161–70.
67. Dilogo IH, Canintika AF, Hanitya AL, Pawitan JA, Liem IK, Pandelaki J. Umbilical cord-derived mesenchymal stem cells for treating osteoarthritis of the knee: a single-arm, open-label study. Eur J Orthop Surg Traumatol. 2020;30(5):799–807.
68. Matas J, Orrego M, Amenabar D, Infante C, Tapia-Limonchi R, Cadiz MI, et al. Umbilical cord-derived mesenchymal stromal cells (MSCs) for knee osteoarthritis: repeated MSC dosing is superior to a single MSC dose and to hyaluronic acid in a controlled randomized phase I/II trial. Stem Cells Transl Med. 2019;8(3):215–24.
69. Chen G, Yue A, Ruan Z, Yin Y, Wang R, Ren Y, et al. Human umbilical cord-derived mesenchymal stem cells do not undergo malignant transformation during long-term culturing in serum-free medium. PLoS One. 2014;9(6):e98565.
70. Chen YR, Yan X, Yuan FZ, Ye J, Xu BB, Zhou ZX, et al. The use of peripheral blood-derived stem cells for cartilage repair and regeneration in vivo: a review. Front Pharmacol. 2020;11:404.
71. Kassis I, Zangi L, Rivkin R, Levdansky L, Samuel S, Marx G, et al. Isolation of mesenchymal stem cells from G-CSF-mobilized human peripheral blood using fibrin microbeads. Bone Marrow Transplant. 2006;37(10):967–76.
72. Dubey NK, Mishra VK, Dubey R, Syed-Abdul S, Wang JR, Wang PD, et al. Combating osteoarthritis through stem cell therapies by rejuvenating cartilage: a review. Stem Cells Int. 2018;2018:5421019.
73. Wang Y, Yu D, Liu Z, Zhou F, Dai J, Wu B, et al. Exosomes from embryonic mesenchymal stem cells alleviate osteoarthritis through balancing synthesis and degradation of cartilage extracellular matrix. Stem Cell Res Ther. 2017;8(1):189.
74. Takahashi K, Tanabe K, Ohnuki M, Narita M, Ichisaka T, Tomoda K, et al. Induction of pluripotent stem cells from adult human fibroblasts by defined factors. Cell. 2007;131(5):861–72.
75. Zhao J, Jiang WJ, Sun C, Hou CZ, Yang XM, Gao JG. Induced pluripotent stem cells: origins, applications, and future perspectives. J Zhejiang Univ Sci B. 2013;14(12):1059–69.
76. Tsumaki N, Okada M, Yamashita A. iPS cell technologies and cartilage regeneration. Bone. 2015;70:48–54.
77. Lach MS, Rosochowicz MA, Richter M, Jagiello I, Suchorska WM, Trzeciak T. The induced pluripotent stem cells in articular cartilage regeneration and disease modelling: are we ready for their clinical use? Cells. 2022;11(3):529.
78. Jiang S, Tian G, Li X, Yang Z, Wang F, Tian Z, et al. Research Progress on stem cell therapies for articular cartilage regeneration. Stem Cells Int. 2021;2021:8882505.
79. Li Y, Yuan Z, Yang H, Zhong H, Peng W, Xie R. Recent advances in understanding the role of cartilage lubrication in osteoarthritis. Molecules. 2021;26(20):6122.
80. Mehta S, Akhtar S, Porter RM, Onnerfjord P, Bajpayee AG. Interleukin-1 receptor antagonist (IL-1Ra) is more effective in suppressing cytokine-induced catabolism in cartilage-synovium co-culture than in cartilage monoculture. Arthritis Res Ther. 2019;21(1):238.
81. Evans CH, Gouze JN, Gouze E, Robbins PD, Ghivizzani SC. Osteoarthritis gene therapy. Gene Ther. 2004;11(4):379–89.
82. Bulaklak K, Gersbach CA. The once and future gene therapy. Nat Commun. 2020;11(1):5820.
83. Kose S, Aerts-Kaya F, Uckan Cetinkaya D, Korkusuz P. Stem cell applications in lysosomal storage disorders: Progress and ongoing challenges. Adv Exp Med Biol. 2021;1347:135–62.
84. Madry H, Cucchiarini M. Advances and challenges in gene-based approaches for osteoarthritis. J Gene Med. 2013;15(10):343–55.
85. Evans CH, Ghivizzani SC, Robbins PD. Orthopaedic gene therapy: twenty-five years on. JBJS Rev. 2021;9(8):10.2106/JBJS.RVW.20.00220.
86. Steinert AF, Noth U, Tuan RS. Concepts in gene therapy for cartilage repair. Injury. 2008;39 Suppl 1(Suppl 1):S97–113.
87. Szwedowski D, Szczepanek J, Paczesny L, Pekala P, Zabrzynski J, Kruczynski J. Genetics in cartilage lesions: basic science and therapy approaches. Int J Mol Sci. 2020;21(15):5430.

88. Uzieliene I, Kalvaityte U, Bernotiene E, Mobasheri A. Non-viral gene therapy for osteoarthritis. Front Bioeng Biotechnol. 2020;8:618399.
89. Yin H, Kanasty RL, Eltoukhy AA, Vegas AJ, Dorkin JR, Anderson DG. Non-viral vectors for gene-based therapy. Nat Rev Genet. 2014;15(8):541–55.
90. Watson-Levings RS, Palmer GD, Levings PP, Dacanay EA, Evans CH, Ghivizzani SC. Gene therapy in Orthopaedics: Progress and challenges in pre-clinical development and translation. Front Bioeng Biotechnol. 2022;10:901317.
91. Gouze E, Pawliuk R, Pilapil C, Gouze JN, Fleet C, Palmer GD, et al. In vivo gene delivery to synovium by lentiviral vectors. Mol Ther. 2002;5(4):397–404.
92. Cucchiarini M, Madry H, Ma C, Thurn T, Zurakowski D, Menger MD, et al. Improved tissue repair in articular cartilage defects in vivo by rAAV-mediated overexpression of human fibroblast growth factor 2. Mol Ther. 2005;12(2):229–38.
93. Tomita T, Hashimoto H, Tomita N, Morishita R, Lee SB, Hayashida K, et al. In vivo direct gene transfer into articular cartilage by intraarticular injection mediated by HVJ (Sendai virus) and liposomes. Arthritis Rheum. 1997;40(5):901–6.
94. Yao Q, Glorioso JC, Evans CH, Robbins PD, Kovesdi I, Oligino TJ, et al. Adenoviral mediated delivery of FAS ligand to arthritic joints causes extensive apoptosis in the synovial lining. J Gene Med. 2000;2(3):210–9.
95. Robbins PD, Evans CH, Chernajovsky Y. Gene therapy for arthritis. Gene Ther. 2003;10(10):902–11.
96. Frisbie DD, Ghivizzani SC, Robbins PD, Evans CH, McIlwraith CW. Treatment of experimental equine osteoarthritis by in vivo delivery of the equine interleukin-1 receptor antagonist gene. Gene Ther. 2002;9(1):12–20.
97. Bakker AC, Joosten LA, Arntz OJ, Helsen MM, Bendele AM, van de Loo FA, et al. Prevention of murine collagen-induced arthritis in the knee and ipsilateral paw by local expression of human interleukin-1 receptor antagonist protein in the knee. Arthritis Rheum. 1997;40(5):893–900.
98. Gelse K, Jiang QJ, Aigner T, Ritter T, Wagner K, Poschl E, et al. Fibroblast-mediated delivery of growth factor complementary DNA into mouse joints induces chondrogenesis but avoids the disadvantages of direct viral gene transfer. Arthritis Rheum. 2001;44(8):1943–53.
99. Mi Z, Ghivizzani SC, Lechman E, Glorioso JC, Evans CH, Robbins PD. Adverse effects of adenovirus-mediated gene transfer of human transforming growth factor beta 1 into rabbit knees. Arthritis Res Ther. 2003;5(3):R132–9.
100. Korkusuz P, Kose S, Kopru CZ. Biomaterial and stem cell interactions: histological biocompatibility. Curr Stem Cell Res Ther. 2016;11(6):475–86.
101. Bonadio J, Smiley E, Patil P, Goldstein S. Localized, direct plasmid gene delivery in vivo: prolonged therapy results in reproducible tissue regeneration. Nat Med. 1999;5(7):753–9.
102. Samuel RE, Lee CR, Ghivizzani SC, Evans CH, Yannas IV, Olsen BR, et al. Delivery of plasmid DNA to articular chondrocytes via novel collagen-glycosaminoglycan matrices. Hum Gene Ther. 2002;13(7):791–802.
103. Bonadio J. Tissue engineering via local gene delivery: update and future prospects for enhancing the technology. Adv Drug Deliv Rev. 2000;44(2–3):185–94.
104. Pascher A, Palmer GD, Steinert A, Oligino T, Gouze E, Gouze JN, et al. Gene delivery to cartilage defects using coagulated bone marrow aspirate. Gene Ther. 2004;11(2):133–41.
105. Hidaka C, Goodrich LR, Chen CT, Warren RF, Crystal RG, Nixon AJ. Acceleration of cartilage repair by genetically modified chondrocytes over expressing bone morphogenetic protein-7. J Orthop Res. 2003;21(4):573–83.
106. Madry H, Kaul G, Cucchiarini M, Stein U, Zurakowski D, Remberger K, et al. Enhanced repair of articular cartilage defects in vivo by transplanted chondrocytes overexpressing insulin-like growth factor I (IGF-I). Gene Ther. 2005;12(15):1171–9.
107. Gelse K, von der Mark K, Aigner T, Park J, Schneider H. Articular cartilage repair by gene therapy using growth factor-producing mesenchymal cells. Arthritis Rheum. 2003;48(2):430–41.
108. Ahrens M, Ankenbauer T, Schroder D, Hollnagel A, Mayer H, Gross G. Expression of human bone morphogenetic proteins-2 or −4 in murine mesenchymal progenitor C3H10T1/2 cells induces differentiation into distinct mesenchymal cell lineages. DNA Cell Biol. 1993;12(10):871–80.
109. Madry H, Trippel SB. Efficient lipid-mediated gene transfer to articular chondrocytes. Gene Ther. 2000;7(4):286–91.
110. Nixon AJ, Fortier LA, Williams J, Mohammed H. Enhanced repair of extensive articular defects by insulin-like growth factor-I-laden fibrin composites. J Orthop Res. 1999;17(4):475–87.
111. Nixon AJ, Saxer RA, Brower-Toland BD. Exogenous insulin-like growth factor-I stimulates an autoinductive IGF-I autocrine/paracrine response in chondrocytes. J Orthop Res. 2001;19(1):26–32.
112. Shuler FD, Georgescu HI, Niyibizi C, Studer RK, Mi Z, Johnstone B, et al. Increased matrix synthesis following adenoviral transfer of a transforming growth factor beta1 gene into articular chondrocytes. J Orthop Res. 2000;18(4):585–92.
113. Tew SR, Li Y, Pothacharoen P, Tweats LM, Hawkins RE, Hardingham TE. Retroviral transduction with SOX9 enhances re-expression of the chondrocyte phenotype in passaged osteoarthritic human articular chondrocytes. Osteoarthr Cartil. 2005;13(1):80–9.
114. Iwamoto M, Kitagaki J, Tamamura Y, Gentili C, Koyama E, Enomoto H, et al. Runx2 expression and action in chondrocytes are regulated by retinoid signaling and parathyroid hormone-related peptide (PTHrP). Osteoarthr Cartil. 2003;11(1):6–15.
115. Ikeda T, Kubo T, Arai Y, Nakanishi T, Kobayashi K, Takahashi K, et al. Adenovirus mediated gene

delivery to the joints of Guinea pigs. J Rheumatol. 1998;25(9):1666–73.
116. Madry H, Cucchiarini M, Stein U, Remberger K, Menger MD, Kohn D, et al. Sustained transgene expression in cartilage defects in vivo after transplantation of articular chondrocytes modified by lipid-mediated gene transfer in a gel suspension delivery system. J Gene Med. 2003;5(6):502–9.
117. Fortier LA, Mohammed HO, Lust G, Nixon AJ. Insulin-like growth factor-I enhances cell-based repair of articular cartilage. J Bone Joint Surg Br. 2002;84(2):276–88.
118. Kaul G, Cucchiarini M, Arntzen D, Zurakowski D, Menger MD, Kohn D, et al. Local stimulation of articular cartilage repair by transplantation of encapsulated chondrocytes overexpressing human fibroblast growth factor 2 (FGF-2) in vivo. J Gene Med. 2006;8(1):100–11.
119. Madry H, Zurakowski D, Trippel SB. Overexpression of human insulin-like growth factor-I promotes new tissue formation in an ex vivo model of articular chondrocyte transplantation. Gene Ther. 2001;8(19):1443–9.
120. Evans CH, Ghivizzani SC, Robbins PD. Gene delivery to joints by intra-articular injection. Hum Gene Ther. 2018;29(1):2–14.
121. Grol MW, Lee BH. Gene therapy for repair and regeneration of bone and cartilage. Curr Opin Pharmacol. 2018;40:59–66.
122. Lee KH, Song SU, Hwang TS, Yi Y, Oh IS, Lee JY, et al. Regeneration of hyaline cartilage by cell-mediated gene therapy using transforming growth factor beta 1-producing fibroblasts. Hum Gene Ther. 2001;12(14):1805–13.
123. Song SU, Cha YD, Han JU, Oh IS, Choi KB, Yi Y, et al. Hyaline cartilage regeneration using mixed human chondrocytes and transforming growth factor-beta1-producing chondrocytes. Tissue Eng. 2005;11(9–10):1516–26.
124. Mobasheri A. Future cell and gene therapy for osteoarthritis (OA): potential for using mammalian protein production platforms, irradiated and transfected protein packaging cell lines for over-production of therapeutic proteins and growth factors. Adv Exp Med Biol. 2020;1247:17–31.

19 Inflammatory and Metabolic Cartilage Diseases

Bilgehan Çatal

19.1 Introduction

Inflammatory and metabolic cartilage diseases are a group of medical conditions that affect the joint cartilage, cause progressive damage and lead to pain, stiffness, and reduced joint function. Most of these diseases cause systemic involvement and show a wide range of clinical features. Cartilage diseases in this section will be explained under two main headings: inflammatory cartilage diseases and metabolic cartilage diseases.

19.2 Inflammatory Cartilage Diseases

19.2.1 Rheumatoid Arthritis

Rheumatoid Arthritis (RA) is a complex autoimmune condition that primarily targets the joints, resulting in progressive destruction of cartilage and functional impairment. Although the exact etiology remains unclear, genetic, environmental, and immunologic factors have contributed to the pathogenesis of RA.

RA affects approximately 0.5–1% of the global population with a higher prevalence in women than in men [1]. The disease commonly manifests at sixth decade of life, although it can occur at any age [2]. Genetic predisposition, smoking, and exposure to certain environmental factors have been reported as risk factors for developing RA [3]. The most important genetic risk factors that have been identified are the HLA-DRB1 shared epitope alleles [4]. Rheumatoid factor (RF) and anti-citrullinated protein antibodies (ACPA) are types of autoantibodies and exert a critical influence on the progression of the disease by inducing joint inflammation and damage [5].

At the pathophysiological level, RA initiates with an unknown antigen triggering an aberrant immune response. This leads to the activation of T-cells, which in turn stimulates macrophages and synovial fibroblasts, resulting in the production of pro-inflammatory cytokines such as interleukin-1 (IL-1), interleukin-6 (IL-6) and tumor necrosis factor-alpha (TNF-α). These cytokines perpetuate synovial inflammation and drive the proliferation of synovial tissue, forming a pannus. The pannus invades and damages adjacent cartilage, causing the characteristic joint deformities seen in RA. Furthermore, the systemic nature of the disease can result in extra-articular manifestations including cardiovascular, pulmonary, and ocular complications [2].

RA primarily affects the synovial joints, leading to pain, swelling, and stiffness, particularly in the morning. The disease is typically symmetrical and can progress to cartilage damages, joint

B. Çatal (✉)
Department of Orthopedic Surgery, Medipol Mega Hospital Complex, İstanbul Medipol University, Bağcılar/İstanbul, Turkey

M. E. Erdil et al. (eds.), *Current Concept in Cartilage Treatment*,
https://doi.org/10.1007/978-3-032-27099-3_19

deformities, and disability, if left untreated. Extra-articular manifestations, including cardiovascular, pulmonary, and neurological complications, may also occur, contributing to increased morbidity and mortality [6].

The diagnosis of RA is made according to some clinical, laboratory, and radiological criteria and findings. The 2010 American College of Rheumatology/European League Against Rheumatism (ACR/EULAR) classification criteria for RA provide a standardized approach to diagnosis, emphasizing the importance of ACPA and RF, along with clinical features (Table 19.1) [7]. Ultrasound and magnetic resonance imaging (MRI) are vital imaging studies that play an essential part in identifying early joint involvement. Based on the 2010 classification criteria, a diagnosis of RA is confirmed when the total score exceeds six and other potential causes of synovitis are ruled out [7].

The management of RA has undergone significant transformation over the past two decades, with early diagnosis and aggressive treatment now considered essential [2]. Disease-modifying antirheumatic drugs (DMARDs), particularly methotrexate, are the first line of treatment [8]. Biologic agents such as, IL-6 Receptor Inhibitors, IL-1 Receptor Antagonists, TNF Inhibitors, T-cell Activation Inhibitors, B-cell Depleting Agents, and Janus Kinase (JAK) Inhibitors targeting specific immune pathways have revolutionized the management of RA, providing significant improvements in outcomes for many patients [9]. These biologic agents are typically prescribed for patients who have not responded adequately to traditional DMARDs, or in conjunction with them. To optimize function and quality of life necessitates a holistic approach to care, encompassing physical therapy, occupational therapy, and educational support for patients.

Table 19.1 American College of Rheumatology/European League Against Rheumatism (ACR/EULAR) classification criteria for RA

Criteria		Points
Joint involvement	1 large	0
	2–10 large	1
	1–3 small	2
	4–10 small	3
	>10 (at least 1 small)	5
Serology	Negative RF and ACPA	0
	Low positive RF/ACPA	2
	High positive RF/ACPA	3
Acute phase reactants	Normal CRP/ESR	0
	Abnormal CRP/ESR	1
Symptom duration	<6 weeks	0
	>6 weeks	1

Rheumatoid Arthritis remains a challenging condition, with significant impacts on patients' lives. Ongoing research into the pathogenesis, genetics, and treatment of RA is essential to further our understanding and improve patient outcomes. The advent of personalized medicine, targeting specific pathways involved in the disease process, holds promise for more effective and tailored therapies in the future.

19.2.2 Juvenile Idiopathic Arthritis

Juvenile idiopathic arthritis (JIA) is a broad condition that includes several types of arthritis that begin before age 16 and last for at least 6 weeks. The exact etiology of Juvenile Idiopathic Arthritis remains unknown, though it is speculated to arise from an interplay of genetic predispositions and environmental influences [10]. JIA is characterized by joint inflammation, pain, and swelling, and it can also affect the eyes and other organs.

Based on factors such as the count of affected joints, specific blood antibodies, and symptoms exhibited in the initial 6 months, the International League of Associations for Rheumatology (ILAR) has categorized JIA into seven categories [11]. These categories are systemic arthritis, oligoarthritis, polyarthritis (rheumatoid factor-positive), polyarthritis (rheumatoid factor-negative), enthesitis-related arthritis, psoriatic arthritis, and undifferentiated arthritis. Each category shows different frequency, age of onset, and gender distribution (Table 19.2) [12].

Its pathophysiology is multifaceted, involving genetic predisposition, environmental triggers, and immune dysregulation. Central to JIA's

Table 19.2 Epidemiological characteristics of subgroups of JIA

Subgroups	Percentage in total (%)	Peak age	Gender distribution
Oligoarthritis	27–56	2–4 years	F >>> M
Rheumatoid-factor-negative polyarthritis	11–28	2–4 years and 6–12 years	F ≫ M
Undifferentiated arthritis	11–21	..	..
Systemic arthritis	4–17	Throughout childhood	F = M
Enthesitis-related arthritis	3–11	Late childhood or adolescence	M ≫ F
Psoriatic arthritis	2–11	2–4 years and 9–11 years	F > M
Rheumatoid-factor-positive polyarthritis	2–7	Late childhood or adolescence	F ≫ M

pathogenesis is the inappropriate activation of the immune system, leading to persistent inflammation within the joints. This immune response involves both the innate and adaptive immune systems, with key roles played by macrophages, dendritic cells, T cells and B cells. These cells release a cascade of pro-inflammatory cytokines, such as IL-1, IL-6, TNF-α, and others, leading to synovial hypertrophy and joint effusion [10]. Over time, the chronic inflammatory process can lead to cartilage damage, bone erosion, and joint deformity.

Depending on the disease subtype, the clinical manifestation of JIA can be highly variable. Systemic JIA is characterized by fever, joint inflammation, and rash. While joint involvement is four or less in oligoarthritis, joint involvement is five or more in polyarthritis. Enthesitis-related arthritis involves inflammation of the tendons and ligaments, and psoriatic arthritis is associated with psoriasis [13].

The diagnosis of JIA is primarily clinical, based on the characteristic symptoms and signs of the disease. The most distinctive symptom is Joint stiffness, intensifies during periods of inactivity like sleeping or extended sitting. Nonetheless, evaluating this stiffness in young children, especially toddlers with limited communication abilities, can be challenging [13]. On a physical examination, active arthritis manifests as joint effusion, warmth in the joint, restricted movement, sensitivity, and pain. Laboratory tests and imaging studies can help to verify the diagnosis and exclude the other pathologies. Common laboratory tests include total blood count, erythrocyte sedimentation rate, C-reactive protein, rheumatoid factor, and antinuclear antibody test [14]. Radiological studies such as X-rays, ultrasound, or MRI can help to assess the joint involvement and extent of joint damage. Osteoarthritis, which begins at a very early age, is a common clinical feature, especially in JRA patients whose attacks are not well controlled (Fig. 19.1).

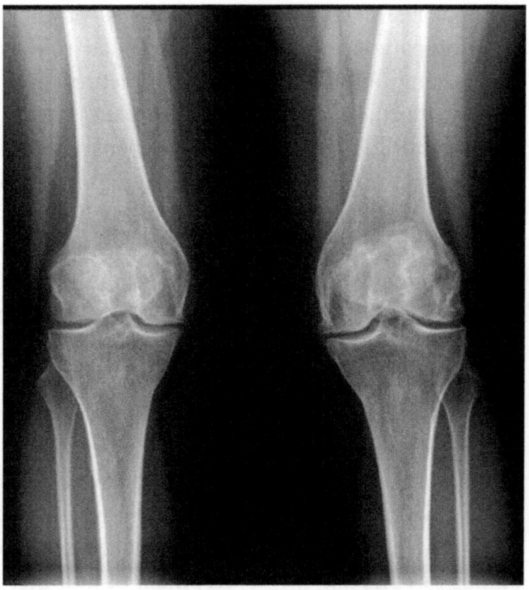

Fig. 19.1 The anteroposterior (AP) knee radiographs of an 18-year-old female patient with JIA, taken in a weight-bearing stance, demonstrate medial joint space narrowing and the presence of osteophytes, indicative of bilateral cartilage damage

The management of JIA necessitates a multidisciplinary approach, aiming not only to improve symptoms but also to preserve joint function and prevent permanent cartilage damage. Nonsteroidal anti-inflammatory drugs (NSAIDs) are frequently the initial line of therapy to reduce pain inflammation. In cases where NSAIDs provide insufficient relief, DMARDs, such as methotrexate, may be introduced. Intra-articular corticosteroid injections are another therapeutic option, particularly beneficial for children with oligoarticular JIA [15]. Biologic agents, specifically TNF inhibitors, have shown to be effective in controlling JIA symptoms and are considered when there is an inadequate response to DMARDs [16]. Beyond pharmacological interventions, physical and occupational therapy play a crucial role in maintaining joint mobility and function [17]. Patient education as well as psychosocial support are integral components of comprehensive care, ensuring that children and their families are well-equipped to manage the disease. The choice of treatment is highly individualized, taking into consideration the JIA subtype, the patient's medical status, and the severity of the disease. Regular follow-ups and monitoring are needed to assess treatment efficacy and adjust therapies as needed.

JIA is a heterogeneous group of chronic arthritis that affects children. The variability in clinical symptoms and progression of the disease adds complexity to both its diagnosis and treatment. Recent advancements in the understanding of the etiology of JIA and the development of new therapeutic agents have improved the prognosis. Future studies are essential for better understanding the etiology of JIA and to create improved therapeutic options.

19.2.3 Systemic Lupus Erythematosus

Systemic Lupus Erythematosus (SLE) is a chronic autoimmune disease leading to chronic inflammation and damage with multisystem involvement. SLE has a broad range of clinical manifestations due to multiorgan involvement [18] The disease predominantly affects women but can occur in both sexes and at any age [19].

SLE is globally distributed, with its prevalence estimated to be between 20 and 150 individuals per 100,000. The incidence of SLE is higher in Hispanics, Asians, Native Americans, and African Americans. The disease is more commonly seen in women, who are affected approximately nine times more often than men [20].

The exact etiology of SLE remains unknown; it is thought to arise from environmental factors and genetic predisposition. Potential environmental triggers may encompass viral infections, exposure to ultraviolet radiation, and some drugs. The hallmark of the disease is a disfunction in the immune system's ability to differentiate between self and non-self, resulting in the creation of immune complexes that trigger inflammation and tissues damage. Central to the disease process is the formation of immune complexes and subsequent deposition in various tissues, including the joints, kidneys, the skin, and the central nervous system. This deposition triggers a chronic inflammatory response, mediated by the activation of complement pathways and recruitment of inflammatory cells, resulting in tissue damage and clinical manifestations. Abnormalities in both the innate and adaptive immunity are evident in SLE, with dysregulation of T cells, B cells, and dendritic cells, leading to an imbalance between pro-inflammatory and regulatory cytokines [21].

SLE is a wide-ranging disease with multiorgan involvement and heterogeneous clinical manifestations. Common symptoms include skin rashes, joint pain and swelling, fatigue, fever, and renal abnormalities [18]. Arthritis is the most common orthopedic manifestation of SLE [22]. Unlike rheumatoid arthritis, the arthritis in SLE is usually less deforming and erosive, but it can still cause significant discomfort and limitation of motion. Three to six percent of patients have Jaccoud's arthropathy which leads to non-erosive deformity in the hand joints [23]. The disease can also affect the heart, lungs, liver, and central nervous system [24].

The diagnosis of SLE is based on a combination of clinical criteria and laboratory tests. The American College of Rheumatology (ACR) has delineated classification standards for SLE that encompass 11 clinical and lab benchmarks (Table 19.3) [22]. At least four of these criteria

Table 19.3 The American College of Rheumatology (ACR) criteria for Systemic Lupus Erythematosus (SLE) diagnosis

Criteria	Description
Malar rash	Butterfly-shaped rash on cheeks and bridge of nose
Discoid rash	Red, scaly patches on skin that cause scarring
Photosensitivity	Skin rash as a reaction to sunlight exposure
Oral ulcers	Painless sores in the mouth or nose
Arthritis	Non-erosive arthritis in two or more peripheral joints
Serositis	Inflammation of lining around lungs or heart
Kidney disorder	Persistent protein or cellular casts in urine
Neurological disorder	Seizures or psychosis without other known causes
Blood disorder	Hemolytic anemia, leukopenia, lymphopenia, or thrombocytopenia
Immunologic disorder	Positive test for anti-double stranded DNA, anti-smith antibodies, positive antiphospholipid antibodies, or a false-positive test for syphilis
Positive ANA test	Generally positive in patients with SLE

are required for a diagnosis of SLE to be established. Typical laboratory assessments for SLE diagnosis comprise tests for antinuclear antibody (ANA), anti-double stranded DNA (dsDNA) antibodies, and complement levels [25].

The therapeutic strategy for SLE is patient-specific to the individual's symptoms and disease severity, due to its multifaceted nature. Treatment primarily aims to reduce inflammation, manage flare-ups, and minimize organ damage. NSAIDs are usually used to manage pain and arthritis symptoms. Antimalarial drugs, particularly hydroxychloroquine, are widely used for skin and joint issues and have been shown to decrease SLE flares [26]. Corticosteroids remain a mainstay for controlling severe acute manifestations, albeit with caution due to their long-term side effects. Immunosuppressive agents, like azathioprine, mycophenolate mofetil, and methotrexate are used in cases of organ-threatening disease. Belimumab, a biologic therapy, has been approved for certain patients with active autoantibody positive SLE [27]. Regular monitoring for adverse effects of treatment is crucial, as is lifestyle modification, including sun protection and diet adjustments. Patient education on symptom management and adherence to treatment regimens is fundamental in improving prognosis and quality of life for those with SLE.

SLE is a complex and challenging disease that requires a multidisciplinary approach to management. Advances in our understanding of the disease and establish new therapeutic agents have improved the prognosis for patients with SLE. However, there is still a need for further research to elucidate the pathogenesis of SLE and develop more targeted and effective treatments.

19.2.4 Seronegative Spondyloarthropathies

Seronegative spondyloarthropathies (SpA) are a group of inflammatory diseases that primarily involves the axial skeleton, entheses, and peripheral joints. They are termed "seronegative" due to the absence of rheumatoid factor; an antibody often presents in rheumatoid arthritis. This group includes ankylosing spondylitis (AS), enteropathic arthritis, reactive arthritis (ReA), psoriatic arthritis (PsA), and undifferentiated spondyloarthropathy [28]. Common clinical features of this group of diseases are peripheral arthritis, enthesitis, tenosynovitis, inflammatory low back pain, extra-articular manifestations, and genetic predisposition [29].

The prevalence of seronegative SpA varies globally, with a higher incidence in populations with a higher prevalence of the HLA-B27 gene [30]. Studies have reported that its global prevalence ranges from 0.2% to 1.6% [31]. The onset of these diseases typically occurs in young adulthood.

The exact etiology of seronegative SpA remains unclear, but it is thought to be a complex interplay of environmental, immunological, and genetic factors. The strong association with HLA-B27, a class I surface antigen, suggests a genetic predisposition. Recent insights suggest that microbial dysbiosis, particularly in the gut, may act as an environmental trigger, altering the immune system's tolerance and leading to chronic inflammation characteristic of SpA. The immune response in these conditions involves both innate and adaptive immunity, with cytokines such as TNF-α playing a key role in the inflammatory process. This results in a cascade of events leading to new bone formation as well as bone erosion, characteristic of these diseases [32].

Ankylosing Spondylitis is characterized by chronic inflammation of the axial skeleton, leading to pain, stiffness, and potential ankylosis. Axial skeletal and sacroiliac joint involvements are often seen simultaneously. Extra-articular manifestations include uveitis (iritis or iridocyclitis), aortic regurgitation, aortic valve insufficiency, skin lesions, enthesitis, tendinitis, fatigue, fever, and pulmonary fibrosis. Ankylosing spondylitis is more common in males [33].

Psoriatic Arthritis is associated with psoriasis and occurs over time in almost 30% of psoriasis patients. It can affect peripheral joints, the axial skeleton, and entheses. Skin and nail changes are common [30].

Reactive Arthritis is an aseptic inflammatory arthritis which follows a genitourinary or gastrointestinal infection, presenting with asymmetric arthritis, enthesitis, urethritis, and conjunctivitis. Women and men are affected equally, with symptoms appearing 1–2 weeks after infection [34].

Enteropathic Arthritis is associated with inflammatory bowel diseases, specifically Chorn Disease and ulcerative colitis, manifesting as peripheral or axial arthritis [35].

Undifferentiated Spondyloarthropathy encompasses patients with SpA features that do not fit into the above categories.

Diagnosis is based on clinical presentation, imaging findings, and laboratory results. The Assessment of Spondylarthritis International Society (ASAS) criteria are widely used (Table 19.4) [36]. HLA-B27 testing and imaging, particularly MRI of the sacroiliac joints, play a key role in diagnosis. In acute sacroiliitis, MRI is more sensitive than X-ray. It reveals bone marrow edema, which appears as high signal intensity on STIR or T2-weighted images, indicative of active inflammation. X-ray findings typically show erosion, joint space narrowing, and subchondral sclerosis. Meanwhile, MRI can detect these changes earlier, showing erosions, fat deposition in place of inflamed marrow, and eventual ankylosis or joint fusion, indicative of the disease's progression (Fig. 19.2).

Table 19.4 ASAS criteria for seronegative SpA

Domain	Criteria
Sacroiliitis on radiological imaging	Plus at least one of the following:
	– Inflammatory back pain – Arthritis – Enthesitis – Uveitis – Dactylitis – Psoriasis – Crohn's disease/ulcerative colitis – Good response to NSAIDs – Family history of SpA – HLA-B27 positive – Elevated CRP
HLA B-27 positivity	Plus at least two of the features listed above

NSAIDs is the first line of the medical treatment, offer symptomatic relief, particularly effective in early inflammatory stages [33]. In cases refractory to first line NSAIDs, DMARDs like sulfasalazine and methotrexate may be considered, primarily benefiting peripheral joint involvement [37]. The advent of biologic agents, especially TNF inhibitors, has revolutionized SpA management, demonstrating substantial efficacy in symptom control, halting disease progression, and improving quality of life [38]. Moreover, recent developments have introduced interleukin 17 (IL-17) inhibitors, expanding the armamentarium for patients unresponsive to TNF blockers [39]. The integration of physical therapy into treatment regimens is essential, promoting flexibility and strength to maintain posture and function.

Seronegative spondyloarthropathies are a group of complex inflammatory diseases with diverse clinical manifestations. Advances in understanding the underlying pathogenesis and the development of biologic therapies have sig-

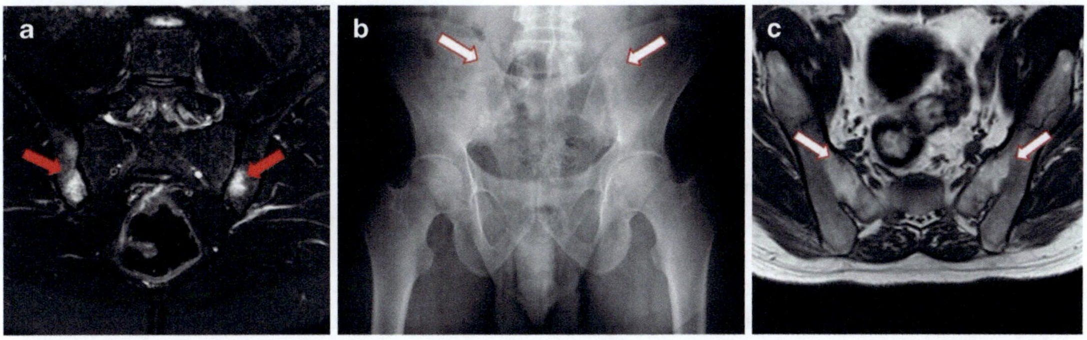

Fig. 19.2 Radiographic Images of Sacroiliitis: T2-weighted coronal plane sacroiliac joint MRI (**a**), red arrows indicate periarticular bone marrow edema in acute sacroiliitis. Pelvis X-ray (**b**) and: T1-weighted coronal plane sacroiliac joint MRI (**c**), white arrows indicate ankylosis of sacroiliac joint in chronic sacroiliitis

nificantly improved patient outcomes. Ongoing research and clinical trials are vital for further elucidating disease mechanisms and optimizing therapeutic strategies.

19.2.5 Relapsing Polychondritis

Relapsing Polychondritis (RP) is a rare multisystemic disorder that primarily targets all forms of cartilaginous tissues, leading to episodic and progressive inflammation. The condition can result in significant morbidity, with potential involvement of the cardiovascular, renal, and auditory systems [40].

RP estimated incidence is 3.5 cases per million individuals per year [41]. It can affect individuals of any age, though it most commonly presents in the fourth and fifth decades of life. There is no clear gender predilection.

The precise pathophysiology of RP remains incompletely understood, but it is believed to be an autoimmune disorder, where the immune system mistakenly attacks the body's own cartilage. This autoimmune reaction leads to recurrent episodes of inflammation in the cartilaginous tissues, resulting in their degradation and destruction over time. The disease process involves both cellular and humoral immunity, with evidence of autoantibodies against type II collagen, cartilage matrix proteins, and other cartilage-related antigens. Cytokines, such as IL-1 and TNF-α, are thought to play a significant role in mediating the inflammatory response. Clinically, this manifests as painful, red, and swollen cartilaginous structures, with potential for severe complications such as airway collapse and arthritis. The episodic and progressive nature of the disease often leads to cumulative damage and deformity [42, 43].

Clinical manifestations of this condition are diverse, reflecting its ability to affect various organ systems. The most involved sites are the ear cartilage, nose, and tracheobronchial tree, leading to characteristic signs such as painful, red, and swollen auricles, saddle nose deformity, and respiratory difficulties. Auricular chondritis, presenting as unilateral or bilateral inflammation of the pinna, spares the earlobe and is considered pathognomonic for the disease [44]. Ocular involvement, observed in a significant number of cases, can result in conjunctivitis, scleritis, or uveitis, potentially leading to vision impairment if not promptly addressed. Articular involvement is also prevalent, presenting as polyarthritis, which tends to be non-erosive and non-deforming, although it can significantly impact the quality of life due to pain and limited mobility [45]. Additionally, costochondritis may occur, causing chest wall pain and tenderness, further complicating the clinical picture. Over time, the recurrent inflammation can lead to cartilage destruction, fibrosis, and calcification, resulting in permanent anatomic changes and functional impairments [40]. Given the potential for significant morbidity, early recognition and appropriate management of orthopedic manifestations in relapsing polychondritis are crucial for optimizing patient outcomes and preserving joint function.

Diagnosis of Relapsing Polychondritis according to the modified McAdam criteria can be made if a patient has at least three of the six clinical signs or one of the clinical signs accompanied by histological confirmation (Table 19.5) [45].

Therapeutic interventions for RP primarily aim at mitigating inflammation and preserving the function of affected cartilaginous structures. First-line medical treatment is NSAIDs, dapsone, and steroids. DMARDs, such as methotrexate or azathioprine, may be employed as steroid-sparing agents or in cases resistant to steroids [41]. Biologic agents, such as TNF inhibitors or infliximab have demonstrated efficacy in some case reports and small series, providing an option for patients who do not respond to conventional therapies [46]. The choice of therapeutic agent often depends on the specific manifestations, the presence of any comorbid conditions, and the severity of the disease.

Table 19.5 Modified McAdam criteria for relapsing polychondritis

Clinical criteria	Description
Recurrent chondritis of both auricles	Inflammation of cartilage in both ears, often sparing the lobule
Non-erosive inflammatory polyarthritis	Inflammation of multiple joints without the erosion seen in conditions like rheumatoid arthritis
Chondritis of nasal cartilages	Inflammation of nasal cartilage
Ocular inflammation	Inflammation of eye structures, including conjunctivitis, keratitis, scleritis, or uveitis
Respiratory tract chondritis	Inflammation of cartilage in the respiratory tract, including laryngeal and tracheal cartilage
Audio vestibular damage	Damage to hearing and balance, manifesting as sensorineural hearing loss, tinnitus, or vertigo
Histological criteria	**Description**
Histologic confirmation	Evidence of inflammation within cartilaginous tissue on biopsy

The prognosis of RP varies widely, depending on the organs affected and the response to treatment. Mortality is primarily due to respiratory and cardiovascular complications. Future studies are required to better recognize the pathogenesis of RP, identify biomarkers for early diagnosis, and develop targeted therapeutic strategies.

19.3 Metabolic Cartilage Disease

19.3.1 Osteoarthritis

Osteoarthritis (OA) is the most common form of non-inflammatory arthritis. It is thought that approximately 18% of women and 10% of men over the age of 60 are affected worldwide [47]. Because of this widespread prevalence, osteoarthritis imposes a significant economic burden. In developed countries, an estimated 1%–2.5% of the gross domestic product is allocated to the management and treatment of OA [48]. The incidence of OA is projected to rise in tandem with the extension of the average human lifespan and the growth of the elderly demographic [49].

The disease predominantly impacts the articular hyaline cartilage of weight-bearing joints; however, it also involves other structures including the joint capsule, synovium, and subchondral bone. Affecting these structures also plays a role in the pathogenesis and progression of the disease [50]. Many studies that have been published indicate that OA is associated with systemic metabolic disturbances [51]. Obesity, dyslipidemia, and diabetes mellitus have been identified as risk factors for OA, suggesting a metabolic component to its pathogenesis [52]. Adipokines and inflammatory cytokines produced by adipose tissue can have systemic effects that promote OA [53, 54]. Furthermore, alterations in mitochondrial function, lipid metabolism, and glucose utilization within chondrocytes have been observed in OA, pointing to intrinsic metabolic dysfunction within the cartilage [55, 56].

Cartilage homeostasis is maintained through a delicate balance between anabolic and catabolic processes. In OA, this balance shifts toward catabolism, driven by both systemic metabolic factors and local joint stressors. The disruption in homeostasis is due to an upsurge in degradative enzymes like matrix metalloproteinases and a decline in the synthesis of matrix components such as type II collagen and aggrecan [57, 58]. This imbalance not only undermines the cartilage's ability to withstand compressive forces but also incites a cascade of inflammatory responses within the joint microenvironment. As the cartilage thins and erodes, the subchondral bone undergoes sclerosis and osteophyte formation occurs, aiming to redistribute loads across the compromised joint but inadvertently contributing to pain and decreased mobility. Thus, understanding the complex interplay between cartilage homeostasis and the pathophysiology of OA is critical for the development of targeted therapeutics aimed at halting or reversing the degenerative processes of this debilitating disease.

The recognition of OA as a metabolic disease opens a host of potential new therapeutic avenues. Impaired AMP-activated protein kinase (AMPK) activity, linked with aging, persistent low-grade inflammation, and metabolic syndrome [59]. Metabolic modulators' agents such as AMPK activators, which can enhance mitochondrial function and improve energy homeostasis, are being explored for their therapeutic potential in OA [60]. In an animal study, metformin, an oral antidiabetic drug, has been shown to have a cartilage-protective effect by activating the AMPK pathway [61]. In a prospective cohort study conducted on obese patients with gonarthrosis, metformin use was shown to reduce the need for total knee prosthesis [62].

The Wingless/Integrated (Wnt) signaling pathway has been identified as a critical regulator of joint homeostasis and has emerged as a promising therapeutic target in the treatment of OA. Aberrant activation of the Wnt pathway contributes to the pathophysiology of OA by promoting cartilage destruction, subchondral bone remodeling, and osteophyte formation [63]. Wnt pathway modulators, therefore, offer a novel approach to modulate disease progression. These modulators such as lorecivivint function by attenuating the Wnt-mediated transcription of pro-inflammatory and catabolic genes, which are pivotal in the degradation of articular cartilage. In a randomized prospective study conducted on patients with knee osteoarthritis, intra-articular lorecivivint treatment was shown to provide better results in terms of both functional and pain scores compared to the placebo group [64].

Transforming growth factor-beta (TGF-β) plays a multifaceted role in the pathogenesis and potential treatment of OA, offering a compelling target for therapeutic intervention. TGF-β is known to exert anabolic effects on articular cartilage, promoting the synthesis of extracellular matrix proteins and inhibiting their degradation, which are crucial processes in maintaining cartilage homeostasis. However, the dysregulation of TGF-β signaling has been implicated in the progression of OA, with altered levels contributing to pathological changes in joint tissues [65]. It has been tried to achieve TGF-B signal modulation through genetic engineering applications and use it in the treatment of osteoarthritis. A study about outcomes of injectable genetically engineered chondrocytes virally transduced with TGF-β1 was reported promising results in the treatment of knee osteoarthritis [66].

Fibroblast growth factor (FGF) 18 signaling plays a critical role in cartilage integrity and joint homeostasis by promoting the proliferation and differentiation of chondrocytes, the cells responsible for cartilage formation and repair [59]. Recent clinical trials have explored the efficacy of intra-articular injections of recombinant FGF18 in patients with knee OA, demonstrating significant improvements in cartilage thickness and joint structure [67]. These findings suggest that FGF18 not only alleviates symptoms but may also modify the disease process. The therapeutic potential of FGF18 is bolstered by its relatively specific action on cartilage and a favorable safety profile, positioning it as a novel treatment modality that could shift the management paradigm from symptom control to disease modification in osteoarthritis. Sprifermin is a recombinant FGF18, used intra-articularly as an OA modifying drug without any specific adverse effects [68].

Treatments targeting subchondral bone, which has an important place in the pathogenesis of OA, have been developed along with drugs that modify microenvironmental cartilage metabolism. Bisphosphonates, traditionally used in the management of osteoporosis, have recently been evaluated for their potential utility in the treatment of OA. These compounds have a high affinity for bone mineral and function primarily by inhibiting osteoclastic bone resorption, which could be beneficial in stabilizing the subchondral bone changes seen in OA. Emerging evidence suggests that by preserving the integrity of the subchondral bone, bisphosphonates may reduce the biomechanical stress on the overlying cartilage, thereby potentially slowing the degenerative process of OA [69]. In a study where Zoledronic acid, a type of bisphosphonate, was used in the treatment of symptomatic knee OA shows that cartilage loss and pain were reduced [70].

Strontium ranelate, a medication historically utilized in osteoporosis treatment, has garnered interest for its potential application in OA management. This dual-action agent is thought to simultaneously promote the formation of new bone while inhibiting bone resorption, potentially offering a unique therapeutic benefit in OA by targeting subchondral bone changes [71]. Strontium ranelate has been shown to reduce cartilage volume loss and bone marrow lesions when used in the treatment of symptomatic knee OA [72].

Teriparatide, a recombinant form of parathyroid hormone (PTH), primarily known for its anabolic effects on bone in the treatment of osteoporosis, is being explored for its potential application in the management of OA. Its mode of action, involving the stimulation of osteoblast activity and enhancement of bone formation, posits a novel approach in addressing the subchondral bone alterations that are implicated in OA pathogenesis [73]. A recently published systemic review about Teriparatide treatment for OA showed that treatment may slow OA, but they also stated that the studies were of low methodological quality [74].

In conclusion, the advancing understanding of OA as not only a degenerative joint disorder but also a metabolic disease has catalyzed the exploration of innovative treatment strategies that target the multifactorial nature of its pathogenesis. The management of OA is poised for transformation, with emerging therapies offering the prospect of not just symptom relief but also of altering the disease trajectory. As the prevalence of OA continues to rise globally, these therapeutic developments hold significant promise for enhancing the quality of life for millions of affected individuals, ultimately alleviating the substantial clinical and economic burden of the disease.

19.3.2 Gout

Gout is a metabolic disorder resulting from the deposition of monosodium urate (MSU) crystals in the joints, leading to acute inflammatory responses. It predominantly affects middle-aged and elderly individuals, particularly men. The male to female sex ratio has been reported to range between 2:1 and 4:1 [75–77]. The surge in prevalence can be attributed to factors such as dietary habits, obesity, and comorbid conditions.

Gout results from the supersaturation of uric acid in the blood, leading to the precipitation of monosodium urate crystals in joints and tissues. Hyperuricemia is the most important risk for gout and defined as blood uric acid concentration of 7 mL/dL and above [78]. Factors contributing to hyperuricemia include overproduction of uric acid, reduced renal excretion, or a combination of both. Genetic predisposition, dietary factors, obesity, hypertension, renal impairment, and certain medications are known risk factors [79–81]. The crystals trigger an inflammatory response, recruiting neutrophils and monocytes to the affected joint, resulting in the classic symptoms of acute gouty arthritis.

The acute attack of gout is characterized by sudden onset of severe pain, swelling, redness, and warmth in the affected joint, commonly the first metatarsophalangeal joint (podagra) [82]. Other frequently involved joints include the ankles, knees, and elbows. Acute attacks typically resolve within a week, even without treatment. However, recurrent attacks can lead to chronic gouty arthritis, with persistent pain and joint stiffness [78]. The deposition of urate crystals can also form tophi—hard, nodular masses in joints, tendons, and surrounding tissues, potentially causing joint deformity and damage.

Diagnosis of gout involves a combination of clinical evaluation, laboratory tests, and imaging. The gold standard for diagnosis is the identification of MSU crystals in synovial fluid or tophi through polarized light microscopy [83]. Serum uric acid levels can be elevated during an attack but are not diagnostic [84]. Imaging modalities such as ultrasound, X-ray, and dual-energy CT (DECT) can provide supportive evidence, showing characteristic signs such as joint effusion, erosions, and tophi.

The management of gout encompasses acute attack treatment, urate-lowering therapy (ULT), and lifestyle modifications. NSAIDs, colchicine, and corticosteroids are the mainstays for acute attack treatment. ULT with medications such as allopurinol or febuxostat is used for long-term management to reduce serum uric acid levels and prevent future attacks. Lifestyle modifications include dietary changes, weight loss, and reducing alcohol consumption [85]. Surgical intervention may be necessary for joint debridement, tophus removal, or joint replacement in cases of advanced joint damage.

Gout is a common and potentially debilitating form of inflammatory arthritis that requires timely and appropriate management to prevent joint damage and improve quality of life.

19.3.3 Chondrocalcinosis

Chondrocalcinosis, also known as pseudogout, is a rheumatic condition characterized by the deposition of calcium pyrophosphate dihydrate (CPPD) crystals in articular cartilage [86]. Chondrocalcinosis is a clinical entity frequently encountered in rheumatology, with prevalence rates increasing with age [87]. Although it can be asymptomatic, the condition often leads to joint pain and inflammation, significantly impacting the quality of life. Understanding the complex interplay of environmental, metabolic, and genetic factors in chondrocalcinosis is crucial for accurate diagnosis and effective management.

The deposition of CPPD crystals in joint cartilage is a hallmark of chondrocalcinosis [88]. There is evidence to suggest a hereditary component to chondrocalcinosis, with several genes implicated in the disease process. Mutations in the ANKH gene, which encodes a transmembrane protein involved in pyrophosphate transport, have been associated with familial forms of the disease [89]. Abnormalities in calcium and phosphate metabolism are thought to contribute to CPPD crystal formation. Hyperparathyroidism, hypomagnesemia, and hypophosphatasia are among the metabolic disorders associated with chondrocalcinosis [90]. Age-related changes in articular cartilage, including reduced water content and alterations in collagen structure, may create an environment conducive to CPPD crystal deposition.

Chondrocalcinosis can manifest in various ways, ranging from asymptomatic crystal deposition to acute inflammatory attacks reminiscent of gout. The knee is the most affected joint, although other joints such as the wrists, shoulders, and hips can also be involved [89]. In many cases, CPPD crystal deposition is discovered incidentally on imaging studies performed for other reasons. These patients may remain asymptomatic or develop symptoms later in life. Some patients with chondrocalcinosis experience acute attacks of joint inflammation, characterized by sudden onset of pain, swelling, and erythema. Unlike gout, acute attacks of Chondrocalcinosis are longer and can last for weeks [91]. These attacks are often triggered by trauma, surgery, or medical illness. In addition to acute attacks, chondrocalcinosis can lead to chronic joint pain and degenerative arthritis, contributing to long-term disability.

The diagnosis of chondrocalcinosis is primarily based on the identification of CPPD crystals in synovial fluid or tissue samples. Radiographic findings, such as chondrocalcinosis and joint degeneration, can also provide supportive evidence. Synovial fluid analysis is the gold standard for diagnosis, with CPPD crystals appearing as positively birefringent rhomboid-shaped crystals under polarized microscopy. Conventional radiography, ultrasound, and MRI can all be utilized to detect crystal deposition and assess joint damage [92].

The management of chondrocalcinosis involves both pharmacologic and non-pharmacologic interventions, aimed at relieving symptoms and preventing future attacks. NSAIDs are the first-line treatment for acute pseudogout attacks. Intra-articular corticosteroid injections can also be effective in reducing inflammation [91]. Systemic interleukin-1β inhibitors were found to be effective in acute pseudogout attacks [93]. For patients with recurrent attacks or chronic symptoms, colchicine can be used for prophylaxis [94]. Joint aspiration and lavage may also be beneficial in some cases.

Chondrocalcinosis is a multifaceted disease with varied clinical manifestations and a complex pathogenesis. Advances in our understanding of the genetic and metabolic underpinnings of the disease have improved diagnostic accuracy and provided new avenues for targeted therapy. Comprehensive patient evaluation, including laboratory investigations and imaging studies, is essential for optimal management. Future research should focus on elucidating the molecular mechanisms of CPPD crystal formation and identifying novel therapeutic strategies to mitigate the impact of this prevalent condition.

19.3.4 Ochronosis

Ochronosis is a rare clinical entity, characterized by the deposition of dark pigments in various connective tissues, including the skin, cartilage, and internal organs [95].

It is most associated with alkaptonuria, a metabolic disorder resulting from a deficiency in the enzyme homogentisate 1,2-dioxygenase (HGD). This deficiency leads to the deposition of homogentisic acid (HGA) in the body. Over time, HGA undergoes oxidation and polymerization, depositing as a dark pigment in connective tissues, a process termed as ochronosis. The ochronotic pigment imparts a characteristic bluish-black coloration to the affected tissues and leads to brittleness and decreased resilience, contributing to cartilage deterioration, osteoarthritic changes, and joint destruction [96].

The clinical manifestations of ochronosis can be categorized into three main areas: dermatologic, musculoskeletal, and cardiovascular. Patients with ochronosis often present with dark pigmentation of the skin, particularly in sun-exposed areas, pressure points, and sites of friction (Fig. 19.3). The ear cartilage is a common site of involvement, leading to a bluish-black discoloration [97]. Ochronotic arthropathy is a hallmark of the disease, with early degeneration of the intervertebral discs and large joints, particularly the spine, hips, and knees. Patients may present with pain, stiffness, and limited range of motion [98]. Deposition of HGA in the cardiovascular system can lead to valvular heart disease, aortic stenosis, and coronary artery disease [99].

The diagnosis of ochronosis is based on clinical presentation, urine analysis, and imaging studies. The presence of dark urine that turns black upon alkalinization or standing is suggestive of alkaptonuria. Radiographic findings include calcification of intervertebral discs and large joints. Histopathological examination of tissue samples can confirm the presence of dark pigments in the connective tissues.

There is no cure for ochronosis, and management is primarily supportive and symptomatic. Pain management, physical therapy, and joint

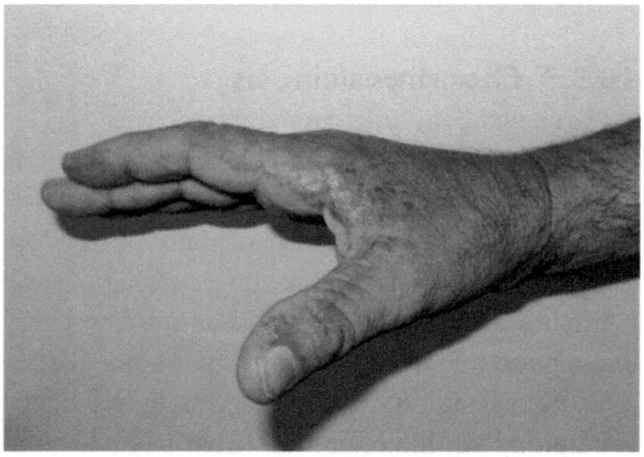

Fig. 19.3 Black pigmentation is observed in the friction area of the hand of a 45-year-old male patient with ochronosis

replacement surgeries may be required for musculoskeletal manifestations. Monitoring and managing cardiovascular involvement are crucial. Nitisinone, an inhibitor of 4-hydroxyphenylpyruvate dioxygenase, has shown promise in reducing HGA levels, but long-term effects and optimal dosing are still under investigation [100].

Ochronosis is a rare and complex disorder with significant impact on the quality of life of affected individuals. Early diagnosis and management are crucial to mitigate the progression of the disease and improve patient outcomes. Further research is needed to develop targeted therapeutic strategies.

In conclusion, the exploration of inflammatory and metabolic cartilage diseases in this chapter provides a thorough understanding of their complex pathologies, clinical manifestations, and the latest therapeutic interventions. Conditions like Rheumatoid Arthritis, Juvenile Idiopathic Arthritis, Systemic Lupus Erythematosus, Seronegative Spondyloarthropathies, Relapsing Polychondritis, Osteoarthritis, Gout, Chondrocalcinosis, and Ochronosis have been discussed in detail, highlighting their unique characteristics and the challenges they pose in diagnosis and treatment. The chapter underscores the significant advances in our understanding of these diseases, largely due to cutting-edge research and clinical insights. This enhanced understanding has led to more effective diagnostic methods, preventive measures, and treatment strategies, offering hope for better patient outcomes. However, the complexity of these diseases, coupled with their diverse manifestations, necessitates ongoing research and a multidisciplinary approach to care. The future of managing these conditions lies in personalized medicine, where treatments are tailored to individual patients based on their specific disease characteristics. This approach, along with continuous research and development of new therapeutic agents, holds promise for improving the quality of life for patients suffering from these debilitating cartilage diseases. The chapter effectively illustrates that while significant progress has been made, there remains a crucial need for continued exploration and innovation in this field.

References

1. Gibofsky A. Overview of epidemiology, pathophysiology, and diagnosis of rheumatoid arthritis. Am J Manag Care. 2012;18(13 Suppl):S295–302.
2. Lin YJ, Anzaghe M, Schülke S. Update on the pathomechanism, diagnosis, and treatment options for rheumatoid arthritis. Cells. 2020;9(4):880. https://doi.org/10.3390/cells9040880.
3. Smolen JS, Aletaha D, McInnes IB. Rheumatoid arthritis [published correction appears in Lancet. 2016 Oct 22;388(10055):1984]. Lancet 2016;388(10055):2023–38. https://doi.org/10.1016/S0140-6736(16)30173-8.
4. van Drongelen V, Holoshitz J. Human leukocyte antigen-disease associations in rheumatoid arthritis. Rheum Dis Clin N Am. 2017;43(3):363–76. https://doi.org/10.1016/j.rdc.2017.04.003.
5. Steiner G. Auto-antibodies and autoreactive T-cells in rheumatoid arthritis: pathogenetic players and diagnostic tools. Clin Rev Allergy Immunol. 2007;32:23–36. https://doi.org/10.1007/bf02686079.
6. De Rycke L, Peene I, Hoffman IE, et al. Rheumatoid factor and anticitrullinated protein antibodies in rheumatoid arthritis: diagnostic value, associations with radiological progression rate, and extra-articular manifestations. Ann Rheum Dis. 2004;63(12):1587–93. https://doi.org/10.1136/ard.2003.017574.
7. Aletaha D, Neogi T, Silman AJ, Funovits J, Felson D, Bingham CO, Birnbaum NS, Burmester G, Bykerk V, Cohen MD, et al. Rheumatoid arthritis classification criteria: an American College of Rheumatology/European League Against Rheumatism collaborative initiative. Ann Rheum Dis. 2010;69:1580–8. https://doi.org/10.1136/ard.2010.138461.
8. Cronstein BN. Low-dose methotrexate: a mainstay in the treatment of rheumatoid arthritis. Pharmacol Rev. 2005;57(2):163–72. https://doi.org/10.1124/pr.57.2.3.
9. van Vollenhoven RF, Geborek P, Forslind K, et al. Conventional combination treatment versus biological treatment in methotrexate-refractory early rheumatoid arthritis: 2-year follow-up of the randomised, non-blinded, parallel-group Swefot trial. Lancet. 2012;379(9827):1712–20. https://doi.org/10.1016/s0140-6736(12)60027-0.
10. Rigante D, Bosco A, Esposito S. The etiology of juvenile idiopathic arthritis. Clin Rev Allergy Immunol. 2015;49(2):253–61. https://doi.org/10.1007/s12016-014-8460-9.
11. Petty RE. Classification of childhood arthritis: a work in progress. Baillieres Clin Rheumatol. 1998;12(2):181–90. https://doi.org/10.1016/s0950-3579(98)80013-7.
12. Ravelli A, Martini A. Juvenile idiopathic arthritis. Lancet. 2007;369(9563):767–78. https://doi.org/10.1016/S0140-6736(07)60363-8.

13. Crayne CB, Beukelman T. Juvenile idiopathic arthritis: oligoarthritis and polyarthritis. Pediatr Clin N Am. 2018;65(4):657–74. https://doi.org/10.1016/j.pcl.2018.03.005.
14. Petty RE, Laxer RM, Lindsley CB, et al. Textbook of pediatric rheumatology. 7th ed. Philadelphia: Elsevier; 2016.
15. Espinosa M, Gottlieb BS. Juvenile idiopathic arthritis. Pediatr Rev. 2012;33(7):303–13. https://doi.org/10.1542/pir.33-7-303.
16. Prakken B, Albani S, Martini A. Juvenile idiopathic arthritis. Lancet. 2011;377(9783):2138–49. https://doi.org/10.1016/S0140-6736(11)60244-4.
17. Cakmak A, Bolukbas N. Juvenile rheumatoid arthritis: physical therapy and rehabilitation. South Med J. 2005;98(2):212–6. https://doi.org/10.1097/01.SMJ.10000146588.22557.A5.
18. Buyon JP. Systemic lupus erythematosus. In: Primer on the rheumatic diseases. New York, NY: Springer New York; 2008. p. 303–38.
19. Borchers AT, Naguwa SM, Shoenfeld Y, Gershwin ME. The geoepidemiology of systemic lupus erythematosus. Autoimmun Rev. 2010;9(5):A277–87. https://doi.org/10.1016/j.autrev.2009.12.008.
20. Rees F, Doherty M, Grainge MJ, Lanyon P, Zhang W. The worldwide incidence and prevalence of systemic lupus erythematosus: a systematic review of epidemiological studies. Rheumatology (Oxford). 2017;56(11):1945–61. https://doi.org/10.1093/rheumatology/kex260.
21. Choi J, Kim ST, Craft J. The pathogenesis of systemic lupus erythematosus—an update. Curr Opin Immunol. 2012;24(6):651–7. https://doi.org/10.1016/j.coi.2012.10.004.
22. Tan EM, Cohen AS, Fries JF, Masi AT, McShane DJ, Rothfield NF, Schaller JG, Talal N, Winchester RJ. The 1982 revised criteria for the classification of systemic lupus erythematosus. Arthritis Rheum. 1982;25(11):1271–7. https://doi.org/10.1002/art.1780251101. PMID: 7138600.
23. Ostendorf B, Scherer A, Specker C, Mödder U, Schneider M. Jaccoud's arthropathy in systemic lupus erythematosus: differentiation of deforming and erosive patterns by magnetic resonance imaging. Arthritis Rheum. 2003;48(1):157–65. https://doi.org/10.1002/art.10753.
24. Lee YH, Choi SJ, Ji JD, Song GG. Overall and cause-specific mortality in systemic lupus erythematosus: an updated meta-analysis. Lupus. 2016;25(7):727–34. https://doi.org/10.1177/0961203315627202.
25. Aringer M. Inflammatory markers in systemic lupus erythematosus. J Autoimmun. 2020;110:102374. https://doi.org/10.1016/j.jaut.2019.102374.
26. Bertsias G, Gordon C, Boumpas DT. Clinical trials in systemic lupus erythematosus (SLE): lessons from the past as we proceed to the future-the EULAR recommendations for the management of SLE and the use of end-points in clinical trials. Lupus. 2008;17:437–42. https://doi.org/10.1177/0961203308090031.
27. Francis L, Perl A. Pharmacotherapy of systemic lupus erythematosus. Expert Opin Pharmacother. 2009;10(9):1481–94. https://doi.org/10.1517/14656560902971003.
28. Moll JM, Haslock I, Macrae IF, Wright V. Associations between ankylosing spondylitis, psoriatic arthritis, Reiter's disease, the intestinal arthropathies, and Behcet's syndrome. Medicine (Baltimore). 1974;53(5):343–64. https://doi.org/10.1097/00005792-197409000-00002.
29. Duba AS, Mathew SD. The seronegative spondyloarthropathies. Prim Care. 2018;45(2):271–87. https://doi.org/10.1016/j.pop.2018.02.005.
30. Brown MA, Kennedy LG, MacGregor AJ, et al. Susceptibility to ankylosing spondylitis in twins: the role of genes, HLA, and the environment. Arthritis Rheum. 1997;40(10):1823–8. https://doi.org/10.1002/art.1780401015.
31. Stolwijk C, van Onna M, Boonen A, van Tubergen A. Global prevalence of spondyloarthritis: a systematic review and meta-regression analysis. Arthritis Care Res (Hoboken). 2016;68(9):1320–31. https://doi.org/10.1002/acr.22831.
32. Jiao Y, Wu L, Huntington ND, Zhang X. Crosstalk between gut microbiota and innate immunity and its implication in autoimmune diseases. Front Immunol. 2020;11:282. https://doi.org/10.3389/fimmu.2020.00282.
33. Taurog JD, Chhabra A, Colbert RA. Ankylosing spondylitis and axial spondyloarthritis. N Engl J Med. 2016;374(26):2563–74. https://doi.org/10.1056/NEJMra1406182.
34. Rihl M, Klos A, Köhler L, Kuipers JG. Infection and musculoskeletal conditions: reactive arthritis. Best Pract Res Clin Rheumatol. 2006;20(6):1119–37. https://doi.org/10.1016/j.berh.2006.08.008.
35. Colìa R, Corrado A, Cantatore FP. Rheumatologic and extraintestinal manifestations of inflammatory bowel diseases. Ann Med. 2016;48(8):577–85. https://doi.org/10.1080/07853890.2016.1195011.
36. Rudwaleit M, van der Heijde D, Landewé R, et al. The development of assessment of SpondyloArthritis International Society classification criteria for axial spondyloarthritis (part II): validation and final selection [published correction appears in Ann Rheum Dis. 2019 Jun;78(6):e59]. Ann Rheum Dis. 2009;68(6):777–83. https://doi.org/10.1136/ard.2009.108233.
37. Coates LC, Gossec L, Ramiro S, et al. New GRAPPA and EULAR recommendations for the management of psoriatic arthritis. Rheumatology (Oxford). 2017;56(8):1251–3. https://doi.org/10.1093/rheumatology/kew390.
38. Ritchlin CT, Daikh BE. Recent advances in the treatment of the seronegative spondyloarthropathies. Curr Rheumatol Rep. 2001;3(5):399–403. https://doi.org/10.1007/s11926-996-0010-x.

39. Blair HA, Dhillon S. Secukinumab: a review in ankylosing spondylitis. Drugs. 2016;76(10):1023–30. https://doi.org/10.1007/s40265-016-0598-8.
40. Sharma A, Gnanapandithan K, Sharma K, Sharma S. Relapsing polychondritis: a review. Clin Rheumatol. 2013;32(11):1575–83. https://doi.org/10.1007/s10067-013-2328-x.
41. Kent PD, Michet CJ Jr, Luthra HS. Relapsing polychondritis. Curr Opin Rheumatol. 2004;16(1):56–61. https://doi.org/10.1097/00002281-200401000-00011.
42. Foidart JM, Abe S, Martin GR, et al. Antibodies to type II collagen in relapsing polychondritis. N Engl J Med. 1978;299(22):1203–7. https://doi.org/10.1056/NEJM197811302992202.
43. Lang B, Rothenfusser A, Lanchbury JS, et al. Susceptibility to relapsing polychondritis is associated with HLA-DR4. Arthritis Rheum. 1993;36(5):660–4. https://doi.org/10.1002/art.1780360513.
44. Trentham DE, Le CH. Relapsing polychondritis. Ann Intern Med. 1998;129(2):114–22. https://doi.org/10.7326/0003-4819-129-2-199807150-00011.
45. Damiani JM, Levine HL. Relapsing polychondritis—report of ten cases. Laryngoscope. 1979;89(6 Pt 1):929–46.
46. Cuestas D, Peñaranda E, Mora S, et al. Relapsing polychondritis, an underestimated dermatological urgency: case report and literature review. Int J Dermatol. 2017;56(12):1379–86. https://doi.org/10.1111/ijd.13755.
47. Glyn-Jones S, Palmer AJ, Agricola R, et al. Osteoarthritis. Lancet. 2015;386(9991):376–87. https://doi.org/10.1016/S0140-6736(14)60802-3.
48. Hiligsmann M, Cooper C, Arden N, et al. Health economics in the field of osteoarthritis: an expert's consensus paper from the European Society for Clinical and Economic Aspects of Osteoporosis and Osteoarthritis (ESCEO). Semin Arthritis Rheum. 2013;43:303–13.
49. GBD 2021 Osteoarthritis Collaborators. Global, regional, and national burden of osteoarthritis, 1990–2020 and projections to 2050: a systematic analysis for the Global Burden of Disease Study 2021. Lancet Rheumatol. 2023;5(9):e508–22. https://doi.org/10.1016/S2665-9913(23)00163-7.
50. Hu W, Chen Y, Dou C, Dong S. Microenvironment in subchondral bone: predominant regulator for the treatment of osteoarthritis. Ann Rheum Dis. 2021;80(4):413–22. https://doi.org/10.1136/annrheumdis-2020-218089.
51. Kluzek S, Newton JL, Arden NK. Is osteoarthritis a metabolic disorder? Br Med Bull. 2015;115(1):111–21. https://doi.org/10.1093/bmb/ldv028.
52. Sellam J, Berenbaum F. Is osteoarthritis a metabolic disease? Joint Bone Spine. 2013;80(6):568–73. https://doi.org/10.1016/j.jbspin.2013.09.007.
53. Conde J, Scotece M, Lopez V, et al. Adipokines: novel players in rheumatic diseases. Discov Med. 2013;15:73–83.
54. Lago F, Dieguez C, Gómez-Reino J, Gualillo O. The emerging role of adipokines as mediators of inflammation and immune responses. Cytokine Growth Factor Rev. 2007;18(3–4):313–25. https://doi.org/10.1016/j.cytogfr.2007.04.007.
55. Loeser RF, Collins JA, Diekman BO. Ageing and the pathogenesis of osteoarthritis. Nat Rev Rheumatol. 2016;12(7):412–20. https://doi.org/10.1038/nrrheum.2016.65.
56. Lane RS, Fu Y, Matsuzaki S, Kinter M, Humphries KM, Griffin TM. Mitochondrial respiration and redox coupling in articular chondrocytes. Arthritis Res Ther. 2015;17(1):54. Published 2015 Mar 10. https://doi.org/10.1186/s13075-015-0566-9.
57. Wang M, Sampson ER, Jin H, et al. MMP13 is a critical target gene during the progression of osteoarthritis. Arthritis Res Ther. 2013;15(1):R5. https://doi.org/10.1186/ar4133.
58. Chang JC, Sebastian A, Murugesh DK, Hatsell S, Economides AN, Christiansen BA, Loots GG. Global molecular changes in a tibial compression induced ACL rupture model of post-traumatic osteoarthritis. J Orthop Res. 2017;35(3):474–85. https://doi.org/10.1002/jor.23263.
59. Gezer HH, Ostor A. What is new in pharmacological treatment for osteoarthritis? Best Pract Res Clin Rheumatol. 2023;37:101841. https://doi.org/10.1016/j.berh.2023.101841.
60. Wang J, Li J, Song D, Ni J, Ding M, Huang J, Yan M. AMPK: implications in osteoarthritis and therapeutic targets. Am J Transl Res. 2020;12(12):7670–81.
61. Li J, Zhang B, Liu WX, Lu K, Pan H, Wang T, Oh CD, Yi D, Huang J, Zhao L, Ning G, Xing C, Xiao G, Liu-Bryan R, Feng S, Chen D. Metformin limits osteoarthritis development and progression through activation of AMPK signalling. Ann Rheum Dis. 2020;79(5):635–45. https://doi.org/10.1136/annrheumdis-2019-216713.
62. Wang Y, Hussain SM, Wluka AE, et al. Association between metformin use and disease progression in obese people with knee osteoarthritis: data from the osteoarthritis initiative—a prospective cohort study. Arthritis Res Ther. 2019;21:127. https://doi.org/10.1186/s13075-019-1915-x.
63. Lories RJ, Monteagudo S. Review article: is Wnt signaling an attractive target for the treatment of osteoarthritis? Rheumatol Ther. 2020;7(2):259–70. https://doi.org/10.1007/s40744-020-00205-8.
64. Yazici Y, McAlindon TE, Gibofsky A, et al. A Phase 2b randomized trial of lorecivivint, a novel intra-articular CLK2/DYRK1A inhibitor and Wnt pathway modulator for knee osteoarthritis. Osteoarthr Cartil. 2021;29(5):654–66. https://doi.org/10.1016/j.joca.2021.02.004.
65. van der Kraan PM. Differential role of transforming growth factor-beta in an osteoarthritic or a healthy joint. J Bone Metab. 2018;25(2):65–72. https://doi.org/10.11005/jbm.2018.25.2.65.

66. Cherian JJ, et al. Preliminary results of a phase II randomized study to determine the efficacy and safety of genetically engineered allogeneic human chondrocytes expressing TGF-β1 in patients with grade 3 chronic degenerative joint disease of the knee. Osteoarthr Cartil. 2015;23(12):2109–18. https://doi.org/10.1016/j.joca.2015.06.019.
67. Lohmander LS, Hellot S, Dreher D, et al. Intraarticular sprifermin (recombinant human fibroblast growth factor 18) in knee osteoarthritis: a randomized, double-blind, placebo-controlled trial. Arthritis Rheumatol. 2014;66(7):1820–31. https://doi.org/10.1002/art.38614.
68. Zeng N, Chen XY, Yan ZP, Li JT, Liao T, Ni GX. Efficacy and safety of sprifermin injection for knee osteoarthritis treatment: a meta-analysis. Arthritis Res Ther. 2021;23(1):107. Published 2021 Apr 9. https://doi.org/10.1186/s13075-021-02488-w.
69. Xing RL, Zhao LR, Wang PM. Bisphosphonates therapy for osteoarthritis: a meta-analysis of randomized controlled trials. Springerplus. 2016;5(1):1704. https://doi.org/10.1186/s40064-016-3359-y.
70. Aitken D, Laslett LL, Cai G, Hill C, March L, Wluka AE, Wang Y, Blizzard L, Cicuttini F, Jones G. A protocol for a multicentre, randomised, double-blind, placebo-controlled trial to compare the effect of annual infusions of zoledronic acid to placebo on knee structural change and knee pain over 24 months in knee osteoarthritis patients—ZAP2. BMC Musculoskelet Disord. 2018;19(1):217. https://doi.org/10.1186/s12891-018-2143-2.
71. Reginster JY, Badurski J, Bellamy N, et al. Efficacy and safety of strontium ranelate in the treatment of knee osteoarthritis: results of a double-blind, randomised placebo-controlled trial. Ann Rheum Dis. 2013;72(2):179–86. https://doi.org/10.1136/annrheumdis-2012-202231.
72. Pelletier JP, Roubille C, Raynauld JP, et al. Disease-modifying effect of strontium ranelate in a subset of patients from the Phase III knee osteoarthritis study SEKOIA using quantitative MRI: reduction in bone marrow lesions protects against cartilage loss. Ann Rheum Dis. 2015;74(2):422–9. https://doi.org/10.1136/annrheumdis-2013-203989.
73. Sampson ER, Hilton MJ, Tian Y, et al. Teriparatide as a chondroregenerative therapy for injury-induced osteoarthritis. Sci Transl Med. 2011;3(101):101ra93. https://doi.org/10.1126/scitranslmed.3002214.
74. Li G, Liu S, Xu H, et al. Potential effects of teriparatide (PTH(1-34)) on osteoarthritis: a systematic review. Arthritis Res Ther. 2023;25(1):3. https://doi.org/10.1186/s13075-022-02981-w.
75. Kuo CF, Grainge MJ, Mallen C, Zhang W, Doherty M. Rising burden of gout in the UK but continuing suboptimal management: a nationwide population study. Ann Rheum Dis. 2015;74(4):661–7. https://doi.org/10.1136/annrheumdis-2013-204463.
76. Zobbe K, Prieto-Alhambra D, Cordtz R, et al. Secular trends in the incidence and prevalence of gout in Denmark from 1995 to 2015: a nationwide register-based study. Rheumatology (Oxford). 2019;58(5):836–9. https://doi.org/10.1093/rheumatology/key390.
77. Chen-Xu M, Yokose C, Rai SK, Pillinger MH, Choi HK. Contemporary prevalence of gout and hyperuricemia in the United States and decadal trends: the National Health and Nutrition Examination Survey, 2007-2016. Arthritis Rheumatol. 2019;71(6):991–9. https://doi.org/10.1002/art.40807.
78. Dalbeth N, Gosling AL, Gaffo A, Abhishek A. Gout. Lancet. 2021;397(10287):1843–55. https://doi.org/10.1016/S0140-6736(21)00569-9.
79. Choi HK, Atkinson K, Karlson EW, Willett W, Curhan G. Purine-rich foods, dairy and protein intake, and the risk of gout in men. N Engl J Med. 2004;350(11):1093–103. https://doi.org/10.1056/NEJMoa035700.
80. Choi HK, Atkinson K, Karlson EW, Willett W, Curhan G. Alcohol intake and risk of incident gout in men: a prospective study. Lancet. 2004;363(9417):1277–81. https://doi.org/10.1016/S0140-6736(04)16000-5.
81. Choi HK, Curhan G. Soft drinks, fructose consumption, and the risk of gout in men: prospective cohort study. BMJ. 2008;336(7639):309–12. https://doi.org/10.1136/bmj.39449.819271.BE.
82. Taylor WJ, Fransen J, Jansen TL, et al. Study for updated gout classification criteria: identification of features to classify gout. Arthritis Care Res (Hoboken). 2015;67(9):1304–15. https://doi.org/10.1002/acr.22585.
83. Zell M, Zhang D, FitzGerald J. Diagnostic advances in synovial fluid analysis and radiographic identification for crystalline arthritis. Curr Opin Rheumatol. 2019;31(2):134–43. https://doi.org/10.1097/BOR.0000000000000582.
84. Zhao T, Lv X, Cao L, et al. Renal excretion is a cause of decreased serum uric acid during acute gout. Int J Rheum Dis. 2018;21(9):1723–7. https://doi.org/10.1111/1756-185X.13348.
85. Richette P, Doherty M, Pascual E, et al. 2016 updated EULAR evidence-based recommendations for the management of gout. Ann Rheum Dis. 2017;76(1):29–42. https://doi.org/10.1136/annrheumdis-2016-209707.
86. Kohn N, Hughes R, Mccarty D Jr, Faires J. The significance of calcium phosphate crystals in the synovial fluid of arthritic patients: the "pseudogout syndrome". II. Identification of crystals. Ann Intern Med. 1962;56:738–45. https://doi.org/10.7326/0003-4819-56-5-738.
87. Felson DT, Anderson JJ, Naimark A, Kannel W, Meenan RF. The prevalence of chondrocalcinosis in the elderly and its association with knee osteoarthritis: the Framingham study. J Rheumatol. 1989;16(9):1241–5.
88. Derfus BA, Rachow JW, Mandel NS, et al. Articular cartilage vesicles generate calcium pyrophosphate dihydrate-like crystals

in vitro. Arthritis Rheum. 1992;35(2):231–40. https://doi.org/10.1002/art.1780350218.
89. Rosenthal AK, Ryan LM. Calcium pyrophosphate deposition disease. N Engl J Med. 2016;374(26):2575–84. https://doi.org/10.1056/NEJMra1511117.
90. Ciancio G, Bortoluzzi A, Govoni M. Epidemiology of gout and chondrocalcinosis. Reumatismo. 2012;63(4):207–20. Published 2012 Jan 19. https://doi.org/10.4081/reumatismo.2011.207.
91. Masuda I, Ishikawa K. Clinical features of pseudogout attack. A survey of 50 cases. Clin Orthop Relat Res. 1988;(229):173–81.
92. Miksanek J, Rosenthal AK. Imaging of calcium pyrophosphate deposition disease. Curr Rheumatol Rep. 2015;17(3):20. https://doi.org/10.1007/s11926-015-0496-1.
93. Ottaviani S, Brunier L, Sibilia J, et al. Efficacy of anakinra in calcium pyrophosphate crystal-induced arthritis: a report of 16 cases and review of the literature. Joint Bone Spine. 2013;80(2):178–82. https://doi.org/10.1016/j.jbspin.2012.07.018.
94. Alvarellos A, Spilberg I. Colchicine prophylaxis in pseudogout. J Rheumatol. 1986;13(4):804–5.
95. Fisher AA, Davis MW. Alkaptonuric ochronosis with aortic valve and joint replacements and femoral fracture: a case report and literature review. Clin Med Res. 2004;2(4):209–15. https://doi.org/10.3121/cmr.2.4.209.
96. Chu P, Cuellar MC, Bracken SJ, Tarrant TK. A mimic of ankylosing spondylitis, ochronosis: case report and review of the literature. Curr Allergy Asthma Rep. 2021;21(3):19. https://doi.org/10.1007/s11882-021-01002.
97. Van Offel JF, De Clerck LS, Francx LM, Stevens WJ. The clinical manifestations of ochronosis: a review. Acta Clin Belg. 1995;50(6):358–62. https://doi.org/10.1080/17843286.1995.11718475.
98. Wu K, Bauer E, Myung G, Fang MA. Musculoskeletal manifestations of alkaptonuria: a case report and literature review. Eur J Rheumatol. 2018;6(2):98–101. https://doi.org/10.5152/eurjrheum.2018.18116.
99. Rey EL, Monzonís AM, Bajula A, Peñaranda JMS, Fernández AL. Aortic valve replacement in alkaptonuric ochronosis. Rev Port Cir Cardiotorac Vasc. 2020;27(2):121–3.
100. Introne WJ, Perry MB, Troendle J, et al. A 3-year randomized therapeutic trial of nitisinone in alkaptonuria. Mol Genet Metab. 2011;103(4):307–14. https://doi.org/10.1016/j.ymgme.2011.04.016.

20 Physical Therapy, Rehabilitation, and Return to Sports After Cartilage Surgery

Defne Kaya Utlu

20.1 Introduction

Cartilage repair/regenerative surgery (CRS), including microfracture (MF), autologous chondrocyte implantation (ACI), and osteochondral autograft transplantation (OAT), has been safely performed in clinics for the last two decades to treat isolated cartilage defects in the knee joint. In addition, the development of ankle cartilage repair surgery has witnessed significant advances in recent years leading to better outcomes for individuals with ankle cartilage injury, particularly osteochondral lesions of the talus (OLT).

Cartilage surgeries involve a range of advanced techniques designed to repair, regenerate, and repair damaged cartilage. These surgical interventions offer a glimmer of hope for athletes who experience cartilage injuries. Procedures such as microfracture, mosaicplasty, and autologous chondrocyte implantation aim to restore joint integrity and function, with a focus on stimulating cartilage growth or replacing damaged tissue with healthy donor cartilage.

While cartilage repair surgeries are a critical step toward recovery, they are only the beginning of an athlete's journey back to sports. Recognizing the multifaceted nature of sports-related injuries, current approaches place greater emphasis on specific rehabilitation protocols. These protocols extend far beyond conventional exercise and timelines; They are individualized plans that are specific to the surgical technique, meticulously designed to adapt to the biomechanics of the sport and the athlete.

The personalized rehabilitation process encompasses several stages, each strategically addressing the evolving needs of the healing joint. The early stages focus on pain management, reduction of swelling, and restoration of basic range of motion. As the athlete progresses, rehabilitation shifts toward strengthening the muscles surrounding the joint, increasing joint stability, and retraining proprioception. Gradually, sport-specific movements are introduced that simulate the dynamic challenges of the athlete's chosen sport.

Limited studies have shown that after cartilage repair, cartilage tissue begins to form in the first 6 weeks, and from the twelfth week, the repair tissue and the formed hyaline-like cartilage become stronger [1]. In light of this information, the restriction of weight-bearing for the first 6 weeks is of great importance in terms of giving time for the newly formed cartilage structure to strengthen against the load. Under this title, rehabilitation after surgery (microfracture, mosaicplasty, osteochondral autologous transfer, and matrix-guided autologous chondrocyte implantation) of cartilage lesions in the knee and ankle joints will be explained.

D. K. Utlu (✉)
Department of Physiotherapy and Rehabilitation, Faculty of Hamidiye Health Sciences, Health Sciences University, İstanbul, Turkey
e-mail: defne.kayautlu@sbu.edu.tr

M. E. Erdil et al. (eds.), *Current Concept in Cartilage Treatment*,
https://doi.org/10.1007/978-3-032-27099-3_20

20.2 Rehabilitation Protocols

20.2.1 Pre-surgery Rehabilitation

Exercise approaches that focus on core stability, strengthen hip abductors, and improve plyometric and dynamic stabilization before cartilage repair surgery increase the long-term outcome success after surgery, reduce the athlete's anxiety, and ensure their participation in the rehabilitation process [2]. Hirschmüller et al. propounded a prehabilitation program including "improving neuromuscular control," "improving muscle strength," "improving general fitness," "reducing joint effusion," and "respect for the pain level of each patient" before cartilage surgery [2].

20.2.2 Rehabilitation After Microfracture

The rehabilitation process after microfracture surgery depends on the anatomical location of the area and the size of the lesion. The age, body mass index, and activity level of patients also play an essential role in designing the treatment program. Rehabilitation guidelines have been established after microfracture treatment for two regions around the knee: (1) Femoral condyles and (2) Patellofemoral. General rehabilitation stages after microfracture are indicated in Table 20.1 [3]. After microfracture surgery, returning to football, skiing, basketball, and football should be 6–9 months later. The rate of returning to sports after microfracture surgery is 66% [4].

Table 20.1 General rehabilitation stages after microfracture (this guide is created for knee pathologies)

Assistive device	Crutches should be used in all lesions The use of knee brace is variable In patellar/trochlear lesions, the use of a 0–30° locking knee brace is recommended for 8 weeks
Weight bearing	**In condylar lesion:** Toe touch walking (0–6 or 0–8 weeks), then walking as a tolerable weight **In patellar/trochlear lesions:** Walking with partial weight bearing in the knee brace (0–2 weeks), then walking as a tolerable weight
Continuous passive motion (CPM) device	**In condylar lesion:** It should be started as soon as possible: It should be started at 6–8 hours/day, 0–60° or 30–70°, it should be increased by 10–20° every day until the full range of motion is reached **In patellar/trochlear lesions:** It should be started as soon as possible: 6–8 h/day, 0–50° should be started, it should be increased by 10–20° every day until the full range of motion is reached **In cases where CPM is not used:** Heel (wall) sliding exercise on the wall: 500 repetitions/3 times/day
Range of motion	Passive joint movement without weight bearing should be done within the limits of CPM
Strengthening exercises	**0–8 weeks:** Quadriceps isometric, four-way straight leg raise, wall slide, ankle pumping exercises, and core stability training. The stationary bike can be used without resistance from the second week **8–12 weeks:** Gait training should be given. Treadmill, elliptical, stationary bike (with resistance), and independent walking in the pool **12–16 weeks:** Standing four-way hip resistance exercises, climbing stairs, forward/backward walking, and cardiovascular training at 75% submaximal level **16+ weeks:** Weight training with moderate load: "Leg-press" 0–90°, knee flexion/extension exercises, squats, and lunges for frontal plane control The agility exercises are given at a light level. The rotation and displacement exercises should not be performed 4–6 months before surgery

20.2.3 Rehabilitation After Mosaicplasty and Osteochondral Autologous Transfer Surgery (OATS)

The location of the lesion often determines the rehabilitation protocol after Osteochondral Autologous Transfer Surgery (OATS) and mosaicplasty. If the lesion is located in a weight-bearing area of the femoral condyles, it should be protected from compressive forces, if it is located on the trochlear/retropatellar face, it should be protected from shear forces. The size and depth of the lesion and the area it covers are also important in terms of determining the progress of rehabilitation [5]. General rehabilitation stages after the osteochondral autologous transfer surgery (OATS) and mosaicplasty are listed in Table 20.2 [3]. After OAT and mosaicplasty surgery, restarting sports activities should be after 6 months. Return to sports such as football and tennis should not be before 8–12 months. The rate of return to sports after osteochondral autologous transfer surgery is 91% [4].

Table 20.2 General rehabilitation stages after mosaicplasty and osteochondral autologous transfer surgery (OATS) (this guide is created for knee pathologies)

Assistive device	Crutches should be used in all lesions. A locked knee brace in full extension should be used in all lesions	
Weight bearing	The decision to partial weight-bearing is given according to the location and size of the lesion **If the lesion is in the posterior or patellofemoral joint:** Partial weight bearing with two crutches should be started in the second week **If the lesion is anterior or central:** Partial weight-bearing with two crutches should be started at week 2 for small lesions, week 3 for medium-sized lesions, and week 4 for large lesions. Walking at full weight should be started in 6–tenth week	
Continuous passive motion (CPM) device	It should be started as soon as possible: 6–8 hours/day, starting from 0–60° and increasing by 10–20° every day **In patellofemoral lesions**, if the lesion is larger than 6 cm^2, it should be started from 0–40° It should be continued until the full joint range of motion is reached **In cases where CPM is not used:** Heel (wall) sliding exercise on the wall: 500 repetitions/3 times/day	
Range of motion	**In condylar lesions:** second week: 90° third week: 105° At week 4: 115° At 6 weeks: 125°	**In patellofemoral lesions:** Third week: 90° fourth week: 105° At 6 weeks: 120°
Strengthening exercises	**0–6 weeks:** Quadriceps isometric, four-way straight leg raise, wall slide, ankle pumping exercises, and core stability training. Active knee extension: While it can be done in the range of 90–40° in condylar lesions, active extension should not be done in patellar/trochlear lesions **6–12 weeks:** In condylar lesion: At 8 weeks: Active knee extension (0–90°), "mini-squat" (0–60°), "leg-press" (0–90°) at 10 weeks. In patellar/trochlear lesions: "Mini-squat" (0–45°) at week 8, "leg-press" (0–60°) at week 10, active knee extension (0–30°) at week 12. **12–26 weeks:** Standing quadrupedal resistance exercises, unilateral steps, progressive active knee extension, step climbing, aerobic training on an elliptical or stationary bike If the patellofemoral joint is the donor site, squats and eccentric training should be avoided for 2–3 months **26–52+ weeks:** Progress should be based on patient condition and tolerance. You can start running on a line in the third month. The start of sports activities should be after 6 months. Return to sports such as football and tennis should not be before 8–12 months	

20.2.4 Rehabilitation After Matrix Guided Autologous Chondrocyte Implantation

The maturation of cartilage after autologous chondrocyte implantation occurs in three phases [6]:

(a) **Proliferation Phase (0–6 weeks) (soft, primitive repair tissue):** The implanted cartilage cells attach to the subchondral bone. In the present phase, the patient should be asked to bear weight as toe-touch. The passive joint movement must be performed for the activation of chondrocytes.
(b) **Transition Phase (6 weeks–6 months) (expansion of matrix puttylike consistency):** Matrix development takes place in the present phase. Partial weight-bearing at 6–10 weeks and full weight-bearing after 10 weeks may be allowed.
(c) **Remodeling Phase (6–18 months) (matrix remodeling, tissue stiffens to normal hardness):** The cartilage becomes suitable for loading near normal (hardening). It should be noted that the maturation of the placed graft continues for up to 3 years.

General rehabilitation phases after matrix-guided autologous chondrocyte implantation are listed in Table 20.3 [3]. Following matrix-guided autologous chondrocyte implantation, the return to sports activities should be after 12 months. The rate of return to sports after autologous chondrocyte implantation applications is 67% [4].

As a result, the rehabilitation program to be applied following the knee cartilage surgery should focus on providing complete restoration of the tissue without stress/load on the tissues to be healed. With the joint cooperation of the surgeon, physiotherapist, and patient, a smooth gliding motion in the knee joint should be achieved. It should not be forgotten that the character of the lesion is important in determining the athlete's return to sports. Athletes with a lesion area of less than 2 cm^2 have a high rate of return to high-intensity sports after microfracture and osteochondral autologous transfer [7]. No relationship was demonstrated between autologous chondrocyte implantation and lesion size. This situation is also related to the preference of microfracture and osteochondral autologous transfer for smaller lesions, and autologous chondrocyte implantation for both small and large lesions [4]. You can find some examples of exercises performed after cartilage knee surgeries in Fig. 20.1.

As a result, the rehabilitation program to be applied following the knee cartilage surgery should focus on providing complete restoration of the tissue without stress/load on the tissues to be healed. With the joint cooperation of the surgeon, physiotherapist, and patient, a smooth gliding motion in the knee joint should be achieved. It should not be forgotten that the character of the lesion is important in determining the athlete's return to sports. Athletes with a lesion area of less than 2 cm^2 have a high rate of return to high-intensity sports after microfracture and osteochondral autologous transfer [7]. No relationship was demonstrated between autologous chondrocyte implantation and lesion size. This situation is also related to the preference of microfracture and osteochondral autologous transfer for smaller lesions, and autologous chondrocyte implantation for both small and large lesions [4].

Table 20.3 General rehabilitation stages after matrix guided autologous chondrocyte implantation (this guide is created for knee pathologies)

Assistive device	Crutches should be used in all lesions A locked knee brace in full extension should be used in all lesions Crutches should be left at 8 weeks
Weight bearing	**In condylar lesion:** Toe touch walking (0–6 weeks) **In patellar/trochlear lesions:** Toe walking (0–2 weeks), then walking with 50% of body weight in the third week, 75% of body weight at 4–5 weeks, full weight bearing at 10 weeks
Continuous passive motion (CPM) device	4–6 h/day, starting from 0–40°, increasing by 10–20° every day until the full range of motion is reached
Range of motion	Passive knee flexion: 0–90° by week 2, 120° by week 4, and full flexion by week 6
Strengthening exercises	**0–6 weeks:** Quadriceps isometric, four-way straight leg raise, and ankle pumping exercises. The stationary bike can be used without resistance from reaching 100° of knee flexion. Closed kinetic chain exercises (with light weights) from the third week, isometric "leg-press" from the fourth week. Active knee extension: It should be done 90–40° (without using weight) in the condylar lesion. Active knee extension should not be performed during these weeks in patellar/trochlear lesions **6–12 weeks:** "Mini-squat" (0–45°), "leg-press," squat on the wall, and walking training on the treadmill/pool should be started. Open kinetic chain exercises should be started after the eighth week. **In condylar lesions:** Open kinetic chain exercises and stepping forward/sideways (week 8) **In patellar/trochlear lesions:** "Leg-press" (0–60°) is still prohibited when starting at 8 weeks **12–26 weeks:** Leg-press (0–90°), squat (0–60°), forward/sideways stepping, strengthening for hip stabilizers, gait program, elliptical and stationary bike. In condylar lesions: Forward lunge and open kinetic chain knee extension (0–90°), In patellar/trochlear lesions: Backward lunge and open kinetic chain knee extension (start with 0–30°) Light jogging can be started at 24–26 weeks. **26–52+ weeks–6 months:** Golf, swimming, skating **8–9 months**: Light jogging, jogging, aerobics **12th month:** Tennis, basketball, football and baseball

Important notes applicable to all surgeries:
* Knee flexion should be gained as soon as possible after surgery
* Crutches and knee brace must be dropped as soon as the following criteria are met:
1. Full knee extension
2. 0–100° knee flexion
3. No loss of extension
4. Ability to walk without pain and in an appropriate pattern

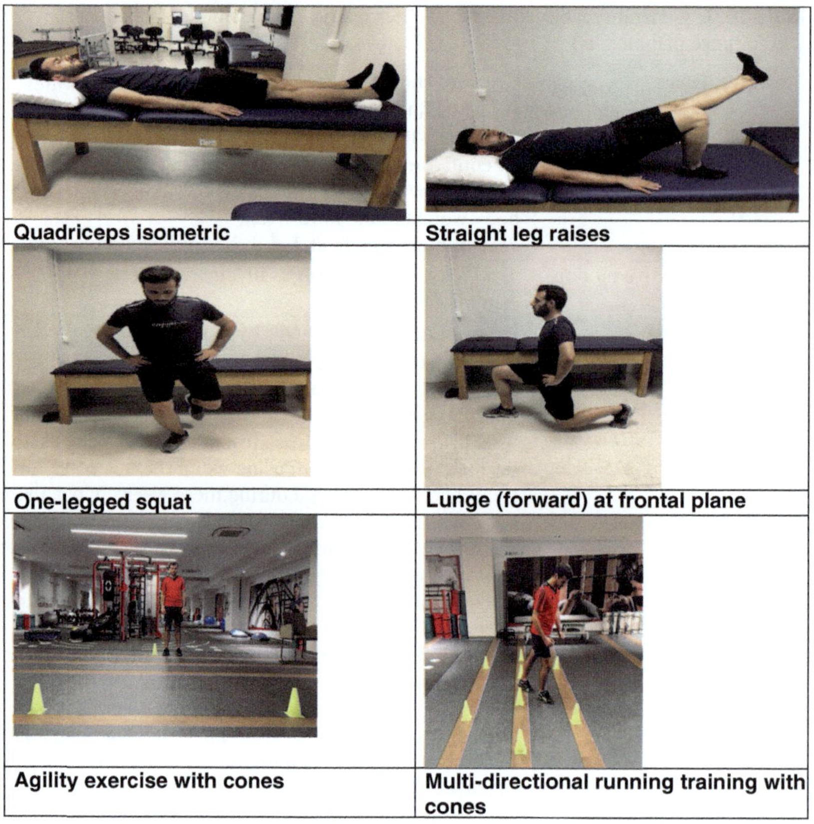

Fig. 20.1 Examples of exercises performed after cartilage knee surgeries

20.3 Return to Sports

Due to the limited number of studies in the literature on rehabilitation and return to sports after cartilage surgery, a return-to-sports protocol example will be given for talus osteochondral lesions in this section. In a study describing the return to sports after surgery in osteochondral injuries of the talus, it was suggested to use a protocol consisting of four activity levels and also used in the Achilles tendon rupture [8]. The four levels and protocol layout created according to this protocol are shown in Table 20.4.

The main point is that if patients are now able to return to higher levels of activity and sports, it is the responsibility of both the surgeon and the physiotherapist to ensure that technically sound surgery be performed and biological recovery takes place, as well as that the athlete is quantitatively and qualitatively prepared to meet such high-level demands. Therefore, it is important to determine the level of mental, physical, and biological well-being and readiness [9]. In return to sports, motion scanning can be applied to identify the lack of recovery and residual/established faulty patterns in the athlete because it can be as easy as a simple video capture to a more complex motion capture system.

In the selection of methods that can be used in rehabilitation after cartilage surgery, individual factors such as age, gender, and physical condition, as well as pathomechanical reasons such as the size and location of the lesion, and surgical technique should not be taken into consideration. Joint range of motion exercises, load transfer, strengthening, and balance training in the rehabilitation process, although there is no clear consensus on the criteria, form the basis of rehabilitation [10]. In light of this information, it is recommended that the treatment program to be prepared for the patient should be by diversifying the exercises mentioned in this section.

The evolution of cartilage surgery has made great strides in the last 3 years, making it possible

Table 20.4 Return to sports (this guide is created for talus osteochondral lesions)

Level	Aim	Training	Examples
1	To be able to walk with normal weight bearing	Gait training with weight bearing Training of active ankle joint movements	Activities under all weight-bearing levels should be selected in the easy to difficult order of the following criteria: – Non-weight bearing- > toe-touch- > heel touch – Intact lower extremity only - > two lower extremities together - > affected extremity only – Intermittent light loading- > intermittent normal loading- > static loading- > intermittent high-intensity loading
2	To perform and maintain the running activity on a flat surface	Running	Jogging, training on a flat surface
3	To return to non-contact sports	Strength and agility training in sport-specific activities	Skipping rope Pivot turns on foot Sudden acceleration and sprint on level ground
4	To return to contact sports	Speed, muscle strength, endurance, explosive strength, and sport-specific training	
		Agility training	Runs with left-right and reverse direction changes with command
			8 figure run The distance between the two cones should be decreased
			Short interval shuttle run The distance between the two cones should be decreased
			Sudden pivots on one extremity. The rotation frequency should be increased
		Proprioceptive training	Running with textured and/or foam insoles Running on uneven ground (sandy ground, soil ground)
			The floor on which the activity takes place should be uneven ground (sandy ground, soil ground)
		Sport-specific training	Basketball: Crab running, vertical jump, forward-right-left lunge, and pivot turn
			The sprinter: Block breakout training
			American football: Field goal training

to return to high levels of activity and sports. It has been proven that cartilage implants are more durable and show much more durability than when they were first used. However, although mentioned in this chapter, post-surgical rehabilitation guidelines seem to have developed very slowly relative to the development of surgical techniques.

References

1. Gill TJ, McCulloch PC, Glasson SS, Blanchet T, Morris EA. Chondral defect repair after the microfracture procedure: a nonhuman primate model. Am J Sports Med. 2005;33(5):680–5.
2. Hirschmüller A, Schoch W, Baur H, Wondrasch B, Konstantinidis L, Südkamp NP, et al. Rehabilitation before regenerative cartilage knee surgery: a new prehabilitation guideline based on the best available evidence. Arch Orthop Trauma Surg. 2019;139(2):217–30.
3. Tyler TF, Lung JY. Rehabilitation following osteochondral injury to the knee. Curr Rev Musculoskelet Med. 2012;5(1):72–81.
4. Mithoefer K, Hambly K, Della Villa S, Silvers H, Mandelbaum BR. Return to sports participation after articular cartilage repair in the knee: scientific evidence. Am J Sports Med. 2009;37(Suppl 1):167S–76S.
5. Lahav A, Burks RT, Greis PE, Chapman AW, Ford GM, Fink BP. Clinical outcomes following osteochondral autologous transplantation (OATS). J Knee Surg. 2006;19(3):169–73.
6. Jones DG, Peterson L. Autologous chondrocyte implantation. J Bone Joint Surg Am. 2006;88:2502–20.
7. Mithoefer K, Williams RJ, Warren RF, Wickiewicz TL, Marx RG. High-impact athletics after knee articular cartilage repair: a prospective evaluation of the microfracture technique. Am J Sports Med. 2006;34:1413–8.
8. van Eekeren IC, Reilingh ML, van Dijk CN. Rehabilitation and return-to-sports activity after debridement and bone marrow stimulation of osteochondral talar defects. Sports Med (Auckland, NZ). 2012;42(10):857–70.
9. Patel S, Marrone W. The evolution of rehabilitation and return to sport following cartilage surgery. Int J Sports Phys Ther. 2023;V18(3):551–7.
10. D'Hooghe P, Murawski CD, Boakye LAT, Osei-Hwedieh DO, Drakos MC, Hertel J, Lee KB, Popchak A, Wiewiorski M, van Dijk CN. International consensus group on cartilage repair of the ankle. Rehabilitation and return to sports: proceedings of the international consensus meeting on cartilage repair of the ankle. Foot Ankle Int. 2018;39(1_suppl):61S–7S.

Atlas of Cartilage

21

Mehmet E. Erdil and Bahattin Kemah

See Figs. 21.1, 21.2, 21.3, 21.4, 21.5, 21.6, 21.7, 21.8, 21.9, 21.10, 21.11, 21.12, 21.13 and 21.14.

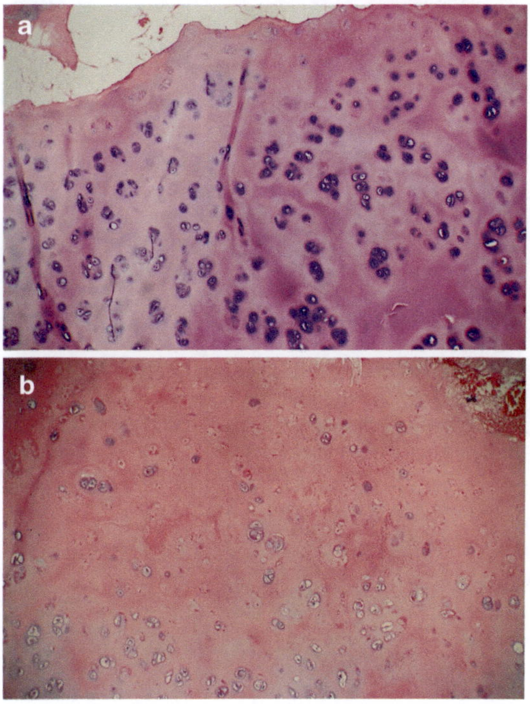

Fig. 21.1 Histological section through the developing lower limb; ankle joint, surrounding the developing bone is cartilage, skeletal muscles, and connective tissue of the limb. Histologic specimen of hyaline cartilage (**a**) With H&E staining (**b**) With eosinophilic staining

M. E. Erdil (✉)
Private Orthopaedic Practice, Istanbul, Türkiye

B. Kemah
Department of Orthopedics & Traumatology, Umraniye Training & Research Hospital, Istanbul, Turkey

M. E. Erdil et al. (eds.), *Current Concept in Cartilage Treatment*,
https://doi.org/10.1007/978-3-032-27099-3_21

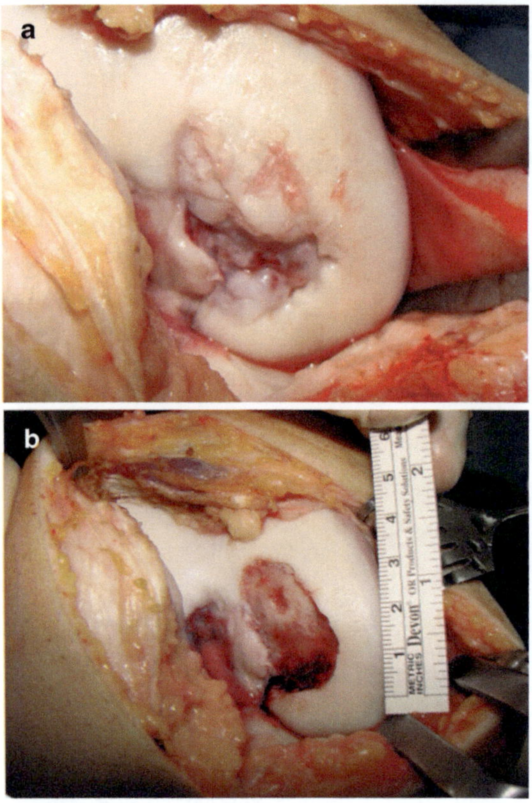

Fig. 21.2 (**a**) Focal cartilage lesion; Localized damage of the cartilage covering joint surfaces. (**b**) After preparing the lesion for cartilage surgery, defining borders and curetting to subchondral bone

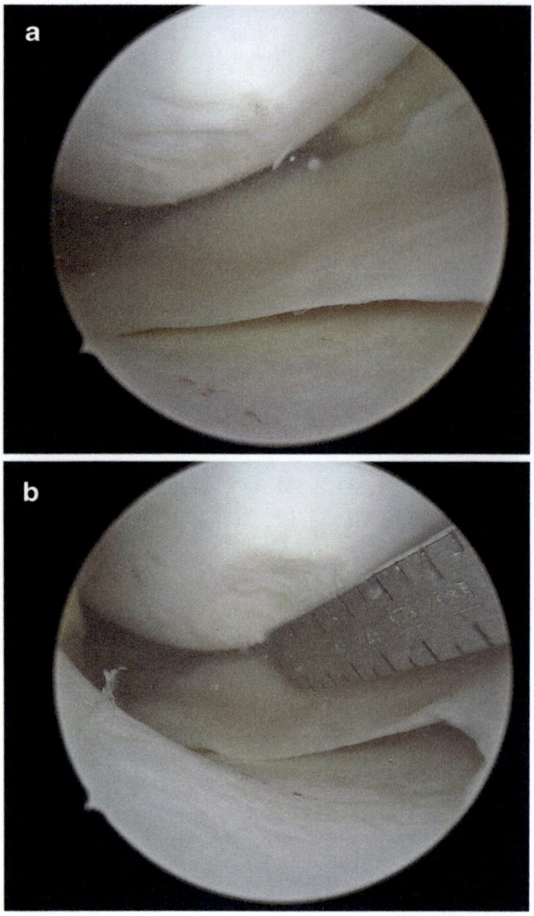

Fig. 21.3 (**a**) Early stage focal cartilage lesion Outerbridge stage II lesion; referring osteochondral lesion extending down to less than 50% of cartilage depth. (**b**) Measurement of the lesion size after debriding the lesion

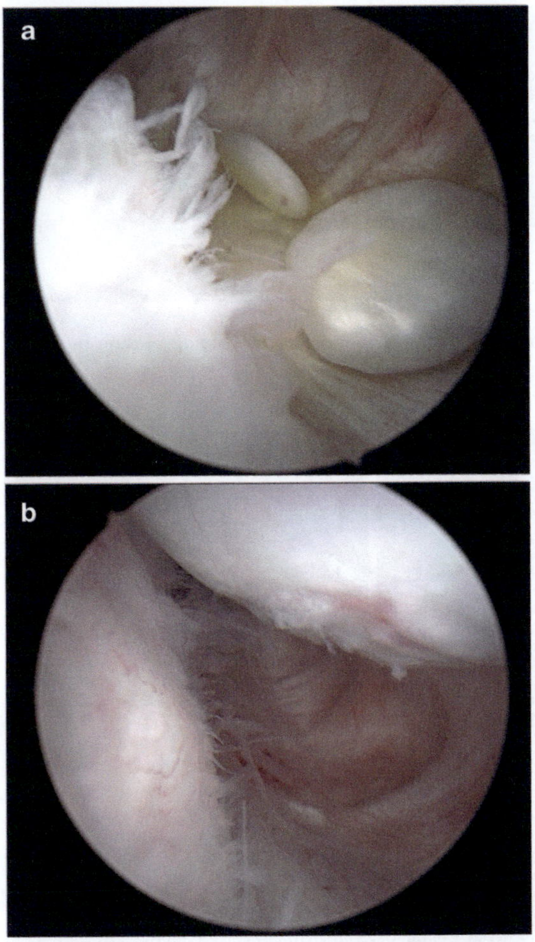

Fig. 21.4 (**a**) Osteochondral loose bodies in posterior pouch of the glenohumeral joint. (**b**) Humeral osteochondral lesion (origin of loose bodies)

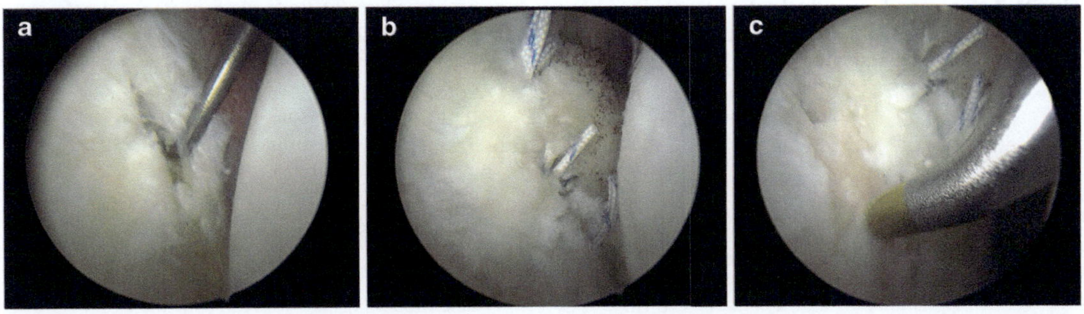

Fig. 21.5 (**a**) Bankart lesion with focal cartilage lesion Outerbridge stage II lesion; referring osteochondral lesion extending down to less than 50% of cartilage depth. (**b**) Bankart repair with suture anchors. (**c**) Bone marrow stimulation; microfracture technique of chondral lesion

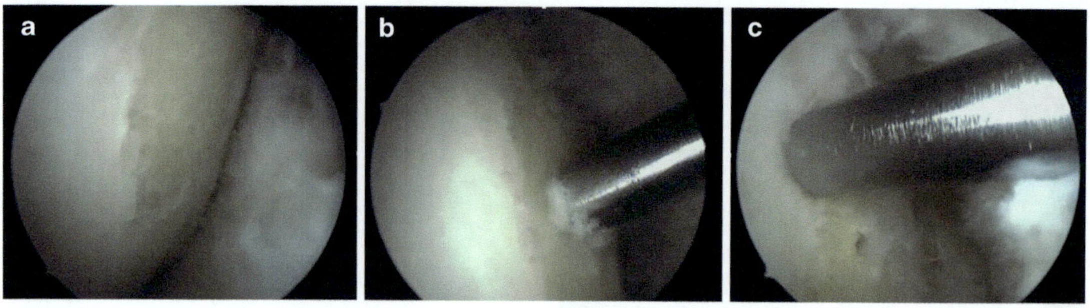

Fig. 21.6 Nanofracture is another technique of bone marrow stimulation (**a**) Stage 4 osteochondral lesion in medial femoral condyle. (**b, c**) Performing nanofracture

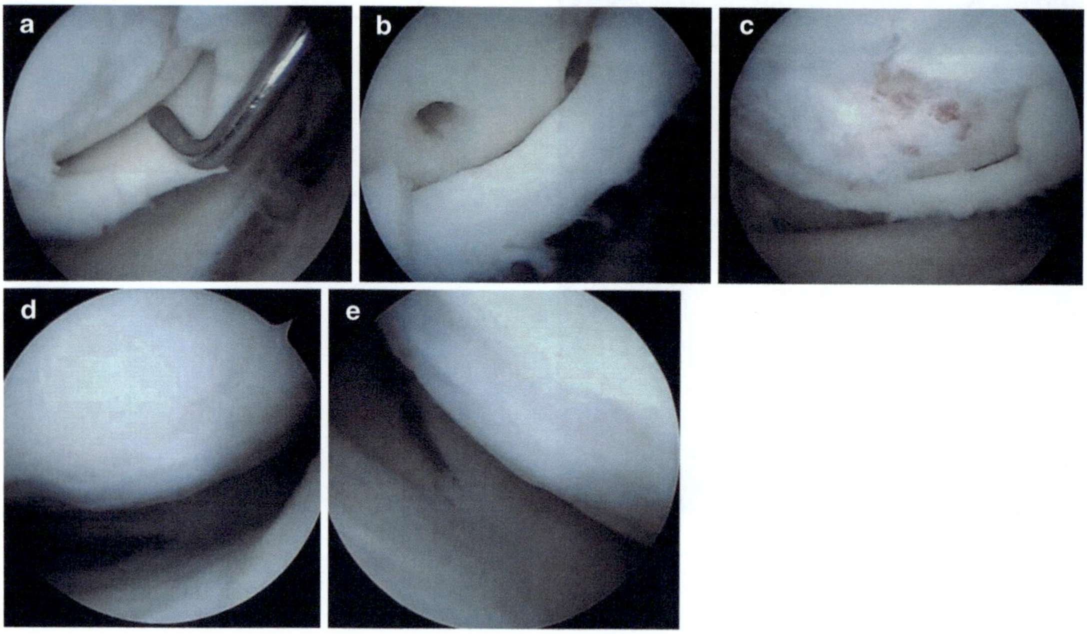

Fig. 21.7 Fibrocartilage is the healing tissue after bone marrow stimulation. (**a**) Exposing grade 4 osteochondral lesion in medial femoral condyle (**b**) Performing microfracture procedure (**c**) Bone marrow from microfracture holes. (**d, e**) Evaluating healing in second look arthroscopy at the 33rd month of the surgery

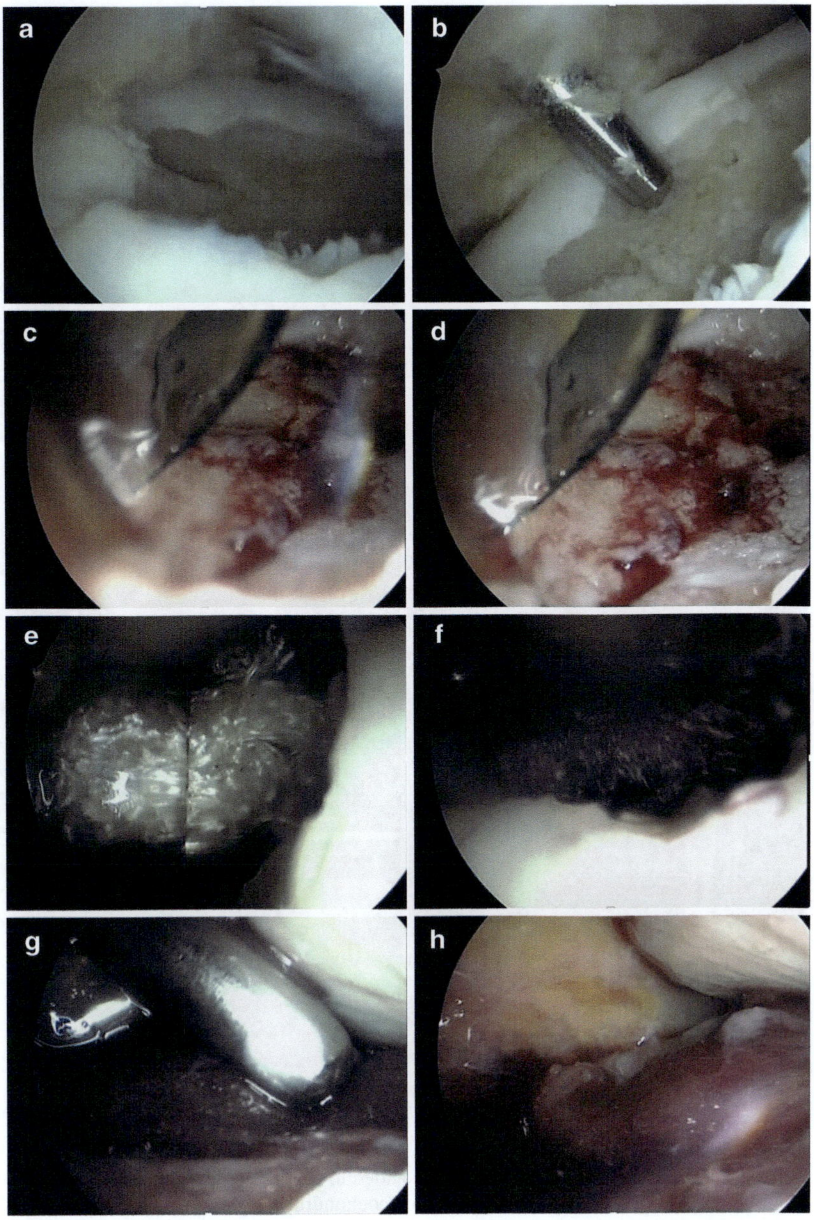

Fig. 21.8 In addition to bone marrow stimulating techniques, scaffolds can be used for bigger lesions for stabilizing the clot and obtaining a good environment for the mesenchymal stem cells coming from subchondral bone. (**a**) Exposing 2 × 2 cm grade 4 osteochondral lesion in trochlea (**b**) Performing nanofracture procedure. (**c, d**) Blood coming from nanofracture holes (gas arthroscopy) (**e, f**) Placing the hyaluronic acid based scaffold to the osteochondral lesion. (**g**) Positioning the scaffold to the osteochondral lesion. (**h**) Fixing the scaffold with fibrin glue

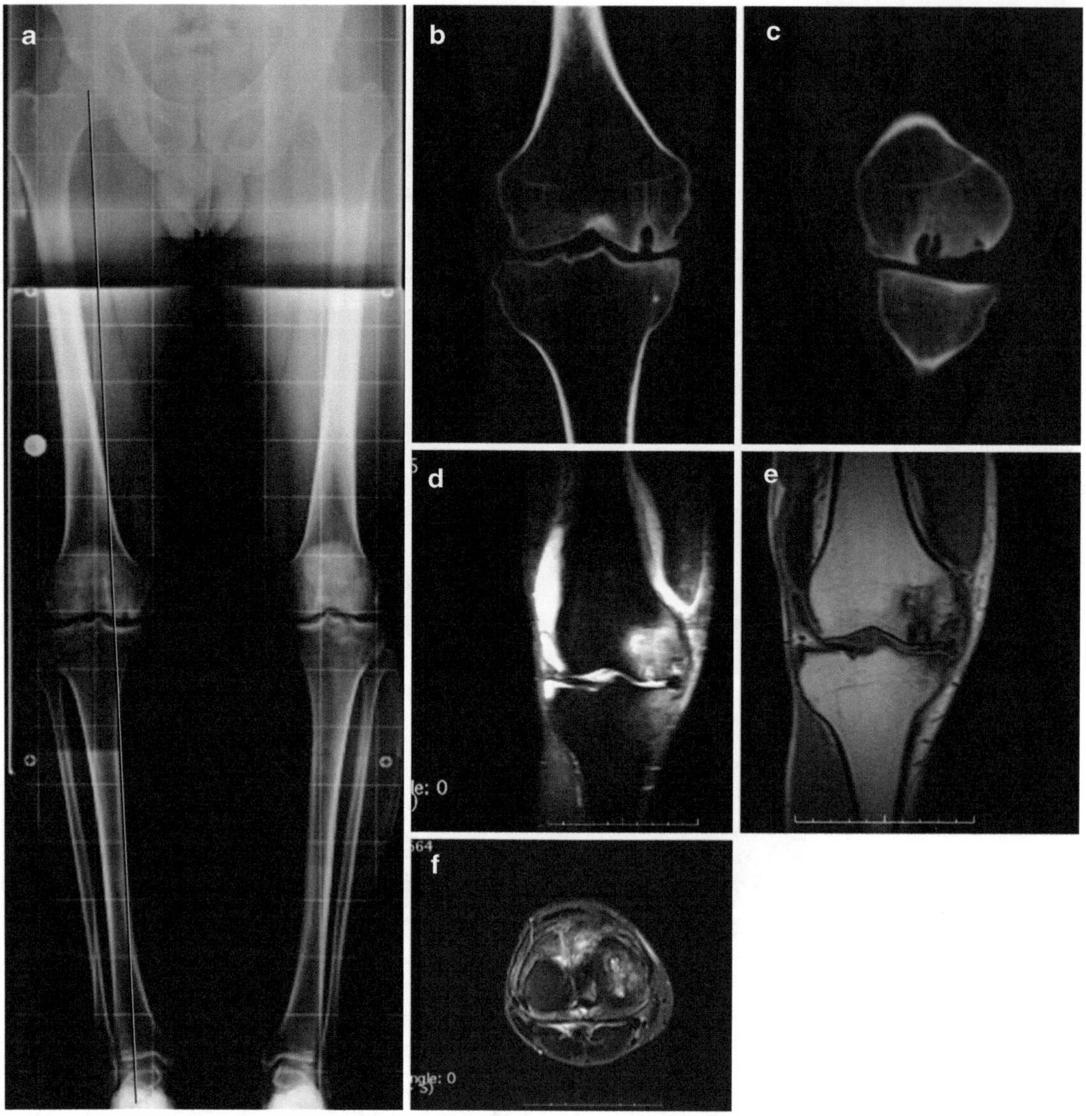

Fig. 21.9 Malalignment should be treated in cartilage lesions. Re-alignment procedures should be added to cartilage surgery. (**a**) Radiography of grade 4 osteochondral lesion in medial femoral condyle in right knee. Genu varum was detected. (**b, c**) CT scan of the lesion for determining the size and depth. (**d–f**) MRI depicts the soft tissues. (**g**) Exposing the osteochondral lesion after performing high tibial osteotomy. (**h**) Preparing the lesion for cartilage surgery. (**i**) Bordering the osteochondral lesion. (**j**) Placing the multi-layered matrix, composed of collagen and hydroxyapatite (**k**) Postoperative radiography showed normal alignment of lower limb

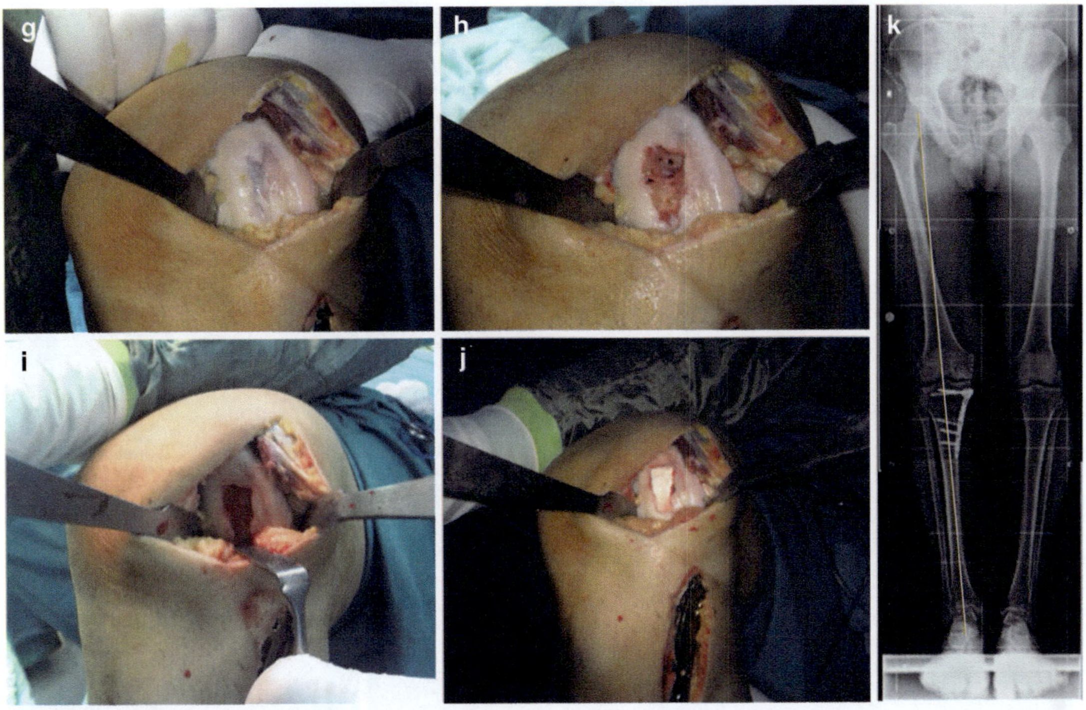

Fig. 21.9 (continued)

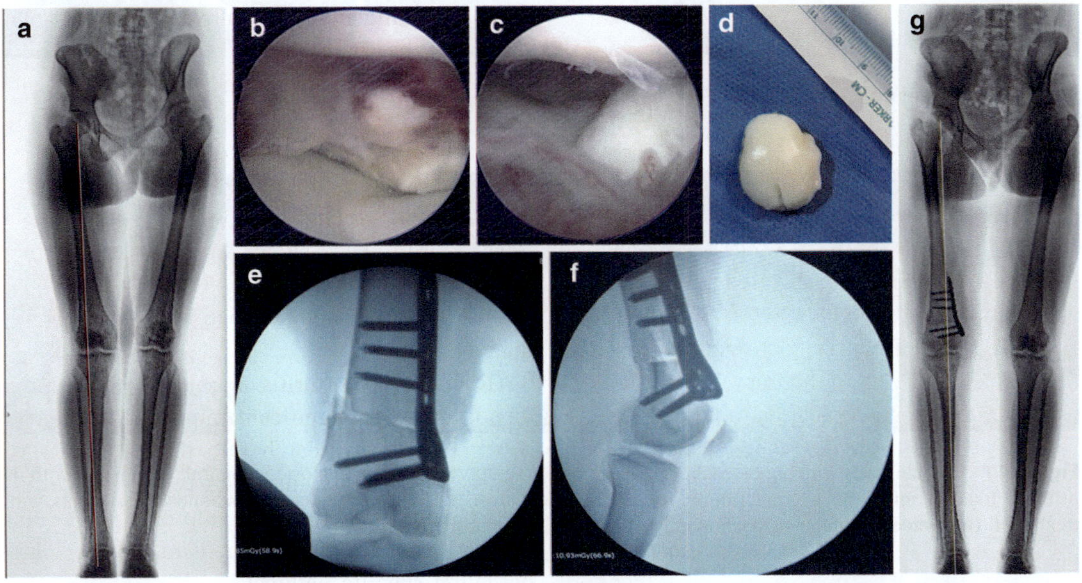

Fig. 21.10 Autologous chondrocyte implantation is a 2-stage surgery. Re-alignment procedures and biopsy should be performed in the first stage. (**a**) Radiography of grade 4 osteochondral lesion in lateral femoral condyle in right knee. Genu valgum was detected. (**b, c**) Osteochondral loose body in the arthroscopic procedure (first stage surgery). (**d**) Removing and measuring osteochondral loose body (first stage surgery). (**e, f**) Fluoroscopic views of femoral varization osteotomy (first stage surgery).(**g**). Postoperative orthoroentgenographic view showing realignment after first stage surgery. (**h, i**) Second stage surgery; measuring osteochondral lesion in lateral parapatellar arthrotomy of the knee. (**j**) Grafting the lesion with autologous bone graft harvesting from iliac crest (second stage surgery). (**k**) Scaffold of which autologous chondrocytes were reproduced in laboratory and implanted. (**l**) Templating for scaffold (second stage surgery). (**m**) Placing and fixing the scaffold (second stage surgery)

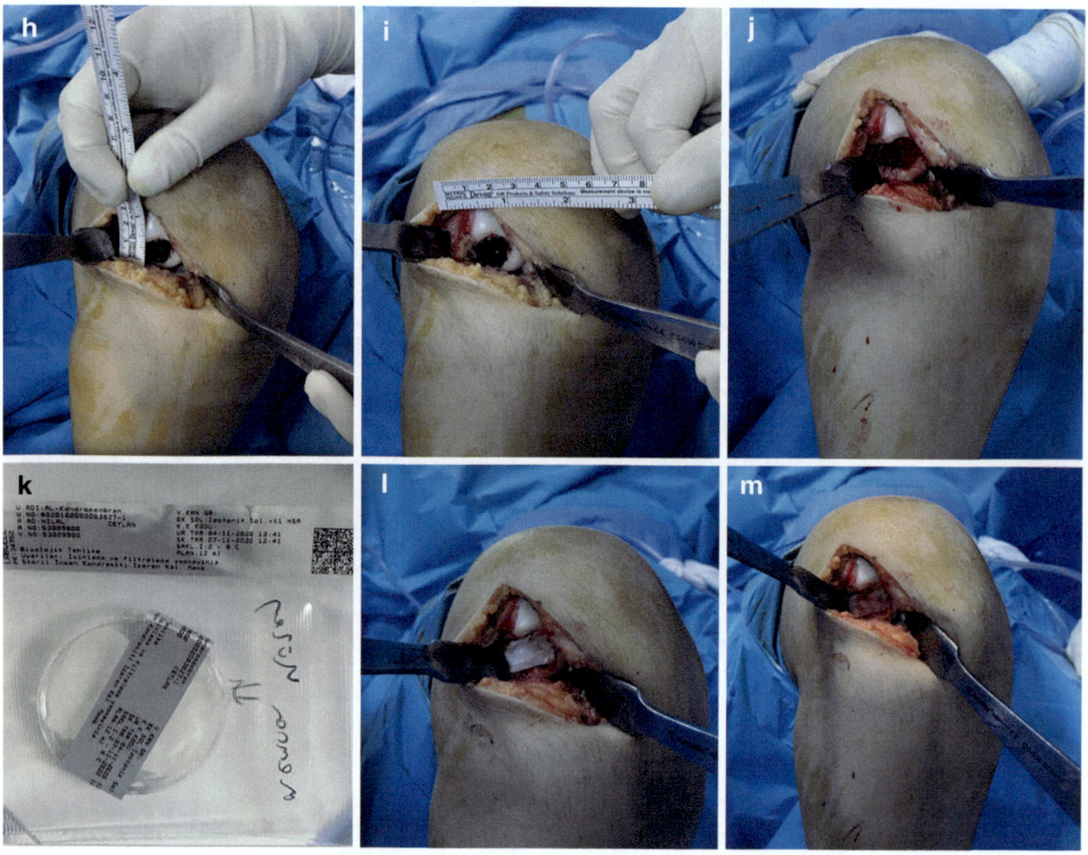

Fig. 21.10 (continued)

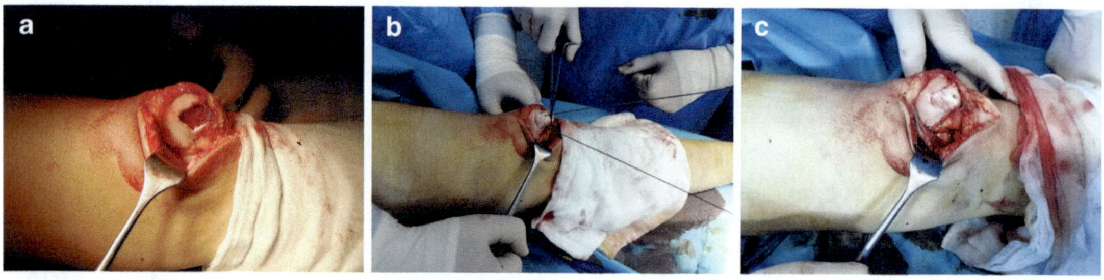

Fig. 21.11 In acute cases with big osteochondral lesions, primary fixation might be a good option for cartilage treatment. (**a**) Grade 4 patellar osteochondral lesion. (**b**) Temporary fixing the osteochondral fragments with K wires. (**c**) Fixation of the osteochondral fragments with bioabsorbable screws

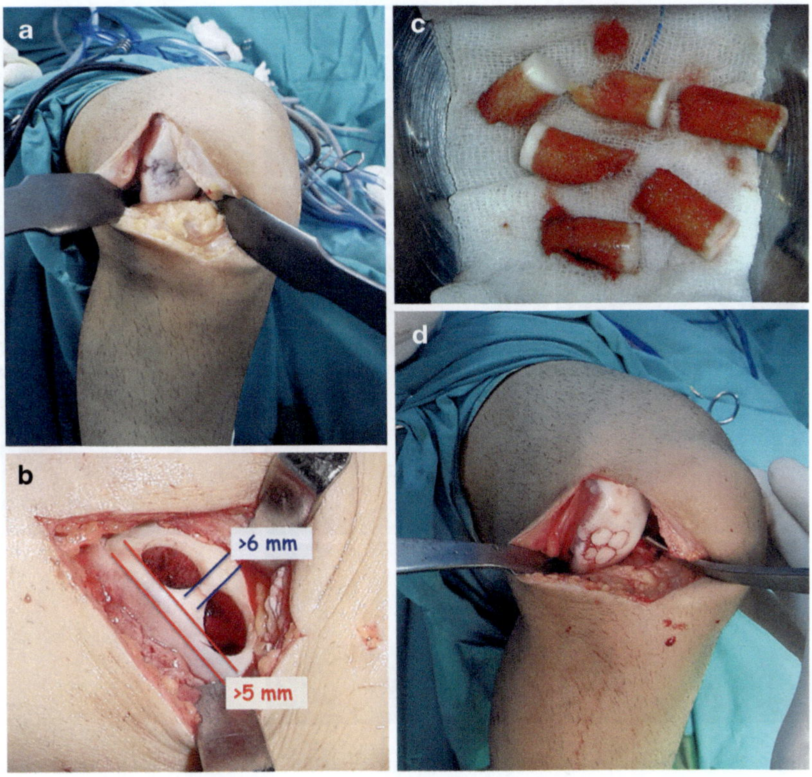

Fig. 21.12 Mosaicplasty is autotransplantation of osteochondral plugs which are harvested from non-weight-bearing regions of the joint, and implanting the plugs to the osteochondral lesion. (**a**) Mosaicplasty is a good option for big size osteochondral defects. (**b**) While harvesting from non-weight bearing regions of the joint; the distance between two holes should be more than 6 mm, and there should be more than 5 mm from the edge of the joint. (**c**) Measurement is the most important step of the procedure. (**d**) Joint surface congruence is the key for the success of the surgery

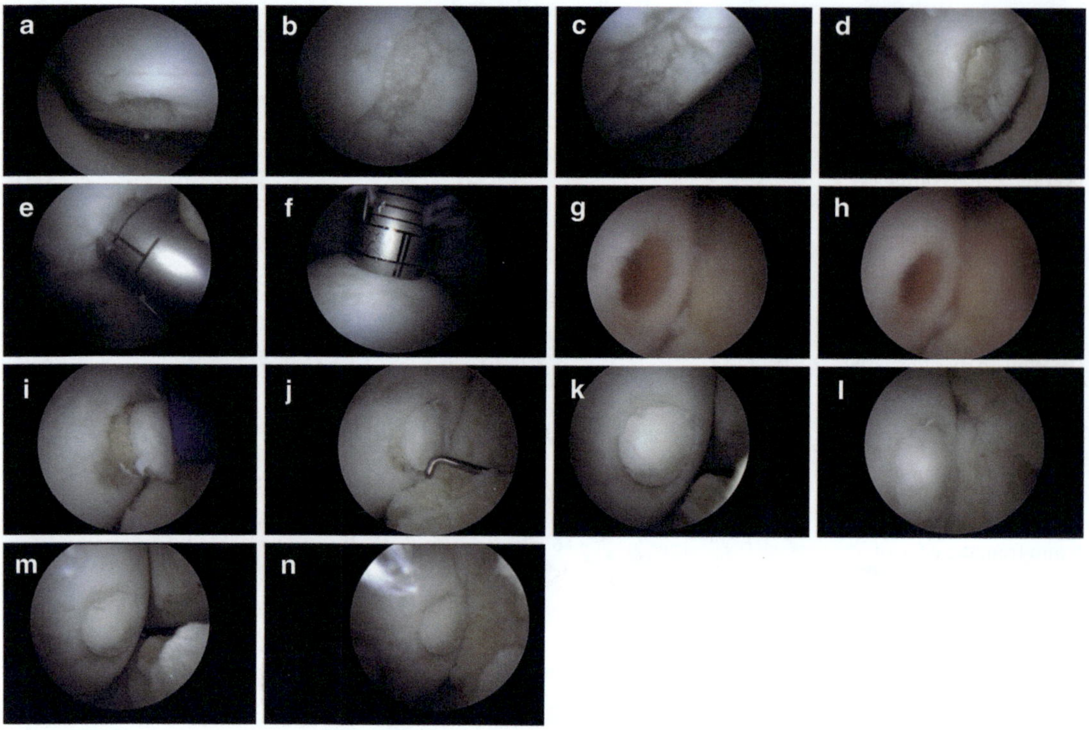

Fig. 21.13 Mosaicplasty or OAT (Osteochondral Autograft Transplantation) can be performed arthroscopically. (**a–c**) Exposing the osteochondral lesion in medial femoral condyle. (**d**) Preparing and bordering the lesion. (**e**) Creating the hole in the lesion area with special instruments. (**f**) Harvesting osteochondral plug from non-weight-bearing area, anterior part of lateral femoral condyle. (**g, h**) The hole in the lesion area. (**i**) Implanting the osteochondral plug in defect area. (**j**) Checking the joint congruency. (**k**) Adjusting the plug for joint congruency. (**l–n**) Defect was filled with single osteochondral plug

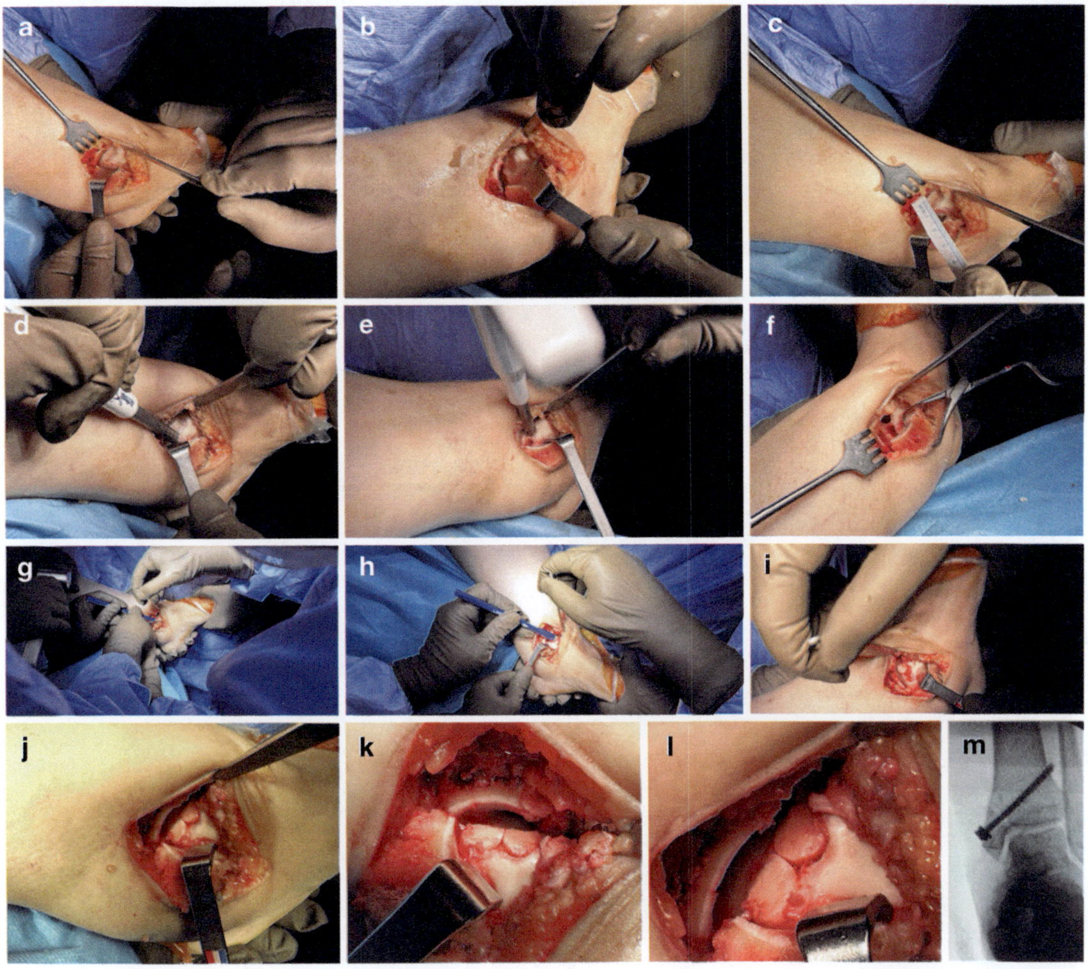

Fig. 21.14 Malleolar osteotomy is usually required for the treatment of talus osteochondral lesions. (**a–c**) Exposing, preparing, and measuring the osteochondral lesion after malleolar osteotomy. (**d–f**) Creating the holes for preparation of the lesion with special instruments. (**g–i**). Harvesting osteochondral plugs to the lesion area from non-weight bearing area of the ipsilateral knee. (**g–i**). The hole in the lesion area. (**j–l**) Checking the joint congruency of talar dome. (**m**) Fluoroscopic view after fixation of malleolar osteotomy with cannulated screw

GPSR Compliance

The European Union's (EU) General Product Safety Regulation (GPSR) is a set of rules that requires consumer products to be safe and our obligations to ensure this.

If you have any concerns about our products, you can contact us on ProductSafety@springernature.com

In case Publisher is established outside the EU, the EU authorized representative is:

Springer Nature Customer Service Center GmbH
Europaplatz 3
69115 Heidelberg, Germany

Batch number: 10731385

Printed by Printforce, the Netherlands